SAVING LIVES

SAVING LIVES

Why the Media's Portrayal of Nursing Puts Us All at Risk

Sandy Summers, RN, MSN, MPH

Harry Jacobs Summers

UPDATED SECOND EDITION

OXFORD
UNIVERSITY PRESS

OXFORD
UNIVERSITY PRESS

Oxford University Press is a department of the University of Oxford. It furthers the University's objective of excellence in research, scholarship, and education by publishing worldwide.

Oxford New York
Auckland Cape Town Dar es Salaam Hong Kong Karachi
Kuala Lumpur Madrid Melbourne Mexico City Nairobi
New Delhi Shanghai Taipei Toronto

With offices in
Argentina Austria Brazil Chile Czech Republic France Greece
Guatemala Hungary Italy Japan Poland Portugal Singapore
South Korea Switzerland Thailand Turkey Ukraine Vietnam

Oxford is a registered trademark of Oxford University Press in the UK and certain other countries.

Published in the United States of America by
Oxford University Press
198 Madison Avenue, New York, NY 10016

Library of Congress Cataloging-in-Publication Data
Summers, Sandy, author.
Saving lives : why the media's portrayal of nursing puts us all at risk/Sandy Summers, Harry Jacobs Summers.—Updated edition.
p. ; cm.
Why the media's portrayal of nursing puts us all at risk
Includes bibliographical references and index.
ISBN 978–0–19–933706–4 (paperback : alk. paper)
I. Summers, Harry, author. II. Title. III. Title: Why the media's portrayal of nursing puts us all at risk.
[DNLM: 1. Nurses—standards. 2. Nursing—standards. 3. Mass Media. 4. Nurse's Role. 5. Nurse-Patient Relations. 6. Public Relations. WY 16.1]
RT82
610.73—dc23
2014019488

9 8 7 6 5 4 3 2 1
Printed in the United States of America
on acid-free paper

For our children Cole and Simone
And their future nurses

There comes a time when you swim or sink
So I jumped in the drink
Cause I couldn't make myself clear
Maybe I wrote in invisible ink
Oh I've tried to think
How I could've made it appear.

But another illustration is wasted
'Cause the results are the same
I feel like a ghost
Who's trying to move your hands
Over some Ouija board
In the hopes I can spell out my name.

What some take for magic at first glance
Is just sleight of hand
Depending on what you believe
Something gets lost when you translate
It's hard to keep straight
Perspective is everything.

Aimee Mann and Clayton Scoble
from "Invisible Ink"
Aimee Mann, *Lost in Space* (2002)

CONTENTS

FOREWORD

Some years ago, I was invited to be a guest on a national talk show to discuss a popular television drama I'll call *Hospital*. Also on the panel of guests were the actors who played physicians on the drama, a physician who wrote for the show, and two other physicians. The producers of the talk show suggested that if I'd never seen the series (I had not) I should watch a couple of episodes before coming to Los Angeles.

I complied, watched several episodes, and was disappointed not to be surprised by the way they'd chosen to depict nursing. In the episodes, nurses were a nebulous, silent presence in the background. They never actually did anything other than stand around watching the doctors, who were busy single-handedly saving lives.

These Hollywood superdocs did it all—including the nursing duties that I, in my short twenty-year nursing career, never witnessed any physician perform. The only featured nurse role was the most dysfunctional character of all. Portrayed as a brooding, damaged nurse, she was tortured not by overwhelming responsibilities to the patients or by understaffing or burnout, but rather by having to decide which physician to sleep with next.

As with most Hollywood-generated medical shows, I found myself asking the same question I've been asking since my first Dr. Kildare episode: Where are the real nurses?

According to the Gallup polls, nurses are the most trusted professionals. Still, that has not changed Hollywood's hackneyed, one-dimensional portrayals of nurses as sex objects, handmaidens, psychopaths, and worse. In fact, the entertainment industry has done very little to present nurses in a positive light.

Consider my experience on the talk show. After arriving at the Los Angeles studio, I was taken to a small room obviously intended for storage of extra equipment and maintenance supplies, and I was told to wait there until someone came to get me. Thinking I had been mistaken as an applicant for a janitorial position, I explained that I was actually a guest on the show and asked to be taken to the Green Room. I was told the Green Room was not available and left to stare at the walls.

After two hours of staring at brooms and discarded stage lights, I wandered to the floor below. There I found the Green Room where a party for the show's other guests was in full progress. When asked who I was, I replied that I was the nurse author who had been asked to be a guest on the show.

Apparently that answer didn't cut it because I was told that the event in the Green Room was a private party for the show's other guests, and I would have to return to my special waiting area upstairs, or, as I had named it, the "nurses only" closet.

When taping began, I was seated next to *Hospital's* scriptwriting emergency room (ER) physician. The show was taped in front of a live audience, and what should have been a two-hour taping session turned into a seven-hour fiasco. Taping was stop and go, and the retaping had tempers and egos running high.

During one of the numerous breaks, an audience member fell from the bleachers, having a full-blown seizure. I'd unhooked my microphone and was on my way to see what could be done when I realized the scriptwriting ER physician had not moved. Over my shoulder I said, "Come on doc. Man down. Let's go."

He looked at me as if I were insane and replied, "No way. You're the nurse—you take care of it."

So, being an ER nurse, I did.

The show host, dumbstruck that none of the physicians present had offered their assistance, asked me off-camera what the hell that was all about. In a few words I explained that in the real world, it was the nurses who provide most of the care to the patients—a fact that was never brought up during the taping.

After I returned to my place on the stage, I asked the writer/physician if there were any nurses on the show's writing staff.

He answered—and I quote here—"Why in God's name would we ever consider such a thing as that?"

I counted to ten and replied: "Because, as an ER physician you know full well that it is the nurses who run the ER. The nurses triage, make the initial decisions, do most of the work, provide emotional support to both the patient and the family, and at times save the doctor's butt. That's why."

I tried to reason with him that the writers needed to make the nurses' roles more realistic, or the show could not be seen as an accurate portrayal of a real hospital setting.

Of course nothing I said made a dent (me being just a nurse and all), and Hollywood in general is still reluctant to change its attitudes about nurses.

Recently, a producer for a popular hospital reality show asked me to write a script for an episode. I was pretty excited about the prospect until he added that the script had to showcase a heroic ER physician. I told him that if I did agree to write a script, it would have to showcase a heroic ER nurse, since in my personal experience, nurses were the heroes.

Faced with that novel idea, he assured me that viewers were only interested in stories about doctors, not nurses. I finally directed him to the previously-mentioned scriptwriting ER physician who I was sure could give him exactly what he wanted.

It seems that the entertainment industry cannot, or will not, accept nurses as the autonomous, highly-educated health professionals they are. Thus, the subtle demeaning of the nursing profession continues. Unless they already have learned by firsthand experience, the public needs to be shown a true portrayal of the nurse as a professional rich in compassion, skill, and knowledge. This is a rare combination of traits to possess and maintain, especially when considering that nurses work in environments that most people would liken to war zones.

Saving Lives takes a hard look at what is wrong with the way Hollywood and other media have gone about undermining the nursing profession. The chapters in this book instill an awareness that will forever change the way people view nurses in the media.

But take warning: you may be left with a strong desire to change the system. Luckily, the authors tell you how.

Echo Heron, RN, author of *Intensive Care: The Story* of *a Nurse, Tending Lives: Nurses on the Medical Front*, and the Adele Monsarrat medical mystery series

ACKNOWLEDGMENTS

Many people helped us write this book. We thank those who have been with us from the beginning, Truth About Nursing board members Gina Pistulka, Rich Kimball, Kelly Bower-Joffe, and Christine Stainton, as well as our advisor Pat Woods. We also appreciate the vital contributions of the Truth About Nursing's supporters and staff, especially Sandy's mother Joan Summers and brother Jack Summers, Havely Taylor, Saniya Tildon, Hope Keller, Barbara Chamberlain, Carolyn Yucha, Mona Shattell, Kathleen Bartholomew, Donna Cardillo, Ruth DiMarzo, Sara Kozup, and Rose Teskie.

We salute the nursing leaders who have inspired us and given us tireless support over the years, especially Claire Fagin, Diana Mason, and Linda Pugh. We also owe much to others who have explored how the media treats nursing, particularly scholars Beatrice Kalisch and Philip Kalisch.

Our children Cole Summers and Simone Summers graciously tolerated our absences and the stresses associated with this book. They also performed valuable research and analysis of children's television programming, particularly *Doc McStuffins*.

We thank our editor Chad Zimmerman and assistant editor Meredith Keller for their support, insights, and understanding. We are also grateful to everyone else at Oxford University Press who helped us complete this project. And as always we appreciate the efforts of Shannon Berning, the editor of our first edition, who suggested we write the book.

Finally, we thank everyone who has helped us tell the public what nurses really do.

INTRODUCTION

Nurses save lives every day. But the media usually ignores their vital role in health care. That contributes to a lack of respect and resources for the profession, putting many lives at risk.

In 2005 US Army Sergeant Tony Wood was riding in a Humvee in Iraq. A roadside bomb exploded. Metal tore into Wood's internal organs. A month later he woke up at Walter Reed Army Medical Center in Washington, DC. Wood's story appeared in an August 2008 *New York Times* article by Lizette Alvarez about traumatic brain injuries in combat veterans.[1] Once Wood arrived at a hospital, expert nurses led the 24/7 effort that helped him survive, as they do with any patient whose injuries are so severe. But here is how Alvarez summed up that effort: "Doctors patched up most of his physical wounds over five months."

In a similar incident, a roadside bomb blew up near a Humvee in which US Army Sergeant Nick Paupore was riding in Kirkuk City. Paupore lost his leg and an enormous amount of blood, but he too survived. In March 2008 the CNN website posted a story by Saundra Young about a Walter Reed neurologist's use of a promising new mirror therapy to help amputees like Paupore cope with phantom limb pain.[2] Once again, nurses no doubt provided the great majority of the care that helped Paupore live. But in describing the care Paupore received in Germany on his way to Walter Reed, the article reported simply that "doctors fought to save his life."

Of course, sometimes the media is merely repeating without question what it hears from those with influence. In November 2013 remarks reported around the world, French Foreign Minister Laurent Fabius called for intervention in the Central African Republic because that nation was in "complete chaos" and "on the verge of genocide." What was most worrisome, specifically? "You have seven surgeons for a population of five million, an infant mortality rate of 25 percent in some areas and 1.5 million people who have nothing, not even food, and armed gangs, bandits, etc."[3] It sure sounded like *surgeons* were the nation's most pressing need. But in fact, to resolve the grave public health problems lurking behind the Minister's comment—poverty, malnutrition, malaria, pneumonia, birth trauma, social conflict—the African nation's critical shortage of nurses and midwives would be far more important.

Meanwhile, over the last decade, a new wave of television hospital dramas has become popular around the world. On ABC's *Grey's Anatomy*, fifteen elite surgeon characters agonize adorably about love 'n' stuff and in their spare moments handle every meaningful aspect of patient care. On Fox's *House*, a witty, misanthropic genius led a team of hospital physicians in diagnosing mysterious diseases, work that the show seems to equate with restoring patients to health. Once again, physician characters provide all important care. Fox's more recent sitcom *The Mindy Project* focuses mainly on the personal lives of quirky but skilled obstetrics/gynecology physicians. It also includes three minor nurse characters that display virtually no skill and might be described charitably as kooky, less charitably as punchlines.

When nurses appear on most hospital shows and other popular Hollywood products, it is generally to mutely absorb physician commands, to move things or convey messages, or to serve as disposable romantic foils. The nurses are dramatic mirrors, reflecting light back on the beautiful physicians. And physician characters on hospital shows have repeatedly mocked nursing, making clear that they see it as a job for pathetic losers.

In 2009, although no nurse-focused shows had appeared in more than 15 years, three such shows premiered: Showtime's *Nurse Jackie*, NBC's *Mercy*, and TNT's *HawthoRNe*. At times each show wrongly suggested that physicians are really in charge of nurses, but each also featured a strong, smart central character that fought for patients and saved lives. Jackie Peyton in particular has displayed true clinical virtuosity. But *Mercy* lasted only 22 episodes and *Hawthorne* 30 total episodes over three seasons. The recent Channel 4/PBS drama *Call the Midwife* has shown London nurses to be tough, skilled, and autonomous—in the 1950s.

In this anxious post-9/11 world, we have found our high-tech heroes, and for the most part they aren't nurses. Sadly, the media often ignores nurses' real contributions to health. Instead, it presents nurses as low-skilled handmaidens, sex objects, or angels. In countless media products, only "doctors" receive credit for care that is actually provided by a team of nurses and other skilled health professionals. These misconceptions are widespread in global society, but the media strongly reinforces and even exacerbates them.

Who cares?

You should. In reality, nurses are science professionals who save lives and improve patient outcomes every day. They monitor patients 24/7, provide high-tech treatments, advocate for patients, and teach them how to live with their conditions. But since the late 1990s, the world has suffered from a deadly nursing shortage—the worst in modern history. A key element underlying many of the immediate causes of the shortage is poor public understanding of what nurses really do. That ignorance undermines nurses' claims to adequate staffing, nursing faculty, and other resources in our era of ruthless cost cutting. A critical nursing role is to prevent healthcare errors, but data collected between 2008 and 2011 showed that there were roughly 400,000 deaths per year in the United States from healthcare errors,[4] making it the third leading cause of death.[5] These deaths happen in large part because the nurses who could prevent most of them are undervalued and underfunded. It is true that the shortage of nurses needed to fill open nursing positions has declined in some places as a result of the Great Recession. But the shortage of nursing *care* due to an insufficient number of funded nursing positions remains rampant.

Saving Lives explores what the public is told about the nurses who are fighting to save your life. We focus on the most universal source of information: the media. We wrote the book to expand upon our work to improve public understanding of nursing. In 2001, Sandy and other graduate nursing students at Johns Hopkins—Gina Pistulka, Kelly Bower-Joffe, Richard Kimball, and Christine Stainton—started a nonprofit organization called the Center for Nursing Advocacy to improve nursing's image. After the Center decided to close in 2008, we founded the Truth About Nursing (www.truthaboutnursing.org) to continue our work, and Gina, Kelly, Rich, and Christine stayed with us. When we first started, Sandy had practiced nursing for fifteen years in emergency and critical care units at leading trauma centers in Washington, DC, San Francisco, and New Orleans. Sandy's husband, Harry, a lawyer and media junkie, agreed to help her stir things up. Many nurses, nurse educators, and advocates rely on us to monitor and analyze what the media is doing, to push for more accurate portrayals of nursing, and to be a resource for media creators with an interest in what nurses really do. We often use an approach we have called "entertainment advocacy," which aims to stimulate thinking in some of the same ways the media itself does, including irreverent and satirical elements.

Our advocacy has had a real impact on media creators. We have persuaded major corporations to reconsider advertising campaigns that relied on nursing stereotypes, such as a global Skechers campaign featuring Christina Aguilera as a "naughty nurse." We have helped companies rework advertising campaigns to avoid nursing stereotypes. In 2005 we convinced the US government to revise the name of an annual minority health care campaign to one that would not exclude the nurses who actually provide much of that care. News stories about our advocacy have appeared on major television networks and in print sources from the *Los Angeles Times* to the *Times of India*. Even Hollywood has reacted, grudgingly, to our analysis of its mostly poor portrayal of nursing. We interact with producers and executives, and some have been receptive to our concerns. In 2013, the Truth About Nursing and other nurses prevailed upon MTV to take several steps to lessen the damage caused by the partyin' portrayal of young nurses on the "reality" show *Scrubbing In*. But far more needs to be done.

Of course, we also create controversy. Some people, including some nurses, cannot accept criticism of their favorite media products or challenges to the status quo generally. That criticism seems especially unwelcome when it comes from females in a traditionally female profession. Nurses are supposed to serve in silence! Nursing is about hearts and bedpans, not aggressive public advocacy, so shut up! Rock star Jack White accused us of "metaphorical ignorance" when we pointed out that one of his songs used nursing as a lazy metaphor for unskilled romantic care. Other critics deny that the popular media could affect the real world ("It's just a television show. Get over it!"). That attitude persists despite research to the contrary. It happens even though other fields (such as education, politics, and advertising) rely on the same basic concept: what we see affects what we think and what we do, even when what we see is fiction. Still other critics insist that nursing can be helped only in some particular way other than what we do. Therefore, we must stop what we're doing.

Because the global media has a keen interest in the many life-and-death issues in health care, the media that relates to nursing is vast. So this book is not comprehensive. It presents some basic ideas and notable recent examples. For in-depth treatment of the subjects discussed here, please consult the Truth About Nursing's website, www.truthaboutnursing.org.

Here is a short summary of what you will find in *Saving Lives*. As we explain in Chapter 1, nursing is a distinct scientific field and an autonomous profession. Nurses follow a holistic practice model that emphasizes preventive care and overall well-being. Virtually all US nurses are now educated at colleges by nursing scholars. Nurses report to senior nurses, not physicians. Nurses practice in high-tech urban trauma centers and in vital health programs for poor mothers in bayou swamps. They work in leading research centers and in disaster zones. Nurses manage patient conditions, prevent deadly errors, teach and advocate for patients, and work for better health systems. But patients die when nurses are understaffed or underempowered and when nursing care is assigned to those who are not nurses in order to cut costs. The current nursing shortage kills thousands, if not millions, of people every year.

Chapter 2 shows how the media affects nursing. Research confirms that even entertainment television affects popular attitudes about health care generally and nursing specifically. At times, the media offers an insightful look at what nurses really do. But usually nurses are portrayed as the peripheral servants of heroic physicians. Despite the introduction of a few nurse-focused television shows in recent years, physicians and physician characters have continued to dominate most health care depictions. Hollywood has often presented nursing as a job in a sad time warp. As Meredith Grey snapped at a male colleague in a 2005 *Grey's Anatomy* episode: "Did you just call me a *nurse*?!" In a 2013 episode of *The Mindy Project*, the female lead character was offended for the same reason. Key factors in Hollywood's nursing problem include entrenched stereotypes, insufficient support from physicians, and nursing's own overall failure to represent itself well. Unfortunately, poor understanding limits the resources available for nursing practice, education, and research, which in turn leads to worse patient outcomes, including death.

The media often portrays nursing with a mix of toxic female stereotypes. As we discuss in Chapter 3, most media portrayals fail to convey that nurses are college-educated professionals who save lives. A few media items, particularly in the print press, have conveyed something of advanced nursing skills. Occasionally, this has even happened on television, particularly on *Nurse Jackie* and the other recent nurse-focused shows. The most influential media, however, regularly sends the message that physicians are the sole masters of health knowledge and the only important staff in hospitals, even though hospitals exist mainly to provide nursing care. Contempt for nursing remains common. In a 2012 segment of Comedy Central's *The Daily Show with Jon Stewart* about reintegrating military veterans into the civilian workforce, the host suggested that school nursing basically involves "kickball" and "tummy aches." On Hollywood shows, physician characters often do exciting things in which nurses would actually take the lead, like defibrillation, triage, and psychosocial care. Many news accounts assign credit for nurses' work to physicians, "hospitals," or machines. Some media ignore nursing even when nurses play a central role in the relevant topic, such as responding to mass casualty events. Nurses are rarely recognized as health experts or important scholars.

Of course, nurses may get credit for an isolated save outside their usual workplaces, which is news because it's a shock (Nurse passerby saves life?! Dog dials 9-1-1?!). Other items suggest that any helpful person or piece of healthcare technology is a "nurse." Some call newborn nannies "baby nurses," but those caregivers are no more nurses than they are babies.

Chapter 4 explores the prevailing media view of nurses as the faceless crew of a healthcare ship captained by charismatic physicians. Contrary to that view, nursing is an autonomous profession. Nurses train and manage themselves. They have independent legal duties to patients and a unique scope of practice, including special expertise in such areas as pain management and lactation research and practice. Hundreds of thousands have at least a master's degree in nursing. Occasionally media products have given some sense of nursing autonomy. These include infrequent news items about nursing leaders or pioneering nursing research, and a few fictional portrayals, such as *Call the Midwife*. But the most influential entertainment media presents nurses as physician handmaidens. Major Hollywood hospital shows have done so regularly, including *Grey's Anatomy, House*, and *The Mindy Project*. The paradigmatic nurse-physician interaction is a physician "order" followed by a meek nurse's "Yes, doctor!" And although all of the 2009 US nurse shows have shown nurses pushing back against poor physician care, every one of them—even *Nurse Jackie*—has at times wrongly suggested that nurses report to physicians.

The media often presents nurses as half-dressed bimbos. In Chapter 5 we examine the staggering global prevalence of the "naughty nurse" image. It appears in television shows, music videos, sexually-oriented products, and even the news media. In 2007, on *LIVE with Regis and Kelly*, Kelly Ripa promised to be a "sponge bath nurse" in her "little nursey costume" for cohost Regis Philbin, who was undergoing heart bypass surgery. At half-time during a televised 2012 basketball game, the Dallas Mavericks Dancers donned naughty nurse outfits and did a sexually-oriented dance to the tune of Robert Palmer's "Bad Case of Loving You." Major corporations have used the naughty nurse to sell alcohol, razor blades, cosmetics, shoes, and even milk. The naughty image encompasses more subtle messages that nurses are mainly about the romantic pursuit of men, particularly physicians. Of course, the creators of naughty nurse imagery are "just joking"! But such social contempt discourages practicing and potential nurses, undermines nurses' claims to adequate resources, and encourages workplace sexual abuse—a major problem for real nurses.

Not surprisingly, nursing remains more than 90 percent female. Yet as we explain in Chapter 6, a lot of media created by "feminists" has been hostile to nursing. Many popular Hollywood hospital shows of recent years, particularly *Grey's Anatomy*, have sent the message that nursing is not good enough for smart modern women. Films like *Akeelah and the Bee* (2006) and *Gracie* (2007) have celebrated the idea that promising girls, unlike their bitter mothers, do not have to settle for nursing. This same media can be open to the idea of men in nursing, particularly in news stories. But the entertainment media has mocked male nurses. TNT's *Rizzoli & Isles* spent a 2010 episode jeering at a male nurse for wanting to be a "stay-at-home-daddy" and for being an ugly caricature of a traditional woman. On ABC's *Private Practice*, nurse Dell was a clinic *receptionist*. He became a midwife, then proudly announced that he had been admitted to medical school just before the show killed him off in 2010. Too much of the media defines success solely in terms of traditionally male jobs, such as medicine.

The media commonly presents nurses as angels of mercy or loving mothers, as we explain in Chapter 7. Even many nurses and their supporters embrace the angel image. Johnson & Johnson's Campaign for Nursing's Future, which aims to address the nursing shortage, has aired gooey, soft-focus television advertisements about "the importance of a nurse's touch." For Nurses Week in 2011, Kaiser Permanente ran a radio advertisement that relentlessly portrayed nurses as selfless angels, as exemplified by a reference to a nurse's "gargantuan heart all squishy with compassion thumping away." Compassion and caring are important parts of nursing, but the extreme emphasis on "angel" qualities reinforces the sense that nursing is not about thinking or advanced skills. It implies that nurses, as virtuous spiritual beings, need very little education, clinical support, or workplace security. Nursing was traditionally seen as a religious vocation. But today, angel imagery suggests that nursing is not a serious modern profession and deters nurses from advocating for themselves and their patients.

Chapter 8 shows that the media often views nurses who do exert authority as battle-axes. The classic manifestation was the sociopathic Nurse Ratched in *One Flew Over the Cuckoo's Nest*, but the 2012 film *Cloud Atlas* included Nurse Noakes, the oppressive, violent supervisor of a nursing home that held older people against their will. The battle-axe has survived on prime time television as a vindictive bureaucrat enforcing oppressive, trivial hospital rules—even on *Nurse Jackie*. The battle-axe image seems to be the opposite of both the angel and the naughty images. But it is yet another one-dimensional female extreme. So while today's society may be ambivalent about punishing women *generally* for exercising power, it's still cool to punish women for trying to be powerful *nurses*. Sure, modern women are allowed to be tough and independent—as long as they pursue a traditionally male career.

As we discuss in Chapter 9, advanced practice registered nurses (APRNs) provide care that includes tasks traditionally done by physicians. APRNs combine the holistic nursing care model with additional practitioner training, offering a hybrid approach that is changing health care. Contrary to the claims of some physicians, research shows that APRN care is *at least as effective* as that of physicians. Hollywood has offered a few well-meaning depictions of APRNs, but these tend to wrongly suggest that APRNs are skilled assistants to physicians. Other portrayals show disdain, as in a mocking suggestion on Disney's *Lab Rats* in 2013 that one character could be called a nurse practitioner because he had flunked out of medical school. Some shows, including TNT's *The Glades* and even *Mercy*, have suggested that really ambitious nurses aim for medical school. A number of news stories have given a good sense of actual APRN practice, but APRNs are usually ignored as health experts. Many press accounts have wrongly suggested that APRNs can treat only minor problems. The news and advertising media constantly reinforce the idea that practitioner care is provided only by "doctors."

Chapter 10 explains what *everyone*—not just nurses—can do to improve understanding of nursing. We can all look closely at the role nurses play in the healthcare system and consider whether our language reflects that role; for instance, some use the word "nurse" to refer to any untrained caregiver. The media can convey a sense of what nursing really is. The news media should consult nurses when they have the expertise it needs. To learn more, journalists might shadow nurses. Hollywood should include characters to reflect the nurses who actually provide the compelling health care it has shown physicians providing. Governments and foundations must recognize the value of nursing. Hospital managers should promote nursing as they do medicine. Hospitals and universities should consider launching nurse shadowing programs, in which medical students and physicians follow nurses in the clinical setting to learn about nursing. When more physicians learn about the skill and autonomy that nurses have, the physicians can use their social power to communicate that reality to the public. Lack of understanding by medical professionals has led to many workplace conflicts and serious healthcare errors.

But as we argue in Chapter 11, nurses themselves must play the leading role in improving their image. Nurses should recognize that they have the power—and the responsibility—to foster change in their profession. They can start by projecting a professional image in everyday interactions, from how they deal with patients to the way they dress (we suggest fewer cartoon characters on scrubs). Nurses can also show that they are serious professionals by offering health advice to others and by becoming more engaged in health policy issues. Nurses must work to help the media create more accurate depictions and persuade the media to reconsider harmful existing portrayals. In that respect, nurses can think globally by following the Truth About Nursing's media analyses and campaigns online and by signing up to receive our free news alerts. They can act locally by starting chapters of the Truth About Nursing to reach out to local media makers. Nurses should also consider creating their own media to explain the value of nursing to the public directly. Modern media technology offers nurses many options, including letters to the editor, op-eds, blogs about health care issues, children's books, online radio shows, and even television shows and films.

Nurses are the critical front-line caregivers in modern health care. For millions of people worldwide, nurses are the difference between life and death, self-sufficiency and dependency, hope and despair. Yet a lack of true appreciation for nursing has contributed to a shortage that is one of our most urgent public health crises. Many nurses feel that they've written in invisible ink, that their hard work is not understood, and the result is a lack of resources for their practice, education, and research. The shortage of nurses and nursing is overwhelming the world's health systems. It is no exaggeration to say that our future depends on a better understanding of nursing.

Changing the way the world thinks about nursing may require a superhuman effort. But as the philosopher Albert Camus once wrote, "tasks are called superhuman when humans take a long time to complete them, that is all. The first thing is not to despair."[6]

We can do it—if you help.

Notes

1. Lizette Alvarez, "War Veterans' Concussions Are Often Overlooked," *New York Times* (August 25, 2008), http://tinyurl.com/myjwg2g.
2. Saundra Young, "For Amputees, an Unlikely Painkiller: Mirrors," CNN (March 19, 2008), http://tinyurl.com/26r9h2.
3. Reuters, "France Says Central African Republic on Verge of Genocide" (November 21, 2013), http://tinyurl.com/n5oj2nc.
4. John T. James, "A New, Evidence-based Estimate of Patient Harms Associated with Hospital Care," *Journal of Patient Safety* 9, no. 3 (September 2013): 122–128, http://tinyurl.com/lfbmbeq.
5. Centers for Disease Control and Prevention, "Leading Causes of Death" (2011), http://tinyurl.com/6js8e.
6. Albert Camus, "The Almond Trees" (1940), http://tinyurl.com/mg9xr2g.

DANGEROUS IGNORANCE: WHY OUR UNDERSTANDING OF NURSING MATTERS

1 WHO ARE NURSES AND WHERE HAVE THEY GONE?

One night our friend Dan Lynch had a patient who had just undergone a mechanical replacement of the aortic valve—the exit valve of the heart. As a cardiac surgical intensive care unit (ICU) nurse at a major hospital in Florida, Dan was monitoring the patient's heart that night with an arterial blood pressure line, among other ways. The "art line," as it's called, is a tube that runs from an artery in the patient's wrist to a monitor, which displays in waveforms how well the heart is pumping blood through the arteries. Dan noticed that about every fifteen minutes the patient's art line waveform became flat. That could indicate that the patient's heart had stopped. Or, less dramatically, it could indicate that the art line's interior catheter had simply become kinked or stuck next to the arterial wall. After some moments, the patient's waveform returned to normal.

During the episodes, the heart monitor continued to indicate that the heart was beating normally. But Dan also noted that when the art line waveform became flat, the patient's central venous pressure monitor that measured the pressure of the blood coming into the heart failed to fluctuate in the expected waveform. Because the patient was still on the ventilator and heavily sedated, Dan was not able to measure whether he got dizzy or his level of consciousness dropped during these episodes. But Dan could not find a pulse at these times. Dan surmised that when the waveforms went flat, blood was not being pumped from the heart.

Dan concluded that the new aortic valve was sticking closed during the episodes. He called the surgeon at home and woke him up. The surgeon said that he had "never heard of such a thing" and that the art line was probably positioned incorrectly. Dan confirmed that this was not the case, and noted that even if it were, it would not explain the lack of pulse and lack of central venous pressure waveform. The surgeon, unconvinced, hung up the telephone.

Then the surgeon called the nursing supervisor, who was overseeing the whole hospital's nursing staff that night, to report Dan for bothering him at home with unfounded telephone calls. Neither she nor the charge nurse supervising the ICU nurses that night would back Dan up because they too had "never heard of such a thing."

Despite this adversity, Dan continued to call persistently, over the course of hours, until the surgeon finally came in to prove him wrong. But Dan wasn't wrong. It turned out that one of the stitches holding the valve in place was periodically obstructing its opening and closing—a problem that, left unaddressed even for a short time, could have killed the patient. The surgeon removed the stitch and resewed it. The patient survived.

The surgeon did not thank Dan for saving the patient, but he did allow that it was "the craziest thing" he'd ever seen. As far as Dan knows, neither the patient nor his family ever learned what Dan had done to save his life.

Nurses save lives every day by using advanced skills and fighting for patients. But few people know it or even know what nursing is: a distinct scientific field. Nurses promote health and prevent illness. They follow a holistic practice model emphasizing a wide-angle view of health, with a strong focus on preventive care.

Nurses confront some of the most exciting challenges in health care. Their work settings range from the high-tech of teaching hospital ICUs to chaotic urban level-one trauma centers, from major research centers to community projects, war zones, and humanitarian relief projects around the world.

Nurses teach and advocate for patients. Nurses monitor and manage patient conditions, prevent deadly errors, provide skilled emotional support, perform key procedures, and work for better health systems. But if nurses are understaffed or underempowered, or if they simply make an error under pressure, patients can die.

Nursing is an autonomous profession.[1] Hospital nurses collaborate with physicians, but they are not managed by physicians. Instead, senior nurses manage nurses. Some nurses lead hospitals. Of course, physicians receive substantial medical training, and there is certainly an overlap with what nurses learn, as well as knowledge unique to physician training. But nursing also encompasses a great deal of unique health expertise that physicians as a class do not have. Therefore, contrary to popular belief, physicians as a class cannot do or manage nursing work.

Nurses are educated at colleges by nursing scholars who conduct cutting-edge research. Hundreds of thousands of nurses have graduate degrees in nursing. An increasing number have doctorates in nursing science. Nurses take rigorous examinations to secure the government licenses they need to practice. Once licensed, nurses are bound by their own legal and ethical practice codes.

In addition to using the physiological expertise Dan Lynch displayed, nurses save lives in other ways. In a 2004 *American Journal of Nursing* article titled "Two Cups: The Healing Power of Tea," Hanne Dina Bernstein described how she cared for an emaciated leukemia patient who had recently had a bone marrow transplant.[2]

The patient was depressed, refusing soup, grimacing at his medication, and turning down a newspaper. Bernstein took a pot of tea and two cups to the patient's room and declared, "I would like to watch the news." The patient was "clearly taken aback." He closed his eyes. Bernstein turned on the news and sat down.

Some time later Bernstein noticed that her patient was watching the television. She told him that she had brought an extra cup of tea. The patient said he might have half a cup. The next night the patient had two cups of tea and a piece of toast, "his first solid food in a month." The following night the patient told Bernstein about his family, who lived too far away to visit. The fourth night the patient got out of bed.

A few days later he left the hospital, able to recuperate closer to home. Months later, while Bernstein was shopping, a "booming voice" greeted her. It was the now vigorous patient. He gave the nurse a hug and introduced her to his wife: "This is Hanne. She saved my life with a cup of tea."

She did. The story may bring a tear to readers' eyes, and at the most basic level, this kind of intervention is something that even lay people may understand nurses do. Consider US Vice President Joe Biden's June 2013 half-compliment that physicians "allow you to live" but nurses "make you want to live"—implying that nurses do not save lives with physiological skill.[3] But let's look at the depth and importance of what Bernstein did. She quickly saw that the patient was depressed, alone, not eating—all of which could spell decline in a frail, critically ill patient. Although Bernstein initially felt "defeated," she decided to politely barge into her patient's life. At first the patient did not seem interested, but through her presence and the television, Bernstein reminded him of his connection to other humans. At the same time, she started him on the path to physical recovery with a cup of tea. She followed up in the ensuing days. The patient started eating and gaining strength. Of course almost anyone could physically do these things. But what average person would insist on "watching the news" in the room of a tired and depressed postoperative cancer patient?

However, when nurses make mistakes, patients can die. Nurses have so many complex judgment calls to make—calls like Dan Lynch made with his heart patient or Bernstein with her leukemia patient—that it is easy to miss something, especially when a nurse is responsible for too many patients.

In 2006 veteran Wisconsin obstetrics nurse Julie Thao mistakenly gave a pregnant patient an epidural anesthetic through her intravenous line, thinking the drug was penicillin prescribed for a streptococcus infection. The anesthetic stopped the mother's heart and she died. (Her son was delivered alive by cesarean section.) Fatigue from excessive overtime and medication packaging problems may have contributed to the error. The case received national attention because Wisconsin for a time unwisely pursued a felony neglect charge against the nurse. Julie Thao herself expressed great remorse, started a support group for nurses involved in serious errors, and has since devoted her time to changing hospital systems that lead to nursing errors.[4] She also promotes post-error hospital policies that focus less on narrow financial concerns and more on learning from the error and allowing nurses to help affected families heal.

Such high-profile cases are rare. In general, nurses operate under the radar, making health care function if they can. There are an estimated 16 million registered nurses (RNs) worldwide.[5] In the United States, there were about 2.8 million RNs practicing or teaching nursing[6] and another half million not employed in nursing in 2012.[7] By comparison, there are about 690,000 physicians,[8] a ratio of about four nurses to one physician. RNs in the United States must have at least an associate's degree in nursing, which can require up to three years of rigorous college science work—one year of prerequisites plus two years of nursing courses. About 60 percent of US RNs have at least a bachelor of science in nursing degree.[9] More than 375,000 hold at least a master's degree in nursing and 50,000 hold doctoral degrees.[10] In 2012 there were more than 260,000 employed advanced practice nurses and nursing educators in the United States, including 106,000 nurse practitioners, 70,000 clinical nurse specialists, 34,000 nurse anesthetists, 5,700 nurse midwives, and 56,000 nursing educators.[11] Advanced practice nurses play leadership roles in clinical nursing and assume some duties traditionally performed by physicians. For example, nurse anesthetists now outnumber physician anesthesiologists by 53–47 percent.[12] Just fewer than 10 percent of US nurses are men, but their numbers have grown as barriers to their entry decrease.[13] Nursing schools often refused admittance to men before the US Supreme Court ruled such practices illegal in 1981.[14] The number of men is higher in some nursing specialties; more than 40 percent of nurse anesthetists are men.[15]

What exactly do all these nurses do?

- Nurses identify and address life-threatening infections.
- Nurses coordinate the care provided by other health professionals, including physicians, social workers, and physical therapists.
- Nurses advocate for patients and protect them from instances of inferior care; some nurses risk their careers to blow the whistle on incompetence.[16]
- Nurses found and run new health systems for underserved communities, providing care to patients confronting obesity, prenatal difficulties, violence, and substance abuse.
- ICU nurses diagnose patients' wide-complex tachycardia, call codes, and defibrillate—saving the patients' lives.
- Emergency department nurses triage patients based on their own expert evaluation of who needs care first.
- Military nurses, as commissioned officers, manage complex military care operations around the world.
- Nurses provide most of the professional health care given by aid groups, such as Doctors Without Borders.[17]
- Nurses manage violent, intoxicated patients alone until hospital security arrives—which sometimes does not happen at all, because of resource issues—and so nurses are most at risk for assault in a hospital setting.
- Nurses are the caregivers most likely to be present when patients are screaming, crying, laughing, or dying.

Real nursing is exciting. That's why major hospital shows on television, such as *Grey's Anatomy, House*, and *ER*, have spent so much time showing work that real nurses do. Sadly, they have shown physician characters doing it. But more on that later.

A Few Notes on Nursing History

The origins of nursing depend on what one thinks nursing is. Is it skilled professional health care or just any care? Family members have always cared for the sick. But calling that care "nursing" suggests that anyone is qualified to be a nurse.

Even in ancient times, groups of people cared for those who could not care for themselves. In the third century B.C.E., a school for male caregivers was established in India.[18] Its practitioners focused on moral purity and skill, especially in cleaning beds. In the third century C.E., the Parabolani order in Greece began caring for plague victims. The name Parabolani referred, aptly, to those who took a risk.[19]

The roots of modern nursing are in religious and military settings. In the Middle Ages, European religious orders began to establish groups of trained caregivers. Saint Benedict founded such an order around 500 C.E. Christian deacons and deaconesses cared for the sick in order to serve God.[20] In the sixteenth century the Italian priest Saint Camillus worked to improve care in facilities for the ill and in the wider community.[21] He developed the first ambulance and invented the sign of the red cross to represent care for the sick. In the seventeenth century, Saints Vincent de Paul and Louise de Marillac established the Sisters of Charity (though de Paul preferred "Daughters of Charity") in France to provide health care to the poor. The Sisters did their nursing in patients' homes, on battlefields, and in their own facilities.[22]

But by the nineteenth century, basic care was often provided by less religious individuals. In Europe a "nurse" was commonly thought of as a drunken woman of uncertain morality, such as Sairey Gamp in Charles Dickens's satirical 1844 novel *Martin Chuzzlewit*. In a sense, modern nursing has been caught between the "angel" and the "naughty" images from the beginning.

By the mid-nineteenth century, reformers in Europe and the United States sought to improve the horrific conditions the sick endured, in part by developing a cadre of dedicated female caregivers: nurses. In Bernice Buresh and Suzanne Gordon's *From Silence to Voice* (3rd ed. 2013) and in Gordon's *Nursing Against the Odds* (2005), the authors show that when these reformers professionalized nursing, they sought to establish a respectable job for women outside the home.[23] They had to steer clear of the Gamp image, to enable the nurses to provide intimate care to strangers. The authors, relying in part on the work of nursing scholar Sioban Nelson, show that the reformers used a moral or "virtue" script—first Christian, later civic.[24] This script strongly reinforced nursing's "angel" image. The reformers also assured male physicians that the female nurses would not challenge their authority over care or their scope of practice. Those assurances are important roots of nursing's "handmaiden" image.

The best-known of the reformers was Florence Nightingale, the fierce, brilliant British nurse. Nightingale's wealthy parents initially refused to let her become a nurse. But she managed to receive some hospital training, and in 1854, during the Crimean War, she led a group of nurses in providing care to wounded British soldiers near Constantinople. She soon became revered for her tireless efforts to improve conditions.[25] Back in England, Nightingale tried to reform hospitals, military and civil, particularly in the area of sanitation. In 1860 she established the hospital-based Nightingale Training School for Nurses and published *Notes on Nursing*, which presented nursing as a distinct scientific profession. It is arguably the most influential book ever published about nursing. Nightingale's *Nursing Notes*, the first nursing journal, appeared in 1887. Nightingale also pioneered reforms in care delivery structures and the use of health statistics. Her work had a profound effect on health worldwide. Her nickname—the "Lady with the Lamp"—does not do justice to her accomplishments. But it does at least call attention to her use of light for close 24/7 surveillance and intervention—the hallmark of nursing that may distinguish the profession most clearly from other health care work. Figure 1.1 shows how nurses save lives by using this continuous cycle of monitoring, decision-making, and action.

Other nineteenth century figures also played key roles in the development of nursing, although not all had nursing training. In the middle decades of the century, Dorothea Dix worked to reform US institutions caring for the mentally ill. Clara Barton organized and provided care to soldiers on the

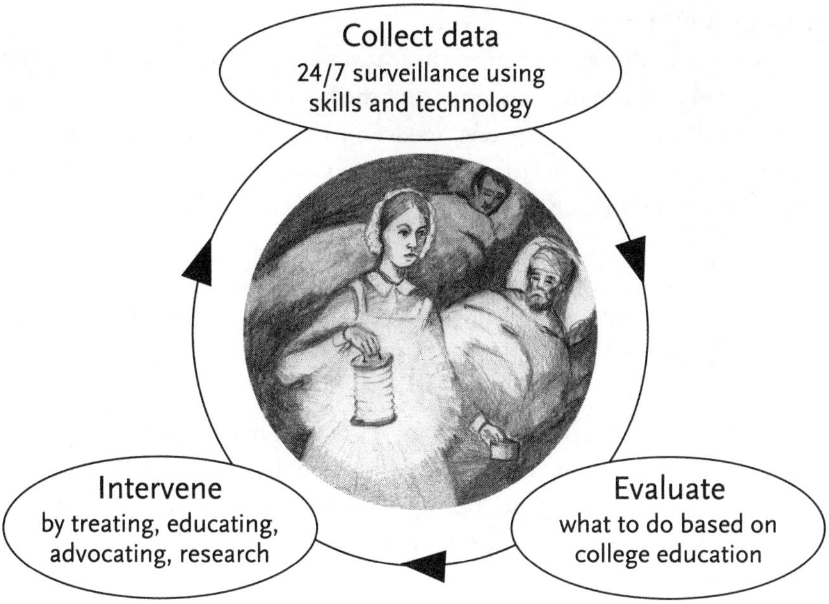
Collect data
24/7 surveillance using skills and technology
Evaluate
what to do based on college education
Intervene
by treating, educating, advocating, research

FIGURE 1.1 How Nurses Save Lives.

battlefields of the Civil War and later founded and led the American Red Cross.[26] She was known as the "Angel of the Battlefield" ("Visionary Disaster Relief Leader" must not have caught on). Linda Richards was the first nurse to graduate from a US nurse training school, at Boston's New England Hospital for Women and Children, in 1872. Richards later established several nurse training schools, including the first in Japan.[27] In 1893, nurse Lillian Wald established New York's Henry Street Settlement, the first visiting nurse institution in the United States.[28] Wald effectively created public health nursing, invented school nursing, and influenced care across the globe.

Although many very early caregivers were male, modern nursing has struggled from the beginning with its gender imbalance. Some men were considered to be acting as nurses during the American Civil War—most famously the poet Walt Whitman—but men were prevented from serving as US military nurses or joining some nursing professional associations until well into the twentieth century.[29]

In the last century, nations began to license nurses, nursing education gradually moved from hospitals to universities, and nursing journals began to flourish. The University of Minnesota granted the first bachelor's degree in nursing in 1909.[30] Yale established the first autonomous school of nursing in 1923.[31] Columbia University first offered a doctorate in education for nurses in 1924, and New York University established the first doctoral program in nursing in 1934.[32]

Meanwhile, nurses were improving care in ways that cut against the grain of accepted practice. In the early part of the last century, Mary Breckinridge established the Frontier Nursing Service in Kentucky, effectively founding US nurse-midwifery. The Frontier Nursing Service has saved the lives of many mothers and children, and it has served as a global model for rural health care delivery.[33]

In the 1960s New York nursing leader and theorist Lydia Hall established an influential nurse-centered rehabilitation hospital, the Loeb Center, where RNs provided all hands-on care. Physicians and other staff played only minor roles.[34]

As understanding and technology advanced, nurses managed increasingly complex patient conditions and care technologies. In the 1960s nurses began training as advanced practitioners in fields that included tasks traditionally done by physicians, although the nurses used their own holistic approach. These advanced practice nurses, most with at least master's degrees in nursing, now provide high-quality care in many health care specialties, but they are especially prominent in family practice, anesthesia, and midwifery. At the same time, graduate-prepared clinical nurse specialists began providing clinical leadership to bedside nurses. In 2004 Columbia established the first doctorate of nursing practice program to award more comprehensive clinical degrees to advanced practice nurses.[35] Nurses have taken the lead in developing better end-of-life care,[36] reducing domestic violence,[37] and improving pain management.[38] Nurses have pioneered cutting-edge fields, such as health informatics, which focuses on managing the increasingly complex body of information in patient care. The American Medical Informatics Association has video interviews of 34 nurse pioneers on its website.[39] And sexual assault forensic nurses represent the state of the art in caring for victims and assembling court evidence.[40]

In recent years nursing leaders have improved public health worldwide through research and innovation. Korean Susie Kim has pioneered new psychiatric treatments and cost-effective mental health centers for the developing world.[41] Kenyan Elizabeth Ngugi has saved countless lives by changing how AIDS care is delivered and studied in ostracized communities.[42] University of Pennsylvania professor Loretta Sweet Jemmott, one of the world's leading experts in preventing HIV transmission to youth, has led efforts to improve the health of underserved urban communities.[43] Jemmott's Penn colleague, prominent scholar Linda Aiken, has published a series of groundbreaking studies linking better working conditions for nurses, including higher staffing levels, with better patient outcomes.[44] Tennessee nurse Carol Etherington has worked to secure the health and human rights of vulnerable populations worldwide, creating effective programs for survivors of natural disaster, war, and other abuses.[45] Johns Hopkins nursing professor Jacquelyn Campbell is one of the world's leading experts in understanding and reducing domestic violence.[46] Ruth Lubic and other nurses have led the struggle to increase US use of nurse midwife-centered childbirth care, which the rest of the developed world uses to achieve better outcomes at a lower cost.[47]

For nursing, the future should be wide open. Nurses have more expertise and in some ways are more empowered than ever, and their holistic approach to public health is sorely needed. But a perfect storm of economic and social factors now poses a threat to nurses and their patients that may be unparalleled in modern times: the global nursing shortage.

The Nursing Shortage

Since the late 1990s, the world has experienced one of the longest and worst nursing shortages in modern history. The shortage has had a devastating effect on patient outcomes—literally killing millions of people every year. While the number of open nursing *positions* has declined in some places as a result of the Great Recession of recent years, the shortage of nursing *care* due to understaffing and undervaluation remains a critical issue worldwide. At its core, the shortage stems from a lack of understanding that nurses are needed to do vital work that could greatly improve global health and prevent costs from spiraling out of control.

Too few nurses are practicing today, and tomorrow may be worse. A 2010 report by the American Hospital Association estimated that US hospitals needed about 4 percent more RNs simply to fill currently vacant positions.[48] A May 2012 poll by National Public Radio, the Robert Wood Johnson Foundation, and the Harvard School of Public Health found that about one-third of hospitalized patients in the United States said nurses were not available when needed or did not respond quickly to requests for help.[49] In January 2012 the US Department of Labor estimated that more than 712,000 new and replacement nurses will be needed by 2020 to create an RN workforce of 3.5 million—a 26 percent increase.[50] A June 2009 report by nursing scholars estimated that the shortage of US nurses could reach 260,000 by 2025.[51] Other developed nations are experiencing similar shortfalls.[52] Meanwhile, as developing nations struggle to finance their meager health care systems, many of their best nurses are emigrating to developed nations eager for their skills.

Immediate causes of the shortage are numerous. Many nurses leave the bedside because of nurse short-staffing or poor working conditions.[53] The nursing workforce is rapidly aging, as too few new nurses are being educated. Inadequate resources are devoted to nursing education, and there is a shortage of qualified faculty. Women in many nations have come to enjoy a far greater range of career choices than in the past. For the most part, women in nursing have not made the gains in workplace empowerment that their counterparts in many other professions have made. At the same time, men are still not entering nursing in significant numbers.[54] Many do not consider the field because they do not know that what nurses do matters. Abusive treatment from physicians and others creates hostile workplaces that continue to drive nurses from the workforce,[55] especially where nurses' status is low.[56] While these problems continue, the demand for nurses has grown because of rapidly aging populations in developed nations and the increasing complexity of health care and care technology.

Short-staffing, driven by the undervaluation of nursing, is central to the crisis. Several key books have explored this, among them *Safety in Numbers*

(2008) by Suzanne Gordon, John Buchanan, and Tanya Bretherton; Gordon's *Nursing Against the Odds* (2005); and Dana Beth Weinberg's *Code Green: Money-Driven Hospitals and the Dismantling of Nursing* (2003).[57] Many nursing positions were actually cut in the 1990s due to managed care, which had curtailed insurance reimbursement, threatening many care facilities. Many hospitals implemented restructuring plans that drastically increased the workloads of RNs. Nurses, who remained underempowered, lacked the resources to resist these threats to their patients and themselves.

At the same time, many care tasks formerly performed by nurses—tasks that enabled nurses to perform critical assessments—were given to less expensive, unlicensed assistive caregivers or not done at all. The job titles of these assistive caregivers include certified nursing assistant (about 6–8 weeks of training), patient care assistant (about 3–4 months), and patient care technician (about 5–7 months).[58] It seems that hospital decision-makers concluded that because tasks like collecting vital signs, walking and bathing patients, and emptying bedpans did not look all that hard to them, facilities could cut costs by having nonnurses do them (while dressed in scrubs like nurses, of course).

But patients pay the price. For example, the vital sign machines upon which such assistive caregivers rely often cannot be trusted; most nurses can attest to seeing these machines report good numbers on patients who were in fact doing very poorly. One of the authors (Sandy) once observed such a machine, still in place after an unsuccessful code, report good numbers on a patient who had died 15 minutes earlier. Imagine if your heart rate was 220 but the machine was only picking up every other heartbeat and reporting it at 110, leading to a lower triage ranking. The author (Sandy) has seen that happen. Consider also that subtle symptoms, such as a tinge of blue color around the mouth, or a little moisture on the skin, or slight retraction of the muscles between the ribs, can signal that a patient is struggling to oxygenate, a condition that could soon lead to death. Wouldn't you want a skilled nurse who could evaluate these tiny cues to your health to determine what was actually going on? And can we talk about poop? Bedpans full of black stool signal intestinal bleeding to nurses, but probably not to assistive caregivers. To nurses, pencil-thin stool sends off warning bells of colon cancer or bowel obstruction; white or light stool suggests possible hepatitis, cirrhosis, or gallbladder obstruction; and mucous stools signal a possible dead bowel. But it's hard to imagine the same analysis from assistive caregivers.

In recent years, austerity policies undertaken in many nations in response to the global recession have resulted in even more pressure to reduce nursing staff. That is why even high nurse vacancy rates do not fully convey the scope of denursification in hospitals. Most hospitals need many more nurses than they are actually seeking.

These conditions have in turn driven away many nurses who could no longer face their growing burnout and the realization that they could not meet their professional responsibilities to their patients.[59] By 2008 roughly half a million US RNs (about one-sixth of the national total) had chosen not to work in nursing.[60]

In recent years many reports have described what short-staffing does to nurses and patients. In February 2004 *Newsweek* ran Michigan emergency department nurse Paul Duke's powerful "If ER Nurses Crash, Will Patients Follow?" Duke's column told how chronic short-staffing was leading him to ask "Did I kill anyone today?" In five years Duke's patient loads had increased from four or five up to ten or twelve. In that environment, he wrote, nurses are "tired and beaten down." Duke vowed to continue with the profession he loved despite feeling "steamrolled," but nurses in general cannot be expected to do so.[61]

In October 2003 *Reader's Digest* published an anonymous ICU nurse's powerful account of one shift in which she was expected, apparently because of staffing decisions made by hospital managers, to do the work of an electrocardiogram technician, nurses' aides, housekeepers, secretaries, and pharmacy delivery people. This overload kept her from giving patients critical medicines on time. Meanwhile, she was responsible for three ICU patients, even though more than one or two is generally regarded as unsafe.[62]

Her patients were an agitated man in restraints suffering alcohol withdrawal, a 300-pound woman with a serious blood infection, and a man with severe cerebral palsy suffering pneumonia and bedsores. The nurse constantly monitored the conditions of these patients and handled their difficult minute-to-minute needs. With the help of other nurses, she adjusted the overweight patient's position so she could breathe. The nurse stopped a dietary worker from giving the patient a meal that would have harmed her. For these key interventions, the nurse received abuse from the patient.

The nurse negotiated a change in a patient's medication to reduce his agitation and the likelihood of complications, despite resistance from junior physicians. The nurse coordinated relations among patients, their families, and other health workers, suffering abuse from family members for not being responsive enough. She also managed to provide skilled support and an Al-Anon referral to a patient's distraught mother. Miraculously, none of the nurse's patients appeared to suffer serious problems. But the nurse ended her piece by describing the physical pain the shift had caused her, noting, "How much longer I can work like this, I just don't know."

In May 2012, National Public Radio reported that understaffing remained widespread in US hospitals. Many nurses were caring for patients nonstop, without breaks, during twelve-hour shifts, while worrying that poor staffing made it impossible to provide safe care. One nurse, declining to give her name because she feared hospital retaliation, gave the example of being unable to respond to one patient's call bell when she had to stay with a different patient while pushing a medication over an extended period, as required to avoid harming the patient. The nurse described driving home at the end of these shifts, her knuckles white on the steering wheel, worrying that she had missed something and thinking that the day she makes a harmful mistake "because the demands exceeded any reasonable capacity on the part of a nurse, that's the day that I never want to be a nurse again."[63]

Sadly, that's not the only thing that can happen on those drives home from work. In November 2013, CNN reported that a man had filed suit against a hospital after the death of his wife, a Cincinnati nurse whose car had veered off the road and hit a tree as she drove home after a long shift. The suit alleged that the nurse's supervisor had expressed fear that she was being "worked to death"; the piece quoted a representative of National Nurses United who argued that "chronic understaffing" remained "rampant" throughout the nation.[64]

A wealth of research links lower nurse staffing levels to nurse burnout and worse patient outcomes, including medication errors, serious complications, longer hospital stays, missed care from surveillance to feedings, and death.[65] Nursing scholar Linda Aiken and colleagues published an influential 2002 study in the *Journal of the American Medical Association* showing that postoperative patients whose nurse had eight patients had a 31 percent higher chance of dying than patients whose nurse had four patients.[66] In 2006 a study in *Health Affairs* showed that raising the number of RNs in hospitals would reduce millions of hospital days and save thousands of lives each year, at a relatively small or no cost.[67] A 2012 follow-up study of hospital data by Aiken and her colleagues found links between poor nurse staffing, nurse burnout, and higher rates of infection, which cost lives and money.[68]

Missed nursing care is a revealing but subtle effect of understaffing, a problem that is so far below the radar that nursing scholar Beatrice Kalisch and colleagues felt the need to explain it in a 2009 concept analysis.[69] In a 2006 study, Kalisch found that the types of care most often left undone were patient education, surveillance, discharge planning, ambulation, turning, feedings, emotional support, hygiene, and intake/output documentation. Eight of those nine critical activities are nurse-prescribed, suggesting that understaffed nurses sacrifice those first. That may be because they view physician-prescribed care, such as medication administration, as more important. Or they may, understandably, want to avoid complaints from a powerful external source.[70]

Globally, the nursing shortage is even more worrisome. A 2009 survey of more than 2,000 nurses across the world by the International Council of Nurses (ICN) and Pfizer found that time constraints prevented 92 percent of nurses from spending the time they thought necessary with patients.[71] The survey also indicated that there were almost twice as many nurses most concerned about heavy workloads (42 percent) as there were nurses most concerned about insufficient pay and benefits (22 percent). Even in highly developed nations, short-staffing can be severe. A 2013 study in the journal *BMJ Quality & Safety*, based on data from hundreds of hospitals in twelve European nations, confirmed that the problem of missed nursing care had become serious and widespread.[72] A 2012 study of staffing at forty-six United Kingdom hospitals by researchers at Kings College London found that nurses had an average of eight patients during the day and eleven at night, in some places fifteen patients at night, and that much nursing care was left undone because of the stressful work environment.[73] The nurse-to-population ratio now varies greatly worldwide. The average ratio in Europe is ten times higher than that in Africa and South East Asia. Some nations, particularly in Central and South America, actually have more physicians than nurses. Bringing the nurse-to-population ratio seen in the most developed nations—roughly 1:100—to the rest of the world would require about 55 million additional nurses, for a total of more than four times the number of nurses we have now. Many nations also have a poor distribution of nurses, with few nurses in rural and remote areas.

In a 2006 report the ICN explained that key factors in the global shortage include the continuing threats of HIV/AIDS, nurse migration, and health sector reform and restructuring.[74] The 2009 ICN report on nurses' socioeconomic welfare noted that gender-based discrimination continues in many countries and cultures, with nursing being undervalued, and that "has resulted in inappropriately low economic and social conditions for many nurses."[75] As the ICN observed, "current compensation structures are often based on gender and not on the value of the job to society."

One of the most alarming global trends is the migration of developing world nurses (and physicians) to much better-paying positions in developed nations with shortages. Notwithstanding the funds these workers send home, this trend has had a devastating impact on already overburdened health systems in poor nations. In a June 2007 article in *Health Services Research*, nursing migration expert Mireille Kingma explained that developed-world shortages had led to aggressive recruiting campaigns overseas. Yet Kingma argued that nurse migration was primarily a "symptom" of larger systemic problems that cause nurses to leave jobs, mainly poor salaries and working conditions. She noted that "no matter how attractive the pull factors of the destination country, little migration takes place without substantial push factors driving people away from the source country." Indeed, in July 2009 CNN reported that Malawi had succeeded in halting its severe nursing "brain drain," at least temporarily, by using international aid funds to give nurses modest pay raises and more educational opportunities. In her 2007 report, Kingma also concluded that "injecting migrant nurses into dysfunctional health systems—ones that are not capable of attracting and retaining domestic-educated staff—is not likely to meet the growing health needs of national populations."[76] Other research has found that foreign-trained nurses working in developed nations tend to practice with less autonomy and to assume less responsibility than their native-born colleagues.[77] In addition, the use of non–US-educated nurses increases patient mortality and failure to rescue.[78]

Although policy makers and thinkers around the world have repeatedly called for measures to strengthen nursing, such as in the landmark 2010 Institute of Medicine report *The Future of Nursing*,[79] legislative efforts to combat the nursing shortage have not yet had a broad impact. Nurse staffing has been a major concern. Following the lead of the Australian state of Victoria, California has been the first US state to impose mandatory minimum nurse staffing ratios, despite fierce opposition from the hospital and insurance industries, which argued that the ratios were impractical and might force hospitals to close. Other jurisdictions that have considered legislation mandating specific minimum ratios include Arizona, the District of Columbia, Florida, Illinois, Iowa, Michigan, Minnesota, Nevada, New Jersey, New York, Pennsylvania, Oregon, Texas, and West Virginia. Fifteen states have passed some sort of staffing legislation, but most of it is weak; only California establishes minimum ratios across all major clinical settings.[80] In June 2014, Massachusetts took a first step by passing legislation for minimum ratios in ICUs.[81] In recent years bills have also been introduced in the US Congress to address staffing ratios, although none has passed. The National Nursing Shortage Reform and Patient Advocacy Act bill, introduced in April 2013, would mandate minimum staffing ratios comparable to those set by California for all hospitals that receive Medicare or Medicaid funds, as well as provide whistleblower protections to nurses. However, passage remains unlikely.[82] The book *Safety in Numbers* argues strongly that mandatory minimum ratios, although not perfect, have proven a cost-effective way to improve working conditions, nurse retention, and patient outcomes in the Australian state of Victoria and in California. The authors show that the horror scenarios predicted by hospitals have not materialized.[83] A 2010 study by Linda Aiken and her colleagues showed that applying the California ratios in Pennsylvania and New Jersey hospitals would save at least hundreds of lives.[84]

Governments have also tried to address some other factors underlying the shortage. By 2010 fifteen US states had prohibited mandatory overtime,[85] but such legislation had yet to pass at the national level. The American Recovery and Reinvestment Act (2009), the massive federal stimulus package passed in response to the economic crisis, did include significant funding for nursing education and community health programs. In addition, the Patient Protection and Affordable Care Act (2010), the major health care reform law known as "ACA" or "Obamacare," includes measures, particularly more insurance coverage, that are likely to increase demand for advanced practice nursing as well as expand federal support for nursing education and community health nursing.[86] But despite these encouraging initiatives, it is not clear whether any current federal legislative measure will have a positive and meaningful long-term impact on nursing.

Hospitals have responded to the shortage in various ways. Many have recruited nurses from overseas[87] and relied on nurse staffing agencies and travel agencies to supplement their staff.[88] Some hospitals have made efforts to improve working conditions, including staffing levels and scheduling policies. In 2012, Philadelphia's Hahnemann Hospital announced that it was adopting an all-RN staffing model.[89] A relatively small number of hospitals, mostly in the United States, have earned Magnet status. The American Nurses' Credentialing Center awards Magnet status to hospitals that satisfy criteria designed to measure the strength and quality of their nursing, including nurses' participation in decision making, job satisfaction, low turnover, and appropriate grievance resolution. Some critics (including nursing unions) have argued that the program is inadequate because it lacks minimum nurse-to-patient ratios, that the nurse empowerment it offers is mostly illusory, and that hospitals have used it mainly as a promotional tool.[90] Recent research has indicated that Magnet hospitals offer some benefits. A 2011 study found that they had "better work environments," with better educated nurses who were less burned out,[91] and a 2013 study found that Magnet hospital patients had lower mortality rates.[92]

Hospital residencies for nurses are a very promising trend. A major residency program involving twenty-eight US care facilities reported a one-year retention rate of 94 percent of new nurses compared to the mere 66 percent who stayed for one year in the absence of the residencies, under the traditional "throw them in and see if they can swim" approach.[93] Yet funding remains elusive. From 2003 to 2008 nursing residencies received roughly $1 of federal funding for every $375 that physician residencies received.[94]

Several media campaigns have aimed to address the nursing shortage. Perhaps the most prominent is Johnson & Johnson's ongoing Campaign for Nursing's Future, launched in 2002. Since then, the drug company has spent tens of millions of dollars on television ads, recruiting videos, a website, and scholarships. Some of these campaign efforts have been positive, but the widely seen television ads have often presented nursing in the same emotional ways in which the public already sees the profession, de-emphasizing nursing skill, and so have done little to enhance real understanding.[95] Nurses for a Healthier Tomorrow, a coalition of health care groups, has tried to interest secondary school students in nursing through focus groups, a website, and other activities. Nurses for a Healthier Tomorrow has also encouraged nurses to become nurse educators. Their media efforts have given specific examples of the life-saving value of nursing.[96]

In recent years, interest in nursing careers has increased somewhat in the United States, due at least in part to a dismal economy and a growing awareness that nursing offers plentiful, diverse positions with the chance to better lives, along with starting pay that is good relative to the amount of formal training required. No doubt this awareness has been driven by extensive media coverage of the shortage and by the previously mentioned media campaigns.

Unfortunately, simply training more nurses, like recruiting from other nations or regions, will do little to address many of the key underlying causes of the nursing shortage. Moreover, a critical shortage of nursing faculty has hampered efforts to educate more nurses, and US nursing schools have turned away many qualified applicants; more than 75,000 such applicants were denied admission in 2011 alone.[97] A 2007 report by the National League for Nursing and the Carnegie Foundation found that nurse educators earn only three-fourths of what faculty in other academic disciplines earn and significantly less than other nurses with the same educational credentials, such as advanced practice nurses.[98] Nursing scholars get relatively little funding from the US government. As of 2014, funding for nursing research made up *less than half of 1 percent* of the budget for the National Institutes of Health.[99]

Recent reports show that the nursing shortage and nurse short-staffing remain critical problems throughout the world. The long-term crisis in the United States is ongoing, although the shortage of nurses seemed to ease temporarily during the Great Recession, as veteran nurses who had left the bedside were forced to return and some care facilities cut staffing even further.[100] In May 2009 the *New York Times* reported that clinics in Prague were offering nurses free plastic surgery in efforts to replace the thousands who had left the Czech Republic for higher-paying jobs in other European nations.[101] Other reports show that the shortage remains critical in nations ranging from Israel to South Korea, where, according to a June 2010 *Korea Times* piece, many nurses face crushing workloads and can think only of sleep.[102]

The picture in poorer nations is often worse. An August 2009 study in *Health Affairs* estimated that the nations of sub-Saharan Africa would be short 551,000 nurses and midwives by 2015.[103] A July 2011 item from the South Africa Press Association reported a "debilitating" brain drain of Zimbabwean nurses not only to developed nations, but also to neighboring Botswana, while nurses who remained had "been reduced to selling tomatoes and other fruit to survive due to poor public sector salaries," according to the health minister.[104] In March 2008 the Indian newspaper *The Hindu* ran a story headlined "India Running Short of Two Million Nurses." The piece reported that nearly 20 percent of "experienced nurses" had left India for the United States or Europe.[105]

If the shortage continues as projected, it will have catastrophic effects. Already it severely hampers our ability to respond effectively to mass casualty events, because nurses would provide the great majority of the care those require. For example, the critical shortage of US school nursing undermines efforts to prevent and contain the H1N1 flu, as a September 2009 Associated Press story reported.[106] In some nations, the shortage is obstructing economic, social, and political development across the board. As the 2006 ICN report stressed, the nursing shortage is a public health crisis.[107]

But as we argue in the chapters that follow, a critical factor underlying the shortage is the huge gap between the *actual* nature and value of nursing, on the one hand, and what policy makers, career seekers, and the public at large *believe* about nursing on the other. Nursing has not received adequate resources because it continues to be seen as a peripheral, menial job for women with few other options. Legislative reforms and better funding will not be enough, vital as those steps are. All the numbers measuring the shortage reflect what starts in our minds. The shortage cannot be resolved until public understanding improves. We must change how the world *thinks* about nursing.

Notes

In these endnotes, The Truth About Nursing is abbreviated "TAN" and the Center for Nursing Advocacy as "CFNA." Please see www.truthaboutnursing.org/references/ for live hyperlinks providing easy online access to virtually all of the references cited below.

1. TAN, "Q: Are You Sure Nurses Are Autonomous? Based on What I've Seen, It Sure Looks Like Physicians Are Calling the Shots," accessed January 28, 2014, http://tinyurl.com/7qfa8zu.
2. Hanne Dina Bernstein, "Reflections: Two Cups: The Healing Power of Tea," *American Journal of Nursing* 104, no. 4 (April 2004): 39, http://tinyurl.com/nqjbyez.
3. Cnet.com, "Biden: 'Doctors Allow You to Live; Nurses Make You Want to Live'" (June 3, 2013), http://tinyurl.com/ks6jlgm.
4. Julie Thao, "Julie Thao's Speech in Pasadena," California, January 28, 2010, YouTube video, http://tinyurl.com/obtuutb.
5. International Council of Nurses, "About ICN" (June 14, 2013), http://tinyurl.com/nxubwo4.
6. US Department of Labor, Bureau of Labor Statistics, "Occupational Employment Statistics: May 2012 National Occupational Employment and Wage Estimates," http://tinyurl.com/q2ywzuv.
7. US Department of Health and Human Services, Health Resources and Services Administration (HRSA), "The Registered Nurse Population: Findings from the 2008 National Sample Survey of Registered Nurses" (2010), http://tinyurl.com/7zgyet7.
8. US Department of Labor, Bureau of Labor Statistics, "Physicians and Surgeons," accessed January 8, 2014, http://tinyurl.com/77ghlzk.
9. David I. Auerbach, Douglas O. Staiger, Ulrike Muench, and Peter I. Buerhaus, "The Nursing Workforce: A Comparison of Three National Surveys," *Nursing Economic$* 30, no. 5 (September-October 2012), http://tinyurl.com/kd63p27.
10. HRSA, "RN Sample Survey" (2010), http://tinyurl.com/7zgyet7; Jane Kirschling, "Designing DNP Programs to Meet Required Competencies—Context for the Conversation" (2012), http://tinyurl.com/oajvwx8.
11. US Department of Labor, Bureau of Labor Statistics, "Query System: Occupational Employment Statistics: Registered Nurses, Nursing Instructors and Teachers, Postsecondary (251072); Registered Nurses (291141); Nurse Anesthetists (291151); Nurse Midwives (291161); Nurse Practitioners (291171); Licensed Practical and Licensed Vocational Nurses (292061)" (May 2012), http://data.bls.gov/oes/;

National Association of Clinical Nurse Specialists, "Clinical Nurse Specialist" (2012), http://tinyurl.com/lcn9eaj.

12. US Department of Labor, Bureau of Labor Statistics, "Occupational Employment Statistics: 29–1151 Nurse Anesthetists; 29–1061 Anesthesiologists" (May 2012), http://tinyurl.com/k4jb5yg and http://tinyurl.com/azxds7v.
13. US Census Bureau, "Men in Nursing Occupations: American Community Survey Highlight Report" (February 2013), http://tinyurl.com/mjxgvue.
14. Michael J. Villeneuve, "Recruiting and Retaining Men in Nursing: A Review of the Literature," *Journal of Professional Nursing* 10, no. 4 (1994): 217–228, http://tinyurl.com/k2jdvsj.
15. US Census Bureau, "Men in Nursing Occupations: American Community Survey Highlight Report" (February 2013), http://tinyurl.com/mjxgvue; Michael J. Villeneuve, "Recruiting and Retaining Men in Nursing: A Review of the Literature," *Journal of Professional Nursing* 10, no. 4 (1994): 217–228, http://tinyurl.com/k2jdvsj.
16. TAN, "Remain in Light" (February 11, 2010), http://tinyurl.com/o9khkr7; CFNA, "Enemy of the People," TAN (June 22, 2005), http://tinyurl.com/o4y7bhs.
17. CFNA, "Infirmières Sans Frontières," TAN (December 3, 2006), http://tinyurl.com/jwa9goe.
18. Bruce Wilson, "The Story of Men in American Nursing," American Assembly of Men in Nursing (November 5, 1997), citing *The Charaka*, Vol. 1, Section xv, http://tinyurl.com/oxrnt38.
19. Patrick Healy, "Parabolani," *The Catholic Encyclopedia*, Vol. 11 (New York: Robert Appleton Company, 1911), http://tinyurl.com/pal4o6o.
20. Christian Classics Ethereal Library, "The Holy Rule of St. Benedict" (1949), Chapter 31, http://tinyurl.com/5w5ely; M. Patricia Donahue, *Nursing, the Finest Art: An Illustrated History*, 3rd ed. (St. Louis: Mosby, 2010): 54.
21. Alban Butler, Donald Attwater, and Herbert Thurston, *Lives of the Saints* (London: Burns & Oates, 1956): 135.
22. AmericanCatholic.org, "St. Louise de Marillac," accessed March 15, 2014, http://tinyurl.com/k2hm3hy.
23. Bernice Buresh and Suzanne Gordon, *From Silence to Voice*, 3rd ed. (Ithaca: Cornell University Press, 2013); Suzanne Gordon, *Nursing Against the Odds: How Health Care Cost-Cutting, Media Stereotypes, and Medical Hubris Undermine Nursing and Patient Care* (Ithaca: Cornell University Press, 2005).
24. Sioban Nelson, "The Image of Nurses – The Historical Origins of Invisibility in Nursing," *Texto & Contexto – Enfermagem* 20, no. 2 (April–June 2011), http://tinyurl.com/ngrw3hs.
25. Florence Nightingale Museum, "Florence's Biography," accessed June 17, 2014, http://tinyurl.com/mppnene.
26. Cole Summers, "Clara Barton," TAN, accessed June 19, 2014, http://tinyurl.com/p3yrayf.

27. American Association for the History of Nursing, "Linda A. J. Richard," accessed June 17, 2104, http://tinyurl.com/2flqy7m.
28. Henry Street Settlement, "Lillian Wald," accessed January 29, 2014, http://tinyurl.com/lqcskyx.
29. Bruce Wilson, "The Story of Men in American Nursing," American Assembly of Men in Nursing (November 5, 1997), http://tinyurl.com/ylecjh4, http://tinyurl.com/yh4mqyh.
30. University of Minnesota School of Nursing, "History" (August 23, 2013), http://tinyurl.com/oeak5qf.
31. Judith Schiff, "Yale's First Female Dean," *Yale Alumni Magazine* (March–April 2011), http://tinyurl.com/k4qmy72.
32. Susan Apold, "The Doctor of Nursing Practice: Looking Back, Moving Forward," *Journal for Nurse Practitioners* 4, no. 2 (2008): 101–107.
33. Gina Castlenovo, "Mary Breckinridge," TAN (2003), www.truthaboutnursing.org/press/pioneers/breckinridge.html.
34. Foundation of New York State Nurses, Inc., Bellevue Alumnae Center for Nursing History, "Loeb Center for Nursing and Rehabilitation Records" (July 2006), http://tinyurl.com/yfkqyh8; Richard Kimball, Mei-Hua Lee, and Sandy Summers, "Lydia Hall, 1906–1969," TAN (2000), http://tinyurl.com/p3fdt25.
35. Columbia News, "First-Ever Clinical Doctorate in Nursing Approved," Columbia University (February 16, 2005), http://tinyurl.com/nfrj67b.
36. Cynthia Adams, "Florence Wald: Pioneer in Hospice Care," TAN (2008), http://tinyurl.com/ouh4ape.
37. Johns Hopkins University School of Nursing, "Jacquelyn Campbell, PhD, RN, FAAN," accessed December 1, 2013, http://tinyurl.com/motvca4.
38. Johns Hopkins University School of Nursing, "Gayle Page, DNSc, RN, FAAN," accessed January 29, 2014, http://tinyurl.com/n8kgvse; TAN, "The Orb of Life" (December 1, 2009), http://tinyurl.com/yeuywam; TAN, "Nurses: Pain Affects Everything Else" (September 14, 2009), http://tinyurl.com/ov2n282.
39. American Medical Informatics Association, "Video Library 1: Nursing Informatics Pioneers," accessed January 29, 2014, http://tinyurl.com/k5ejth4.
40. International Association of Forensic Nurses, "What Is Forensic Nursing?," accessed January 30, 2014, http://tinyurl.com/yh2b9d3.
41. Florence Nightingale International Foundation, "The International Achievement Award: Susie Kim (2001), RN DNSc, FAAN," http://tinyurl.com/pf9qyfy; Carol Findlay, "Susie Kim: Role Model of Excellence," *Journal of Christian Nursing* 19, no. 3 (January 2002): 30–32, http://tinyurl.com/qbheoua.
42. Geoffrey Cowley, "The Life of a Virus Hunter," *Newsweek* (May 15, 2006), http://tinyurl.com/n39ndk9.
43. Dianne Hales, "The Quiet Heroes," *Parade* (March 21, 2004), http://tinyurl.com/lyz5yly.

44. University of Pennsylvania School of Nursing, "Linda Aiken," accessed January 30, 2014, http://tinyurl.com/ygeenrp.
45. Vanderbilt University, "Etherington Honored with MLK Award" (January 24, 2013), http://tinyurl.com/nlt2saj; Florence Nightingale International Foundation, "Awards: Carol Etherington (2003), MSN, RN, FAAN," http://tinyurl.com/yl7gaje.
46. Johns Hopkins, "Jacquelyn Campbell," http://tinyurl.com/motvca4.
47. Phuong Ly, "A Labor Without End," *Washington Post* (May 27, 2007): W20, http://tinyurl.com/ypevt9.
48. American Hospital Association, "The 2010 State of America's Hospitals—Taking the Pulse" (May 24, 2010), http://tinyurl.com/kolwz4l.
49. Robert Wood Johnson Foundation, "Sick in America: Nurses, Other Providers Stretched Thin" (May 29, 2012), http://tinyurl.com/k6otvyt.
50. C. Brett Lockard and Michael Wolf, "Occupational Employment: Employment Outlook: 2010–2020: Occupational Employment Projections to 2020," US Department of Labor, Bureau of Labor Statistics, Monthly Labor Review (January 2012): 89, http://tinyurl.com/ks2t7rr. See also US Department of Labor, Bureau of Labor Statistics, "Occupational Outlook Handbook, 2012–13 Edition, Registered Nurses," http://tinyurl.com/bbabjho.
51. Peter Buerhaus, David Auerbach, and Douglas Staiger, "The Recent Surge in Nurse Employment: Causes and Implications," *Health Affairs* 28, no. 4 (June 2009): w657-w668, http://tinyurl.com/ykfpogv, doi: 10.1377/hlthaff.28.4.w657. For more information see American Association of Colleges of Nursing, "Nursing Shortage Resources," accessed January 29, 2014, http://tinyurl.com/knz7rev.
52. Jane E. Ball, Trevor Murrells, Anne Marie Rafferty, Elizabeth Morrow, and Peter Griffiths, "'Care Left Undone' During Nursing Shifts: Associations with Workload and Perceived Quality of Care," *BMJ Quality & Safety* 23, no. 2 (2014): 116–125 doi:10.1136/bmjqs-2012-001767, http://tinyurl.com/kdhq75w; Bonnie J. Wakefield, "Facing Up to the Reality of Missed Care," *BMJ Quality & Safety* 23 (2014): 92–94, http://tinyurl.com/lrmj793; TAN, "How to Help Nurses Practice at the Top of Their Game" (August 5, 2012), http://tinyurl.com/qamfcof.
53. TAN, "What Happens to Patients When Nurses Are Short-Staffed?," accessed January 29, 2014, http://tinyurl.com/ancmo7r.
54. US Census Bureau, "Men in Nursing Occupations: American Community Survey Highlight Report" (February 2013), http://tinyurl.com/mjxgvue.
55. Alan H. Rosenstein, "Nurse-Physician Relationships: Impact on Nurse Satisfaction and Retention," *American Journal of Nursing* 102, no. 6 (June 2002): 26–34, http://tinyurl.com/yz47l4y.
56. TAN, "Q: What Is Physician Disruptive Behavior and Why Does It Exist?," accessed January 29, 2014, http://tinyurl.com/pwghq62; TAN, "The Weather in My Head" (March 16, 2013), http://tinyurl.com/q6h6fmx; TAN, "Thanking the

Nurse" (August 5, 2012), http://tinyurl.com/pmfs55o; TAN, "Angels on Earth" (October 14, 2012), http://tinyurl.com/or8qhrr.

57. Suzanne Gordon, John Buchanan, and Tanya Bretherton, *Safety in Numbers* (Ithaca: Cornell University Press, 2008); Gordon, *Nursing Against the Odds* (2005); Dana Beth Weinberg, *Code Green: Money-Driven Hospitals and the Dismantling of Nursing* (Ithaca: Cornell University Press, 2003). For more information see TAN, "What Happens To Patients When Nurses Are Short-Staffed?," accessed January 28, 2014, http://tinyurl.com/ancmo7r.
58. Learn 4 Good, "Contact Page - Medical Career School in Plantation, FL," accessed March 8, 2014, http://tinyurl.com/pnyalsg.
59. Jeannie P. Cimiotti, Linda H. Aiken, Douglas M. Sloane, and Evan S. Wu, "Nurse Staffing, Burnout, and Health Care-Associated Infection," *American Journal of Infection Control* 40 (2012): 486–490, http://tinyurl.com/n4cu6p8; Linda Aiken, Sean Clarke, Douglas Sloane, Julie Sochalski, and Jeffrey Silber, "Hospital Nurse Staffing and Patient Mortality, Nurse Burnout, and Job Dissatisfaction," *Journal of the American Medical Association* 288, no. 16 (October 23–30, 2002): 1987–93, http://tinyurl.com/pu6saw9; TAN, "Short-Staffed," http://tinyurl.com/ancmo7r.
60. HRSA, "The Registered Nurse Population: Findings from the 2008 National Sample Survey of Registered Nurses" (2010), http://tinyurl.com/7zgyet7.
61. Paul Duke, "If ER Nurses Crash, Will Patients Follow?," *Newsweek* (February 2, 2004), http://tinyurl.com/kbxxfyt.
62. Anonymous, "One Day in Critical Care: A Nurse's Story," *Reader's Digest* (October 2003), http://tinyurl.com/kd6zph9; CFNA, "Reader's Digest: Burnt-out ICU Nurse 'Blows the Whistle,'" TAN (October 2003), http://tinyurl.com/nb2nv5t.
63. Patti Neighmond, "Sick in America," National Public Radio (May 25, 2012), http://tinyurl.com/7kf9eab; TAN, "Are Your Knuckles White?" (May 25, 2012), http://tinyurl.com/nhdpoas.
64. Dominique Debucquoy-Dodley, "Lawsuit: Ohio Nurse Was 'Worked to Death," CNN (November 13, 2013), http://tinyurl.com/m3krctj.
65. TAN, "Short-Staffed," http://tinyurl.com/ancmo7r.
66. Linda Aiken, Sean Clarke, Douglas Sloane, Julie Sochalski, and Jeffrey Silber, "Hospital Nurse Staffing and Patient Mortality, Nurse Burnout, and Job Dissatisfaction," *Journal of the American Medical Association* 288, no. 16 (October 23–30, 2002): 1987–93, http://tinyurl.com/lf7qr48.
67. Jack Needleman, Peter Buerhaus, Maureen Stewart, Katya Zelevinsky, and Soeren Mattke, "Nurse Staffing in Hospitals: Is There a Business Case for Quality?," *Health Affairs* 25, no. 1 (2006): 204–11, http://tinyurl.com/m7kdm3l; CFNA, "No Magic Number," TAN (January 21, 2006), http://tinyurl.com/qxfjgzu.
68. Jeannie P. Cimiotti, Linda H. Aiken, Douglas M. Sloane, and Evan S. Wu, "Nurse Staffing, Burnout, and Health Care–Associated Infection," *American Journal of Infection Control* 40, no. 6 (August 2012): 486–490, http://tinyurl.com/prg2vzd;

TAN, "How to Help Nurses Practice at the Top of Their Game" (August 5, 2012), http://tinyurl.com/qamfcof.

69. Beatrice J. Kalisch, Gay L. Landstrom, and Ada Sue Hinshaw, "Missed Nursing Care: A Concept Analysis," *Journal of Advanced Care* 65, no. 7 (2009): 1509–1517, http://tinyurl.com/lprkbjh.
70. Beatrice J. Kalisch, "Missed Nursing Care: A Qualitative Study," *Journal of Nursing Care Quality* 21, no. 4 (December 2006): 306–313, http://tinyurl.com/n5vmrlb.
71. International Council of Nurses and Pfizer, "Nurses in the Workplace: Expectations and Needs" (May 2009), http://tinyurl.com/mzsyne2.
72. Dietmar Ausserhofer, Britta Zander, Reinhard Busse, Maria Schubert, Sabina De Geest, Anne Marie Rafferty, Jane Ball, et al., "Prevalence, Patterns and Predictors of Nursing Care Left Undone in European Hospitals: Results from the Multicountry Cross-Sectional RN4CAST Study," *BMJ Quality & Safety* (November 11, 2013), http://tinyurl.com/k3m9mhf.
73. Jane E. Ball, Trevor Murrells, Anne Marie Rafferty, Elizabeth Morrow, and Peter Griffiths, "Care Left Undone," http://tinyurl.com/kdhq75w.
74. International Council of Nurses, "The Global Shortage of Registered Nurses: An Overview of Issues and Actions" (2006), http://tinyurl.com/k45zym6.
75. International Council of Nurses, "Position Statement: Socio-Economic Welfare of Nurses" (2009), http://tinyurl.com/kvl2dkp.
76. Mireille Kingma, "Nurses On the Move: A Global Overview," *Health Services Research* 42, no. 3 (March 20, 2007): 1281–1298, http://tinyurl.com/km738zu. See also Mireille Kingma, *Nurses on the Move: Migration and the Global Health Care Economy* (Ithaca: Cornell University Press, 2006); TAN, "Q: How Is Nurse Migration Affecting Nurses and the Nursing Shortage?," accessed January 28, 2014, http://tinyurl.com/oe3ep66.
77. Paul H. Troy, Laura A. Wyness, and Eilish McAuliffe, "Nurses' Experiences of Recruitment and Migration from Developing Countries: A Phenomenological Approach," *Human Resources for Health* 2007, 5:15, http://tinyurl.com/ljbbelr.
78. Donna Felber Neff, Jeannie Cimiotti, Douglas M. Sloane, and Linda H. Aiken, "Utilization of Non-US Educated Nurses in US Hospitals," *International Journal for Quality in Health Care* 25, no. 4 (2013): 366–372, http://tinyurl.com/n857hxx.
79. Institute of Medicine of the National Academies, "The Future of Nursing: Leading Change, Advancing Health" (October 5, 2010), http://tinyurl.com/2brrusk.
80. American Nurses Association, "Nurse Staffing Plans & Ratios" (December 2013), http://tinyurl.com/par65rs.
81. Gintautas Dumcius, "Governor Signs Nurse-Staffing ICU Bill," *The Lowell Sun*, (June 30, 2014), http://tinyurl.com/qxs3q4j.
82. American Nurses Association, "Safe Staffing," accessed January 28, 2014, http://tinyurl.com/kz4uasu; ANA, "Nurse Staffing" (2013), http://tinyurl.com/par65rs.
83. Gordon, Buchanan, and Bretherton, *Safety* (2008).

84. Linda H. Aiken, Douglas M. Sloane, Jeannie P. Cimiotti, Sean P. Clarke, Linda Flynn, Jean Ann Seago, Joanne Spetz, and Herbert L. Smith, "Implications of the California Nurse Staffing Mandate for Other States," *Health Services Research* 45, no. 4 (April 2010): 904–921, http://tinyurl.com/lkwzvlt.
85. American Nurses Association, "Mandatory Overtime" (January 2012), http://tinyurl.com/lynzoo5.
86. Maria Schiff, "The Role of Nurse Practitioners in Meeting Increasing Demand for Primary Care," National Governors Association (December 2012), http://tinyurl.com/l6f7owb.
87. TAN, "Nurse Migration," http://tinyurl.com/oe3ep66.
88. Dennis O'Brien, "Nurses To Go," *Baltimore Sun* (March 17, 2006), http://tinyurl.com/67vgbw; CFNA, "Would You Like a Krabby Patty with That?," TAN (March 17, 2006), http://tinyurl.com/nr5v4p9.
89. TAN, "America's Top RN Model?" (February 7, 2012), http://tinyurl.com/pk7kjlc.
90. TAN, "Magnet Status: What It Is, What It Is Not, and What It Could Be," accessed January 28, 2014, http://tinyurl.com/79mxv8y.
91. Lesly A. Kelly, Matthew D. McHugh, and Linda Aiken, "Nurse Outcomes in Magnet® and Non-Magnet Hospitals," *Journal of Nursing Administration* 41, no. 10 (October 2011): 428–433, http://tinyurl.com/meyrycv.
92. Matthew McHugh, Lesly A. Kelly, Herbert L. Smith, Evan S. Wu, Jill M. Vanak, and Linda H. Aiken, "Lower Mortality in Magnet Hospitals," *Medical Care* 51, no. 5 (May 2013): 382–388, http://tinyurl.com/mskp4pg.
93. University HealthSystem and American Association of Colleges of Nursing Consortium, "University of Wisconsin Hospital and Clinics Reduces New Graduate Nurse Turnover by 80% With UHC's Nurse Residency Program" (2007), http://tinyurl.com/n5o3adu; Robert Wood Johnson Foundation, Initiative on the Future of Nursing, "The Value of Nurse Education and Residency Programs" (May 2011), http://tinyurl.com/n8t64dp.
94. TAN, "Throw Them Out There" (February 15, 2009), http://tinyurl.com/qfg279h.
95. TAN, "Lucky Charms" (June 2011), http://tinyurl.com/q7xtf2t; CFNA, "Baby We Were Born to Care," TAN (November 2007), http://tinyurl.com/oysyl4t; CFNA, "Touching the World," TAN (May 2006), http://tinyurl.com/lx6k9jy.
96. Nurses for a Healthier Tomorrow, "Careers in Nursing Campaign," accessed January 29, 2014, http://tinyurl.com/paftxzb.
97. American Association of Colleges of Nursing, "New AACN Data Show an Enrollment Surge in Baccalaureate and Graduate Programs Amid Calls for More Highly Educated Nurses" (March 22, 2012), http://tinyurl.com/y9dtqnv.
98. National League for Nursing, "Key Findings of Nationwide NLN-Carnegie Foundation: Study of Nurse Educators Released" (August 29, 2007), http://tinyurl.com/yj8bzct.

99. Department of Health and Human Services, National Institutes of Health, "Overall Appropriations FY 2014," http://tinyurl.com/kwxgg5j.
100. Peter Buerhaus, David Auerbach, and Douglas Staiger, "The Recent Surge in Nurse Employment: Causes and Implications," *Health Affairs* 28, no. 4 (2009): w657–w668, http://tinyurl.com/k8mrzve.
101. Dan Bilefsky, "If Plastic Surgery Won't Convince You, What Will?," *The New York Times* (May 24, 2009), http://tinyurl.com/puoyvl; TAN, "We Are Offering Free Breasts" (July 14, 2009), http://tinyurl.com/l4eylmp.
102. TAN, "Aggravating" (July 6, 2010), http://tinyurl.com/nsusacp.
103. *Health Affairs*, "Sub-Saharan Africa to Face Shortage of Nearly 800,000 Health Care Professionals in 2015" (August 6, 2009), http://tinyurl.com/lv4z54p.
104. TAN, "Saving Lives and Selling Tomatoes" (July 6, 2011), http://tinyurl.com/nk6uv59.
105. Press Trust of India, "India Running Short of Two Million Nurses," *The Hindu* (March 17, 2008), http://tinyurl.com/6zg6n2.
106. TAN, "Crucial, but Not Consulted" (September 2, 2009), http://tinyurl.com/pfmn8la.
107. ICN, "Global Shortage" (2006), http://tinyurl.com/k45zym6.

2 HOW NURSING'S IMAGE AFFECTS YOUR HEALTH

In 2007 a friend of ours got a telephone call. Producers of a popular US prime-time television hospital show that was seen around the world had found her name, presumably in a database of experts. The producers called for a script consultation because our friend is a leading expert in a certain health field. Our friend gave the television producers cutting-edge information to help them develop a plotline.

Our friend said that these Hollywood producers "were *super* surprised I was a nurse—and *super, super* surprised I had a PhD and was one of the leading researchers in the country on this issue." She also "took the opportunity to say quite a bit to them about nursing—both how nurses could be used in the story line and how their general approach to nursing could be substantively improved."

The result? The producers said the show's audience was "interested in doctors not nurses." They said there were no plans to have a nurse character with a significant role: "We have a stable cast and the focus of the show is on physicians." Do not attempt to adjust your television: the stereotypes are in control.

THIS IS A SELF-REINFORCING LOOP: Hollywood tells its audience that physicians' work is dramatic and important, and nursing is not, because that's what the audience expects. And the audience expects to see the stories of physicians rather than nurses in large part because that's what Hollywood presents as compelling entertainment. In fact, as we explained in Chapter 1, real nursing work is highly dramatic and real nurses are much more present in the stories of hospital patients[1]—which is why television physicians spend so much time doing nursing work. Even on the diagnosis-*über-alles* Fox drama *House*, physician characters spent a good deal of time doing what is really nursing work. However, it was presented as the work of physicians. The real physician role alone does not seem to be interesting enough to carry a television drama.

The media has long been fascinated with health care, especially what goes on in hospitals. Countless health items appear daily in the various news media, particularly in light of ongoing national debates over health care financing and technology. Many of the most popular recent television series have been hospital shows, which, like shows about police and lawyers, provide a potentially endless array of cases and characters in conflict, often on the edge of life and death, which tends to make for good television drama. The media's interest in health care, in which nursing plays a central role, is unlikely to wane.

Occasionally the media offers insight into what nurses really do. Examples include an excellent 2012 *New York Times* "Fixes" piece by Tina Rosenberg explaining how clinics run by nurse practitioners can address the shortage of primary care,[2] a 2007 series on the nursing shortage on WBUR (the Boston National Public Radio [NPR] affiliate),[3] and the 2003 HBO film *Angels in America*.[4]

But most of the time nurses are presented as the peripheral and/or sexy servants of the heroic physicians who provide all important care—the care that saves or improves lives. The health sections of major booksellers overflow with titles by or about physicians. Even the elite news media, such as the *New York Times* and NPR, relentlessly equate "doctors" with all of health care. "Doctors are doing all they can," but "doctors say the patient's condition is critical." This is true even in such areas as intensive care, in which nurses actually take the lead in keeping critical patients alive by constantly evaluating them and managing highly complex treatments.

Research has shown that nurses appear in less than 7 percent of health-related newspaper articles. Studies in the United States in the 1990s found that nurses appeared in just 1–4 percent of such articles.[5] More recently, a 2011 study by Pedro Alcântara da Silva of 2,781 articles published between 1990 and 2004 in three Portuguese newspapers found that nurses were sources of information in only 1.1 percent of the news pieces, appeared in 4.4 percent of article titles, and were mentioned in 2.6 percent of the first-page health-related stories.[6] Still, in research published in 2014, Rodrigo Cardoso and colleagues at Coimbra Nursing School found that nurses appeared in 6.6 percent of 1,271 online Portuguese health news items from 2011.[7] Maybe we're making progress! When nurses do appear, it's usually in pieces specifically about nursing's discontents—the nursing shortage, understaffing, abuse of nurses, labor disputes, or extreme misconduct by nurses, like serial killing. It's relatively rare for the media to cover the life-saving work nurses do every day at their jobs or to consult nurses as the health care experts they really are. That contributes to nurses feeling invisible in their work.[8]

The entertainment media is even more troubling. It's true that J. K. Rowling's vastly popular Harry Potter novels, published from 1997 to 2007, include the very minor character Madam Pomfrey. This wizardry school nurse is single-handedly able to cure dragon bites, treat curses, and heal Harry after he falls fifty feet off a flying broom.

But television remains in many ways the dominant global medium. On health-related shows airing during the 2012–2013 prime-time US television season, physician characters outnumbered nurse characters by roughly 47 to 2, unless you count *Call the Midwife*, the United Kingdom show that airs to a limited audience on PBS in the United States. Thus, physician shows continued to dominate. Since 2005 *Grey's Anatomy* has shown its smart, attractive surgeon stars providing all significant care. Although appearances by nurse characters are few and far between, the lives of the nurses who do appear on the show revolve around the physician characters.[9] Over the last decade *Grey's* vied with *House*, which ran from 2004 to 2012, to be the contemporary show most damaging to nursing (the two of us debated which one was worse). *House* also featured a slew of smart, pretty physicians, led by the brilliant, acerbic lead character, Greg House. Again, these physicians provided all important bedside care. The show generally treated the few nurses who appeared—to mutely absorb physician commands—with contempt.[10] These two shows regularly attracted tens of millions of US viewers, and both have been popular around the world.

Other notable contemporary shows have not been much better. The *Grey's* spinoff *Private Practice,* which ran on ABC from 2007 to 2013, focused on another group of pretty, smart physicians. One early character was clinic receptionist Dell, a cute surfer boy—and a nurse studying midwifery, a field the show mocked relentlessly in its first season.[11] Dell appeared in a May 2008 *TV Guide* poll of the "sexiest secretaries" on television. Portrayals of Dell improved somewhat over time, but he was unlikely to be mistaken for a health care expert. And just before the show killed him off in 2010, there was a parting insult to nursing: Dell proudly announced that he had been admitted to medical school, the path Hollywood often suggests that capable nurses ultimately take, even though real nurses are about one hundred times more likely to pursue graduate education in nursing.[12] Similarly, in TNT's summer show *The Glades* (2010–2013), the lead detective character's fiancée Callie Cargill was a nurse who occasionally displayed some skill, but she was also a medical student, again reinforcing the wannabe physician stereotype. Still, those nurse characters are fabulous compared to the idiotic nurses on Fox's sitcom *The Mindy Project* (2012–). That show focuses on a practice of skilled if quirky obstetrics and gynecology physicians, but it also includes three kooky nurses: Morgan, a cheerful but loony ex-convict; the off-kilter Tamra, who at times functions as an office insult comic; and Dorothy, a hostile, inept burnout who the practice fired and later rehired as an office assistant.

Shorter-lived shows have also offered a limited range of physician-centric portrayals. CBS's *Miami Medical*[13] (2010) and the Canadian-based *Combat Hospital*[14] (Global/ABC; 2011) at least included a fairly skilled and authoritative male nurse manager among the trauma physician leads. But the CW's *Emily Owens, MD* (2012–2013), CBS's *A Gifted Man*[15] (2011–2012), and ABC's *Off the Map*[16] (2011) all featured physician characters saving lives by themselves. Producer Terence Wrong's popular ABC documentaries about prominent US hospitals, including *Hopkins*[17] (2008), *Boston Med*[18] (2010), and *NY Med* (2012 and 2014), were largely exercises in physician glorification, presenting surgeons in particular as the moral and intellectual heroes of health care, although nurses did appear sporadically.

In late 2013, two new cable shows did nursing no favors. MTV's "reality" show *Scrubbing In* spent 10 episodes with nine young travel nurses in California. Not surprisingly, the great majority of the show was the nurses' personal dramas, with a focus on partying, romance, and sex. Clinical interactions were very limited and generally unimpressive.[19] HBO's *Getting On* is a dark sitcom adapted from a UK series about the staff at a California geriatric care facility. Virtually every character is a pathetic loser. Nurse Dawn, probably the most prominent character, displays some health knowledge and interest in the patients. But she is a meek, sad soul. Her nursing supervisor Patsy, who uses Dawn for sex, is a weak, ineffective man who either is or pretends to be unsure if he is gay.[20]

Successful health-related shows of the past decade were not much better. NBC's drama *ER*[21] (1994–2009) and the NBC/ABC sitcom *Scrubs*[22] (2001–2010) were overwhelmingly physician-centric, although each did always at least have one major nurse character who could think and talk. But FX's edgy *Nip/Tuck* (2003–2010), which followed the exploits of two ethically challenged plastic surgeons, never had any nurses.

In 2009, an astonishing three new prime-time shows about skilled nurses fighting for their patients appeared in the United States. The most notable was Showtime's compelling "dark comedy" *Nurse Jackie*[23] (2009–), which introduced a tough and expert (though deeply flawed) New York City emergency nurse. This was the first major US prime-time show with a nurse character as the central focus since the early 1990s. Although the portrayal of nursing is not perfect—it has suggested that nurses report to physicians—the show has included many valuable illustrations of nurses' clinical virtuosity and patient advocacy. Also in 2009, NBC began airing *Mercy* (2009–2010), which followed the romantic and work lives of a troubled Iraq war veteran and other New Jersey hospital nurses. Some episodes suggested that nurses report to physicians, but *Mercy* also included some dramatic examples of nursing skill and advocacy.[24] TNT introduced the summer show *HawthoRNe* (2009–2011), whose lead character was a tough, committed chief nursing officer at a Richmond, Virginia hospital. Although some other nurse characters were weak or stereotypical, this show too included strong nursing portrayals, and simply showing the public that chief nursing officers exist has value.[25]

More recently, helpful shows arrived from the United Kingdom. In the drama *Call the Midwife* (BBC/PBS; 2012–), tough, autonomous nurse midwives provide a full range of skilled nursing care to a poor community in London in the 1950s. The show may seem a bit remote from current practice and some critics have found it too sentimental, but it has exposed millions to a strong vision of nursing they would not otherwise see, especially in the United Kingdom, where it has been very popular.[26] The documentary series *24 Hours in A&E* (Channel 4/BBC America; 2011–2013) has given viewers an engaging look at skilled, articulate nurses and other staff working in a busy emergency department at London's King's College Hospital. The show has run at least five seasons in the United Kingdom, although to date only the first season has aired in the United States, as *24 Hours in the ER*.

The appearance of these shows has been encouraging. Possible explanations include a new interest in underdogs and resentment of the health care status quo in a recessionary era. *Nurse Jackie* has lasted at least six seasons, *Call the Midwife* at least three, and *HawthoRNe* three. However, those three shows had far smaller US audiences and far shorter seasons than regular season US shows. *Mercy*, the only one of the new US shows to air on a broadcast network, was canceled after its first season.

The fact is that many shows with accurate nursing portrayals would need to attract large audiences for a long time to counter the huge impact of years of misportrayals in globally successful shows, such as *Grey's Anatomy* and *House*, as well as many short-lived shows like *Emily Owens, MD*. Ironically, the sudden appearance of the 2009 nurse shows generated a backlash from some critics, who reacted to one common theme (skilled nurses challenging physicians to protect patients) with boredom, skepticism, or mockery. For now, the televised health care world remains physician-shaped.

Research confirms that the media plays a key role in forming and reinforcing popular attitudes about health care, including nursing. So it's not surprising that many people still believe nurses are low-skilled physician assistants rather than college-educated professionals who save lives. A 2002 US poll found that only half of respondents knew that RNs must have at least an associate's degree; less than 20 percent knew that nurses must be licensed.[27] In fact, given what people see every day in the media, it would be surprising if most were *not* convinced that health care revolves around brilliant, commanding physicians. This misportrayal undermines the work of all the health professionals who make up the modern healthcare team, including social workers, physical therapists, and respiratory therapists. In particular, physician-centric media undermines nursing practice and education. That, in the end, costs lives.

How did the media get so far from the reality of nursing?

Virtue and Vice: Some Roots of Nursing's Media Stereotypes

Nursing's popular image has long veered among one-dimensional visions of femininity: the angel, the handmaiden, the harlot, or the battle-axe. All of these stereotypes can be traced back to the roots of modern nursing, in which groups of nineteenth-century females began trying to help patients with their most intimate problems at times of great stress. But it's worth taking a brief look at the development of nursing image's since then. In doing so, we rely in part on insightful research on the history of the nursing image that scholars Beatrice and Philip Kalisch produced in the 1980s.[28]

Men and women have long cared for the sick in religious and other settings, as discussed in Chapter 1. But in the period just before the founding of modern nursing, the work was regarded as unskilled drudgery unfit for a respectable person. Nursing was consigned to the likes of the immoral, alcohol-abusing Sairey Gamp in Dickens's *Martin Chuzzlewit*.

Florence Nightingale and her fellow reformers changed that. Kalisch and Kalisch describe the era from Nightingale's mid–nineteenth-century work in the Crimea until the end of World War I as one defined by a female "angel of mercy" image. In this period, popular media tended to see nursing as a noble calling, associated it with the military, and regarded nurses themselves with reverence. Some World War I films featured nurses who volunteered for war duty to be near their soldier boyfriends, then ended up nursing their wounded sweethearts back to health. Kalisch and Kalisch observe that this theme provided a way "to mask the novelty of female independence with traditional female values."

From the 1920s until the end of World War II, nurses were generally seen as pragmatic, even heroic, particularly in war movies. The film *A Farewell to Arms* (1932) presented nurses as noble but relatively unskilled, with strict supervisors who enforced a moral code and deference to physicians.[29] The Dr. Kildare films of the 1930s and 1940s focused on an idealized young physician. Nurse characters were either young love interests or formidable veterans. Kildare also had a crusty, brilliant diagnostician mentor—a forerunner to Greg House, perhaps. Hitchcock's *Rear Window* (1954) included a late example of what Kalisch and Kalisch describe as this era's "private nurse as detective" portrayals. In the film, the older "insurance company nurse" Stella helps the lovely lead characters unravel a mystery. Stella says she is not well educated, but she is autonomous, quick-witted, and tough.[30]

From the end of World War II until the 1960s, nurses tended to be portrayed as maternal helpers to essentially omniscient male physicians. The television show *Ben Casey* (1961–1966), for instance, focused on an idealistic young physician not unlike Kildare. The show's nurse character Miss Wills was motherly and relatively unskilled. *Marcus Welby* (1969–1976) presented physicians as giving all meaningful care, including even the emotional "caring" that many nurses have traditionally regarded as their area. Kalisch and Kalisch refer to depictions of physicians doing everything as "Marcus Welby syndrome," a malady that remains endemic in Hollywood. According to communications scholar Joseph Turow, in the 1950s and 1960s the American Medical Association (AMA) asserted control over network television shows, actually vetting scripts. The AMA helpfully ensured that heroic physician characters generally made no errors and lived morally. Nurses were insignificant.

A few products of the era did focus on nurses. A series of juvenile novels appearing from the 1940s to the 1960s featured Cherry Ames, a virtuous, adventurous, and bright young nurse who moved from job to job solving mysteries (*Cherry Ames: Army Nurse* was a typical title). Cherry Ames inspired many young women to become nurses. A television series called *The Nurses* (1962–1965) actually focused on two hospital nurses, a senior mentor and an inexperienced young nurse. The program even hired a nurse adviser to help the producers develop the show. But already some parents were discouraging talented, ambitious girls from entering nursing.

Then came The Sixties. Sexual liberation and expanding work opportunities for women did not enhance public regard for nursing. As many ambitious women began to contemplate careers in medicine and other fields, the nursing image fled back to the poles of extreme female stereotypes. Naughty nurses became a staple of pornography and exploitation films by B-movie king Roger Corman and others. At times, the free-love nurse characters were balanced with senior battle-axes.

Of course, the most notorious example was Nurse Ratched of *One Flew Over the Cuckoo's Nest* (1975). Milos Forman's film adaptation of Ken Kesey's anti-authoritarian 1963 novel featured the senior nurse as a sociopath who abuses her professional and institutional power over her patients. The film is deeply misogynistic—every female character is a stereotype—with Ratched as a horrific vision of society's repressed Mom.[31]

Robert Altman's antiwar film *M*A*S*H* (1970), based on Richard Hooker's 1968 novel, was less extreme. But it still presented senior US Army nurse "Hot Lips" Houlihan and other nurses as battle-axes, sex objects, and/or handmaidens to cynical but gifted surgeons during the Korean War.[32] The portrayal of nurses on the influential *M*A*S*H* television show (1972–1983) was somewhat more evolved. The show still focused on the male physicians, who were nicer versions of the film characters: irreverent, gifted leaders trying to save lives in impossible situations—a model for countless future shows. Nurses were mostly there to hand the surgeons things or provide casual sex. Houlihan was a repressed martinet, although she did become far more human as the show went on, and she displayed some skill and autonomy.[33]

In the 1980s and 1990s, most television nurses were marginal assistants to the dominant physicians, some of whom were now female. A few shows managed to suggest something of what nursing really was. The influential *St. Elsewhere* (1982–1988) depicted a fairly gritty Boston hospital. The show's physicians were flawed, but they were still the focus, with the occasional formidable nurse character. *China Beach* (1988–1991) was set on a US military base in Vietnam during the Vietnam War. Lead character Colleen McMurphy was a competent, fairly tough Army nurse, but she did not generally display much skill, and the show was mainly about nonhealth subjects. The minor sitcom *Nurses* (1991–1994) treated nurses with some respect. However, the notorious *Nightingales* (1988–1989) featured sexy but vacuous nursing students who spent so much time in states of partial undress that outraged nurses actually managed to chase the show off the air—a historic anomaly.

ER (1994–2009) was one of the most influential healthcare shows in history. It relied on intense, fairly realistic scenes from a tough Chicago emergency department and the romantic interactions of roughly ten major characters. *ER* also presented some of the best depictions of nursing ever to appear on network television, occasionally showing serious nursing skill and even autonomy. But on the whole it featured an evolved handmaiden image: nurses were skilled physician assistants who ultimately had to defer. The show never had more than one major nurse character at a time, and it always relied heavily on physician nursing. Like Marcus Welby, *ER* physicians saved lives using traditional medical skills *and* provided virtually all important bedside care, including key psychosocial care.[34]

At the turn of the millennium, a few other shows had nurse characters of some substance, although no show challenged the idea that only physicians really matter. The Lifetime drama *Strong Medicine* (2000–2006) included hunky, articulate nurse midwife Peter Riggs, a progressive underling set against the female physician stars—probably a model for Dell from *Private Practice*. But the show's other nurses were mute handmaidens.[35] The kooky sitcom *Scrubs* (2001–2010) featured tough nurse Carla Espinosa, who at times displayed real skill. But the show's physicians provided virtually all important care, and the nurses were generally meek assistants with no significant clinical role.[36]

Despite the recent nurse shows, the standard Hollywood nursing portrayal remains the peripheral, low-skilled physician handmaiden with virtually nothing to contribute. *Grey's Anatomy* remains popular and its cute-young-physicians-in-training model has inspired other shows, like *Off the Map*[37] and *Emily Owens, MD. House* continues to air in syndication. Every major character on these shows has been a physician, and the shows' vision of nursing is that of a job in a sad time warp. Now that female physicians are so common, there's no need to include nurse characters at all to have a gender mix that is good for drama. The subtext is obvious: today, no person of substance would even *think* of becoming a nurse. Those who do are pathetic losers unworthy of a second glance from television viewers. Or even a first glance: let's just show their forearms at the edge of the frame, holding something for the smart, interesting physicians as they save a patient's life.

Does What's in Our Brains Matter? How the Media Influences Nursing

At this point, you may be wondering how media portrayals of nurses affect the profession. We often receive skeptical messages on this subject. Here are some of the questions we receive about why the media matters, and our replies.

Come on. Even if the media ignores nursing or presents it inaccurately, how can that possibly affect nursing in real life?

What people see and hear affects what they think, and what they think affects what they do. This is a basic principle of education, religion, art, and any other organized effort to influence people. It is why major corporations spend millions on advertising campaigns to promote their products, and why powerful political advertisements can move polling numbers and affect election results. In 2012, US advertisers spent $140 billion on advertising.[38] Research shows that television can affect conduct greatly. For example, a 2008 study found that the introduction of cable television in rural India resulted in women reporting that they had increased autonomy as well as significant decreases in the acceptability of violence toward them—and in their own preference for having sons.[39]

The same principle applies to health issues. Indeed, in recent years a consensus has emerged in the field of public health that the media affects society's health-related views and behavior. Public agencies, private groups, and scholars now devote substantial resources to analyzing and managing health messages in the media.

The field of health communication addresses how this works. In recent years, health communication has gained prominence[40] and scholars have recognized the growing impact of new media on the public's understanding of key health issues.[41] As public health scholar Deborah Glik noted in "Health Communication in Popular Media Formats," media products "comprise both planned and unplanned content which has the potential to communicate positive, neutral or negative health messages to the public."[42] The inclusion of "unplanned" content means the media influences people whether or not the creators *intended* it, just as a cigarette-smoking parent may influence a child to smoke without intending to do so. The media need not intend to harm nursing to have that effect.

Glik has noted that "from a social marketing perspective, messages in the media that promote specific desirable behaviors have the potential to persuade consumers to change their behavior if messages are viewed as compatible with consumers' own self-interest, competing messages are minimal, and resistance to change is low to moderate." It makes little sense to think that people would learn about substantive health topics like cancer or AIDS from a media product but form no opinions about the health worker who is presenting the information.

In a 2002 report for the Kaiser Family Foundation, scholars Joseph Turow and Rachel Gans noted that "researchers have long recognized that news media coverage affects what the public believes about health care."[43]

Advocates have therefore worked hard to affect the media's coverage of health topics in which they have an interest.

For example, physicians have worked hard for decades to manage their public image. We have noted that the AMA has historically tried to control how physicians are depicted in the media. It has also aggressively promoted coverage of medical research and other physician-centered stories. In general, these efforts have been a resounding success. Today physicians, a critical part of the healthcare team, are generally portrayed by the news media as more or less the *whole* team. The media often consults physicians on issues, such as nutrition and breastfeeding, in which others generally have as much if not greater expertise. Physicians' combination of economic, social, and moral status is unrivaled by any other professional group.

Public health scholars try to increase understanding of what the media is saying, sometimes subtly, about health issues. Glik has explained that, "given the pervasiveness and potential power of the media to shape beliefs, attitudes and behaviors, the media literacy movement has emerged." This movement aims to help children and teenagers understand what the media is really doing, but these skills are also important for adults, especially those whose interests are not served by current media practice. Glik describes the popular media as a "double-edged sword" that may function "as both a tool for progress and a source of ill health that is a reflection of the larger culture it represents."

In particular, we must explore how the media affects one of the most important global health problems: the crisis in nursing. When those without much understanding of nursing get a lifetime of negative stereotypical messages about the profession, they do not consider nursing as a career. Likewise, public officials and healthcare decision makers with little understanding of nursing's real importance do not allocate sufficient funds for nurse staffing, nursing residencies, nursing education, or nursing research. Nurses themselves are not immune. The media's undervaluation can sap nurses' pride, encourage cynicism and self-loathing, and discourage nurses from standing up for themselves and their patients. It can even persuade nurses that physicians really are their masters, rather than colleagues.

On the whole, the nursing crisis can be seen as the result of an entire society's failing to value nursing adequately. But the media is a key factor in that failure.

OK, I can see that some media probably affect how people think about and act toward nursing, like maybe a newspaper article. But how can some television drama, sitcom, or commercial affect people that way? People don't take that stuff seriously!

The effects of fictional media are not always obvious, but they have been felt throughout history in every culture, from Homer to Homer Simpson. These effects have been recognized as important by the health community, the news media, and even Hollywood. Today, more fictional media are more available to more of the world's people than ever before.

To believe that we can disregard everything we perceive in the entertainment media because the scenarios presented aren't literally "true," we would also have to believe that people disregard all messages in advertising, since advertisements often present actors in simulated situations. But that is not how our minds work.

In a recent television advertisement for the Dodge Caravan minivan, a female operating room "nurse" asks a female "brain surgeon" which of two scalpels she wants. The surgeon confidently explains which one she needs. Then, in response to a similarly phrased question from the nurse, the surgeon practically commands the nurse to buy a Caravan rather than a sport utility vehicle. The advertisement also features a goofy male anesthesia professional and a dopey male patient (who drives a sport utility vehicle). Later, the surgeon picks up her kids with the Caravan. The voiceover notes that it "doesn't take a brain surgeon" to know that there's "no smarter choice."[44]

We know we are not seeing real operating room workers. But that does not stop us from absorbing the messages embedded in this clever advertisement. Despite being fiction, the advertisement might influence our views of the vehicle, the ability of women to become authoritative professionals, and the knowledge and roles of physicians and nurses. Some of this result may be "unplanned," but all of it sells the minivan to the target demographic, which is presumably working mothers. Most people would probably admit that this advertisement has some positive influence on society's overall view of women. But that is because there is broad social understanding that women can now become esteemed professionals. Nursing is not well understood, and society has little basis to question the subtext that the brain surgeon is "smarter" than the submissive nurse about health care (and everything else).

The idea that fictional media can influence public views and conduct is not controversial in the field of public health. In their 2002 Kaiser Report, Turow and Gans conclude that "fictional television can . . . play a significant role in shaping public images about the state of our health care system and policy options for improving the delivery of care."[45] Evidently recognizing this, each summer from 2003 to 2007 the Robert Wood Johnson Foundation distributed copies of Turow's DVD essay "Prime Time Doctors: Why Should You Care?" to about 20,000 US medical students.[46]

Glik notes that "an important aspect of health communication today is working with the entertainment media to include or improve health messages in popular programs." A 2004 Kaiser Family Foundation Report confirmed that "many groups have come to believe that entertainment media can play an important positive role in educating the public about significant health messages."[47] Conversely, Glik notes that a good deal of ongoing research has found "unhealthy messages" in entertainment media, for instance smoking in films, which Glik reports has been shown to influence rates of teenage smoking. In fact, a July 2009 Dartmouth study published in the journal *Pediatrics* found that any type of smoking character in movies made teenagers more likely to try smoking, with characters perceived as "bad" actually being most influential.[48]

Turow and Gans explain why entertainment television may actually influence views of health care *even more* than the news media does:

> Certainly TV dramas reach a much wider audience than most news programs. Beyond the size of their audience, some media scholars argue that entertainment TV's impact can be even more powerful than news in subtly shaping the public's impressions of key societal institutions. The messages are more engaging, often playing out in compelling human dramas involving characters the audience cares about. Viewers are taken behind the scenes to see the hidden forces affecting whether there's a happy ending or a sad one. There are good guys and bad guys, heroes and villains and innocent bystanders. Instead of bill numbers and budget figures, policy issues are portrayed through the lives of "real" human beings, often in life-and-death situations. These health policy discussions take place not only in hospital dramas, but also in dramatic storylines on programs like "Law and Order," "The Practice," and "The West Wing."
>
> Hospital dramas provide an opportunity for viewers to learn specifically what goes on at the center of high-intensity medicine. The dramas' fictional presentations open curtains on relationships between doctors and nurses, specialists and generalists. In ways that news reports cannot, they play out various assumptions about how health care ought to be delivered, about what conflicts arise that affect health care, and about how those conflicts should be resolved and why. Doing

> that, hospital dramas represent an important part of viewers' curriculum on the problems and possibilities of health care in America.

Even more to the point, Turow and Gans stress that television hospital dramas' "consistent focus on the relation of doctors and nurses with patients who are in jeopardy make them the source of many viewers' understandings of how the health care system works."[49]

Echoing these ideas, a 2008 report by the Kaiser Family Foundation and the University of Southern California's Hollywood, Health & Society project noted that "entertainment television may be a uniquely powerful health communication tool" because television, particularly prime time shows on major networks, continues to have "enormous reach" and health information "delivered through engaging storytelling—often involving characters the viewer already 'knows' and cares about—is more likely to be attended to than traditional health information sources."[50]

In light of this great influence, Turow and Gans note, public health organizations everywhere "are increasingly turning to entertainment media—from soap operas to sitcoms to reality shows—as a way to reach the public with health messages." This growing effort is often called "entertainment education." Glik defines it as "a way of informing the public about a social issue or concern" by "incorporating an educational message into popular entertainment content in order to raise awareness, increase knowledge, create favorable attitudes, and ultimately motivate people to take socially responsible action in their own lives." Much entertainment education results from what the 2004 Kaiser Report describes as "outreach efforts of special interest groups or health agencies to deliver their message to audiences. These groups often work with Hollywood-based advocacy organizations that serve as liaisons to the entertainment community via industry forums, roundtable briefings, and technical script consultations."

Among the organizations devoting significant resources to entertainment education in recent years are the Harvard and UCLA schools of public health. In addition, USC's Hollywood, Health & Society project has collaborated with television producers to place messages on a wide variety of health topics, including infectious diseases, diabetes, and health care access. That project, part of the school's Norman Lear Center, is a joint venture whose sponsors include the Centers for Disease Control and Prevention (CDC). The Kaiser Family Foundation has worked with various Hollywood shows to place health messages and story lines on subjects including emergency contraception and teenage sexual activity. In an October 2009 episode of *Private*

Practice, the physicians gave free checkups at a shelter for homeless teenagers, as part of the Entertainment Industry Foundation's "iParticipate" project to place storylines promoting community service.[51] In a March 2013 episode of *Grey's Anatomy*, Sarah Chalke played a distraught mother whose son's mysterious ailment was finally diagnosed as Kawasaki disease; the plotline was entertainment education, the result of Chalke lobbying *Grey's* producers after her own son was belatedly diagnosed with the rare condition.[52]

In October 2013 American Public Media's *Marketplace* radio show reported that The California Endowment had given a substantial grant to Hollywood, Health & Society to encourage shows to do plotlines to promote understanding of the Affordable Care Act. The report noted that shows like *Grey's Anatomy* and *Scrubs* had found drama in insurance coverage issues, and it quoted Norman Lear Center director Marty Kaplan: "People learn from TV. Even if they know it is fiction, even if they know that writers can make stuff up, especially in the realm of medicine and public health, if a doctor says something to a patient, people tend to think that someone has checked that, that it's true."[53]

The health community's entertainment education efforts are not confined to the developed world. In December 2004 press reports described a Cambodian soap opera created by British soap guru Matthew Robinson and funded by the BBC World Service Trust to educate Cambodians about disease, especially HIV/AIDS. *Taste of Life* reportedly "follows five student nurses and a student doctor as they move through a nursing college, the local pub and 'Friendship Hospital.' "[54]

On the other hand, public health scholars confirm that Hollywood shows can also cause real harm. Purdue communications professor Susan Morgan is the coauthor of research suggesting that negative entertainment television portrayals of organ donation (including on *Grey's Anatomy*) have contributed to negative views about the vital health practice. Morgan is quoted in a September 2007 *Forbes* article: "It's hard not to get kind of outraged when you see what's going on. You could start drawing this out to real human lives being lost."[55]

Hollywood itself embraces the idea that it can have a *positive* effect on public health. Indeed, many industry figures seem proud to have improved health through entertainment. In presenting former *ER* producer (and physician) Neal Baer with a public service award in December 2003, the Writers Guild of America lauded him for "creating a culture of medical accuracy and groundbreaking realism that revolutionized the primetime landscape."[56] The Writers Guild of America also asserted that the producer's "passion for medical accuracy has paid dividends to the American public, as a recent Harvard study revealed most Americans learn more about health-related problems from series television like *Law and Order: Special Victims Unit* than from their own doctors." In addition to running *SVU* for more than a decade, Baer was responsible for *A Gifted Man*, and he has long cochaired the advisory board of Hollywood, Health & Society. Likewise, in a 2004 issue of *TV Guide*, a medical adviser and an executive producer from *ER* were eager to celebrate the show's apparent influence on the number of women pursuing emergency medicine.[57] In a 2005 NPR interview, *Grey's* creator Shonda Rhimes stressed that her show could help people of color, because "the way people look at people on television is the way they perceive the world. And for me the idea of the show, part of it, is that we can change the assumptions that people have simply by the images they see in the background of the show."[58]

But sadly, those who proclaim the *positive* health effects of Hollywood shows seem unwilling to consider how the industry's inaccurate depiction of nurses as peripheral subordinates could have *negative* effects. Although there is no dispute that the shows affect social views and knowledge of disease, viewers must have some innate filter that blocks even the most compelling media information about health workers' professional roles.

In fact, as we have shown, physicians have long understood the power of entertainment media. In her article "Doc Hollywood," Suzanne Gordon describes the "symbiotic relationship" physicians have with Hollywood, which "has been an active partner in the creation of a heroic medical narrative that has shaped Americans' view of health care . . . and conferred status on medical practitioners and specialists."[59] Today, physicians like Baer provide virtually all significant expert health care advice for entertainment programming other than the recent nurse shows. Nurses may be on set adjusting minor technical details, but physicians are the ones who consult regularly on and even write the scripts that actually drive the shows. Indeed, *ER* was created by physician Michael Crichton, and a number of its key writers have been physicians. At least one *House* writer was a physician. The creator of *Scrubs* based the show on the experiences of one of his best friends, a physician who advised the show.

In 2006–2007, there was a notable burst of US news articles addressing how entertainment programming affects viewers' health-related actions. In October 2006, the *Orange County Register* ran Lisa Liddane's "Paging Dr. Nielsen: TV medical shows." The piece examined how popular hospital dramas like *Grey's Anatomy* reflect and shape real-life health matters. Producers, physician writers, and public health experts confirmed that although such shows are fiction, they affect what the public thinks about health care. Vicky Rideout of the Kaiser Family Foundation noted that "TV medical dramas contribute to agenda-setting—and influence how people look at situations and professions."[60]

Many similar and higher-profile articles followed, all focusing on the accuracy of the shows' technical portrayal of medical conditions. A March 2007 article in *Reader's Digest*, Mary A. Fischer's "Docs in the Box," mentioned one nurse: *Grey's* consultant Linda Klein. Star Ellen Pompeo assured readers Klein "takes the time to show us exactly how something should be done."[61] That is, the nurse consultant shows the actors playing physicians how to do important things nurses really do, and lends an air of realism to a show that portrays her profession as trivial scut work.

A few of the later articles focused on the inaccurate nursing portrayals on these shows. Carol Ann Campbell's excellent "Nurses Urge TV Dramas: Get Real," in the New Jersey *Star-Ledger* in January 2007, had nurses explain how television dramas regularly show physicians doing important work that nurses really do, while showing nurses as peripheral subordinates. *House* creator David Shore admitted to the *Star-Ledger* that his show "ignores" nurses but said that the character Greg House treats everyone badly. In fact, the show generally treated nurses in the same contemptuous way House did and made little effort to rebut House's slurs. Shore even resorted to noting that his mother is a nurse and she "loves" the show.[62] In September 2007 *Forbes* ran Allison Van Dusen's "Playing Doctor: Medical TV Isn't Always Right," which addressed the effects of popular health-related drama, including the concerns of nurses. It noted that nurse characters tend to absorb abuse from physicians like House with no response, reinforcing the image of nurses as meek servants.[63]

More recently, a few helpful articles have focused directly on nurses' concerns with entertainment media. In January 2010, *Baltimore Sun* health reporter Kelly Brewington posted "TV Nurses—The Good and the Bad," a widely reprinted look at the Truth's 2009 awards for best and worst media portrayals of nurses.[64] In April 2010, the Voice of America ran "Nurse, I Need a Reality Check: Hollywood shapes many perceptions of medical professionals but that's a problem for real-life nurses," an in-depth report by Faiza Elmasry with quotes from Sandy Summers and Johns Hopkins nurses.[65] In April 2012, *More* magazine published Jessica Testa's "A Real Nurse Rates the TV Fakes," with critical commentary on major hospital shows then on the air (the "real nurse" was Sandy Summers).[66]

This is an era of media saturation, diverse content, and technological development—an age of virtual reality. It is increasingly difficult to tell what is "real." There is little doubt that today's "fictional" media profoundly affects how we think and act.

Fine, I get that public health and communications scholars, physicians, and even Hollywood believes the entertainment media affects real world health. But does any recent research say so?

Recent research has shown that the entertainment media, especially television, has a clear and powerful effect on viewers' health-related thoughts—and actions. This influence flows not only from prime-time dramas like *Grey's Anatomy* and *ER* but even from sitcoms and soap operas.

Research has directly addressed how the entertainment media affects public views of health care workers, including nurses. In their 2002 Kaiser Report, Turow and Gans noted that their research had found that physicians dominated discussions of health policy issues on US hospital dramas, whereas nurses hardly appeared.[67] The 2008 Kaiser Report evaluated the top 10 scripted prime-time US shows of all types in each year during the period 2004–2006 (including *Grey's, House*, and *ER*) and reported that "popular prime time television conveys a substantial amount of health information." The study concluded that the shows mostly portrayed characters dealing with "a wide range of health issues" and receiving "quality care from physicians with whom they have favorable interactions"—although that conclusion was not an effort to draw attention to the dominance of physician characters, but instead seemed to reflect the same basic assumption seen in the shows themselves: health care = physician care.[68] A 2009 study published in the *Journal of Broadcasting and Electronic Media* by University of Illinois health communication scholar Brian Quick found that regular *Grey's* viewers were more likely to view real physicians similarly to the show's physician characters—as smart, pretty, capable, and interesting.[69]

Some studies have focused on how the popular media affects those who might consider nursing careers. In 2000 the advertising agency JWT Communications conducted a focus group study of 1,800 US youngsters in grades two through ten; respondents said they received their main impression of nursing from *ER*. They knew more about the nurses' love lives than their professional work. Consistent with the show's physician-centric approach, the young people wrongly said nursing was a girl's job, that it was a technical job "like shop," and that it was not a career for private school students, of whom more was expected.[70]

A 2008 University of Dundee (Scotland) study found that media imagery discouraged academically advanced primary school students from pursuing nursing careers by presenting nurses as, in the words of one student, "brainless, sex-mad bimbos" looking to "romance" physicians. Consistent with the earlier JWT research, the Dundee study found that the students' main source of images about nursing was television. Based on all imagery, the students concluded that becoming a nurse would not be "using their examination grades to maximum benefit."[71]

A 2013 study by Roslyn Weaver and colleagues measured the views on health-related television shows held by 484 Australian nursing students, for whom the most-watched show was *Grey's Anatomy*. Most of the nursing students found that the shows presented nurses as handmaidens dithering with unimportant things while physicians did the work that mattered. Most also believed that television lacked role models to inspire the next generation of nurses.[72]

In 2012 a study at University College Dublin (Ireland) found that the most popular videos posted on the YouTube website stereotype nurses as stupid and/or sex objects. The researchers found that, of the ten most popular nurse-related YouTube videos, four portrayed nurses as sex objects, two showed nurses as stupid or incompetent, and only four—all posted by nurses themselves—showed nursing as a skilled and caring profession. All six of the stereotypical depictions were drawn from television products or advertisements.[73]

A May/June 2008 *Nursing Economics* study confirmed that the media affects public understanding of nursing—although the article claimed that nursing is "highly respected."[74] The 2007 public opinion research on which the article relied was funded by drug company Johnson & Johnson, which we had faulted for airing television recruiting advertisements promoting an unskilled angel image of nursing. One survey question asked respondents whether certain broad categories of media made them "respect" nurses more or less. A category consisting of the television shows *ER, Scrubs, House*, and *Grey's Anatomy* reportedly made no difference to 66 percent of respondents but made 28 percent respect nurses more, and only 5 percent respect nurses less. The vague category "advertisements about nursing"—which presumably included the Johnson & Johnson advertisements—had no effect on 60 percent, but supposedly created more respect in 38 percent and less in only 1 percent. In fact, *none* of the media tested had a large negative effect. Evidently, either *every* class of media creates positive views of nurses, or else only the positive media affects people. The *Nursing Economics* survey was too vague and subject to self-reporting bias to provide much useful data. Respondents are unlikely to admit to a pollster that the media makes them "respect" real nurses less. Most people know they are supposed to honor nurses in the abstract. But this generalized affection has not translated into the resources that would show real respect for nurses as professionals. "Respect" can mean different things: is it respect for nurses' life-saving skills, or for their hearts of gold? The study failed to reconcile its shiny happy results with what the media it tested actually said about nursing.

Entertainment television's influence on healthcare views is broad and strong. When the US CDC surveyed prime-time television viewers in 2000, they found that most (52 percent) reported getting information that they trust to be accurate from prime-time television shows.[75] More than a quarter said such shows were among their top three sources for health information. Nine out of ten regular viewers said they learned something about diseases from television, with almost half citing prime-time or daytime entertainment shows. Moreover, almost half of regular viewers who heard something about a health issue on a prime-time show said they took one or more actions, including telling someone about the story line (42 percent), telling someone to do something, or doing it themselves, such as using a condom or getting more exercise (16 percent), or visiting a clinic or health provider (9 percent).[76]

Recent research has also shown that entertainment shows affect public views of specific areas of health care. One 2007 study published in *Health Communication* found that organ donation was presented in a negative or inaccurate way in the great majority of plotlines in fictional prime-time and daytime shows (including comedies and soap operas) in 2004 and 2005.[77] A 2005 study published in *Clinical Transplantation* found that respondents who had negative views of organ donation often mentioned what they had seen on television as a basis for their opinions.[78] A 2007 study by Yale researchers published in the journal *Plastic & Reconstructive Surgery* found that plastic surgery reality shows played an important role in patients' knowledge and decisions about the procedures.[79]

Substantial research has confirmed the influence of specific shows. One striking January 2014 study by two economists found that the MTV reality franchise *16 and Pregnant*, including its *Teen Mom* sequels, had not only sparked more online activity regarding birth control and abortion, but "ultimately led to a 5.7 percent reduction in teen births in the 18 months following its introduction," accounting for "around one-third of the overall decline in teen births in the United States during that period."[80] A 2011 study at the

University of Western Sydney found that about 94 percent of 386 medical students surveyed watched popular health-related entertainment shows, such as *Grey's Anatomy, House*, and *Scrubs*, with 48 percent of female medical students watching *Grey's*.[81] The students reported that they had discussed ethical and medical issues presented on at least one show with their friends "and most believed that medical programs generally portrayed ideals of professionalism well."[82] In September 2008, the Kaiser Family Foundation released a study showing that an embedded *Grey's Anatomy* plotline about maternal HIV transmission had significantly increased audience understanding of the issue.[83] The show's "director of medical research" helped to publicize the study, and she told *TV Guide* that the show took its influence "very seriously."[84]

Many studies have also documented *ER*'s effects on views about health care—even the views of health professionals. A 2009 University of Alberta study published in the journal *Resuscitation* found that many residents and medical students had learned incorrect intubation techniques by watching *ER* and other shows.[85] A 1998 article in the *Journal of the American Medical Association* concluded that medical students' reactions to shows like *ER* suggested that the students "may incorporate the attitudes and beliefs of physicians on television in much the same way they acquire the qualities and behaviors of physicians through their experiences in patient care." The article cited research showing the dramatic growth in emergency department medical residencies since *ER*'s premiere a few years earlier.[86]

A Kaiser Family Foundation survey found that more than half of those who were regular *ER* viewers during the 1997–2000 seasons said they learned about important health issues while watching the show. Almost a third said information from the show helped them make choices about their family's health care. Almost a quarter had sought further information about a health issue, and 14 percent had actually contacted a health care provider because of something they saw in an *ER* episode.[87] According to a 2001 Kaiser Foundation National Survey of Physicians, "one in five doctors say they are consulted 'very' or 'somewhat' often about specific diseases or treatments that patients heard about on TV shows such as *ER*."[88]

ER also affects what viewers think about specific conditions. In September 2007, University of Southern California researchers published a study in the *Journal of Health Communication* that found those who saw an *ER* plotline about teenage obesity and hypertension were 65 percent more likely to report that they had acted in a healthier way.[89] A 2002 study at the Harvard School of Public Health found that regular *ER* viewers were far more aware (57 versus 39 percent) of the need to get a smallpox vaccination right after exposure to the disease following an *ER* episode dealing with the subject.[90]

Entertainment media does not have to be mainly about health care to affect viewers' understanding of health care issues, as the 2008 Kaiser Report's analysis of all types of scripted shows indicated. In 2002 a RAND Health survey of regular viewers of the sitcom *Friends* aged twelve to seventeen found that respondents retained important information from a story line depicting an unplanned pregnancy caused by condom failure. The report concluded that "entertainment television can be most effective as an educator when teens and parents view together and discuss what they watch."[91]

The effects of health-related entertainment programming are also not confined to popular prime-time shows. In 1999 a CDC survey "found that many daytime viewers also report learning about health issues from TV." Almost half of regular daytime drama viewers reported learning something about a disease from watching soap operas. Over one-third reported taking some action after hearing about a health issue or disease on a soap opera.[92] And a 2004 study published in the *Journal of Communication* found that after an episode of *The Bold and the Beautiful* with an HIV subplot, and subsequent display of the CDC's National STD and AIDS hotline, calls to the hotline spiked.[93]

This wealth of research shows that entertainment programming is easily "realistic" enough to affect real world health care—including nursing.

Well, if all that research shows how influential Hollywood is, why won't the industry improve its damaging portrayal of nursing?

So far, despite the minor impact of the recent nurse-focused shows, Hollywood's responses to critics of its nursing portrayal have been inadequate. The industry argues that Hollywood shows are not documentaries and producers must have "dramatic license"; that entertainment media has to focus on physicians because that's what viewers want; that it's just a mean central character who hates nurses, the show really loves them; that there was a shortage of nurses before their show came on the air; that nurses *do* advise the show and they work on set ensuring "medical accuracy"; that the show creator's mother or sister is a nurse and she just loves the show; and that the show works super-hard, really, to present an accurate portrayal of all health professionals. But none of that has prevented the industry from offering hundreds of hours of damaging misportrayals of nursing.

The factors underlying Hollywood's overall failure to portray nursing fairly are complex and varied. In our view, they include:

- entrenched stereotypes about nursing that persist even among the educated media elite, despite the increasing scope and complexity of modern nursing care;
- Hollywood's reliance on conventions and its fairly light focus on the complex realities of society compared to the focus of the news media, which is trained to at least try to report what it actually sees, rather than just what its audience expects to see;
- the fact that nursing remains overwhelmingly female, while men still control most Hollywood programming, and that nursing has not generally enjoyed the respect or understanding of media "feminists" with the power to effect change;
- insufficient support from physicians, who are often the beneficiaries of the misportrayal of nursing, and who provide most meaningful health care advice in Hollywood;
- nursing's own overall failure to represent itself well to the media and the public at large;
- the failure of nurses' concerns, even when assertively presented, to be taken as seriously as the concerns of other groups, perhaps owing to the Catch-22 of the poor image itself (why pay attention to nurses when they're just unskilled handmaidens?); and
- "PC fatigue" and an apparent belief among "progressive" media creators that their work has a positive social impact (e.g., on race, gender, and sexual orientation issues), immunizing them from having to consider whether their work could also be causing harm because they don't actually understand some things as well as they imagine.

At one time, healthcare media creators might have believed they had to include nurses to get a good gender mix and good drama. But today, with so many female physicians, most media creators evidently feel that they need not include any significant nurse characters at all. On serial television, once all the main characters are physicians, the need to constantly sell those characters means they're going to be doing every meaningful act, regardless of what happens in real life.

You might think physicians, who wield so much power in Hollywood, would have a better sense of nursing. Some physicians do. But much physician conduct seems to reflect a narrow, internally focused approach that assumes physicians provide all important health care and need not consider unexpected information. Physicians in general know little about nursing. Some physicians have even said that nurses get "too much education" and that they could "train monkeys" to do nurses' jobs.

But don't nurses bear some responsibility for the poor understanding of their profession?

Yes, of course. But we focus on the media's treatment of nursing because most of it is wildly inaccurate or distorted. Millions are given access to the lives and work of nurses through the media, so the media plays an enormous role in shaping and reinforcing social beliefs, as public health research shows. The popular media also provides an excellent vehicle to engage the public's interest. With its focus on celebrities and compelling characters, the media presents a set of common social reference points in which large parts of the world public already have a deep interest.

Nursing itself has many problems. Far from trying to substitute a positive stereotype of nurses for the negative ones, we simply want people to look at nurses as they really are. We also recognize that nurses often do not present themselves in an ideal way; we discuss that in Chapter 11. From major nursing institutions that continue to embrace unskilled "angel" imagery ("Nurses have a passion for caring!"), to nurses who welcome the idea that people will assess them professionally by how "hot" they are, to nurses who disclaim their own autonomy or won't speak up in clinical or public settings about the work they really do, to nurses who show the Hollywood actors playing physicians how to do things nurses really do—there is plenty of responsibility to go around.

Solving nursing's problems will require a range of strategies. Improving public understanding is one of the most important.

But that television show just happens to be about physicians. Even if it might help nursing to include nurse characters, how can you expect the show to do that?

In mid-2012, as *House* ended its eight-year run, all twenty-seven major characters on the top three US hospital dramas just "happened" to be physicians. In all those hospital shows, in hundreds of hours of programming seen by many millions around the world, the physician characters just "happened" to spend half their time doing key tasks that nurses do in real life.

Those are not random phenomena. Despite the recent appearance of a few nurse-focused shows with limited reach, we see no sign that things will soon even out, that the most popular shows will spend many years with 100 percent nurse characters, who will spend lots of time on tasks physicians really do. Today's healthcare media landscape reflects a critical lack of understanding of nursing and widespread social bias.

What seems to just "happen" in Hollywood is actually driven by the vast gulf between what media creators think and how things really are. In Hollywood, physicians single-handedly save lives. In real life, nurses also save countless lives. In Hollywood, physicians do virtually all critical procedures, like defibrillation. In real life, nurses perform many critical procedures, including most defibrillations. In Hollywood, physicians stay with patients 24/7, providing monitoring, emotional support, and education. In real life, nurses do that. In Hollywood, nurses are mute, deferential physician servants. In real life, they are autonomous professionals with years of college-level education who play the central role in hospitals. Their work is challenging and exciting, and they use their advanced skills to improve patient outcomes every day, often with little or no involvement from physicians.

Sorry, but even if media stereotypes do undermine nursing, I just don't see why I should care. What's in it for me?

You get to live. People sometimes ask journalist Suzanne Gordon why she, not a nurse, has worked so hard to publicize the roots of the nursing crisis and potential solutions. Her response is that it's enlightened self-interest: she wants someone to be there to care for her when she needs it. Having too few nurses leads to worse patient outcomes, suffering, and death.

The effects of the undervaluation of nursing are everywhere. When nurses lack resources, patients do not receive vital care. When nurses lack resources, they burn out and leave the bedside. When nurses lack social power, they cannot advocate for patients, and patients die needlessly from healthcare errors and incompetence. A March 2013 story in *The Washington Post* about efforts to help physicians manage their anger included reports of deaths in California because nurses were too scared of physicians to alert them to worrisome fetal monitor readings.[94] A March 2011 *New York Daily News* piece reported that a local hospital nurse had allegedly been fired for trying to expose her colleagues' refusal to treat a homeless man who was later found dead outside the hospital.[95] A November 2007 Associated Press article reported that operating room nurses at a Rhode Island hospital had repeatedly failed to stop life-threatening surgical errors—like operating on the wrong side of a patient's head—because they lacked the social power to do so.[96] A March 2009 feature in the *Sunday Times* (U.K.) told the story of a tormented nurse in India who regularly gave injections with used needles because she could not question the revered physicians and hospital managers who insisted on the potentially deadly practice.[97]

When nurses lack social power, they also suffer abuse from patients and colleagues. Although data about the extent of that abuse varies, Rose Chapman and colleagues found in a 2010 study of Australian hospital nurses that more than half had been physically assaulted at work in the past year, with an average of twenty-one incidents of assault *per nurse* per year![98] A 2002 study by May and Grubbs found that 74 percent of all nurses and 82 percent of emergency nurses surveyed at one Florida hospital had been physically assaulted in the preceding year.[99] The 2010 Australian study found that nurses do not tend to report the violence unless they have been injured—96 percent of incident reports revealed nurse injury. In fact, the nurses did not report five of six assaults because they believed violence "was just part of the job"; perhaps that had something to do with the fact that 50 percent of the reports to senior managers were met with inaction.[100] The research shows that triggers for abuse generally relate to some dysfunction in the health system, including the enforcement of hospital policies and long wait times, which, of course, often result from understaffing.[101]

Abuse doesn't come only from patients. Visitors and family members are just as likely to be the assailant as are the patients.[102] A 2009 study of Canadian nurses in the *Journal of Nursing Management* found that 77 percent of the nurses had been bullied by coworkers.[103] A 2008 study by the Joint Commission that accredits hospitals found that more than half of US nurses had been bullied on the job.[104] Common effects on the nurses include severe distress, depression, insomnia—and nurses themselves continuing the cycle of abuse.

These are the people who hold your life in their hands.

Notes

1. TAN, "Q: Nurses Are Just Wonderful, but You Really Can't Expect Hollywood to Focus on Them, Can You? After All, Popular Media Products Have to Be Dramatic and Exciting. Why Don't You Just Focus on Getting a Nursing Documentary on PBS or Basic Cable?," accessed January 24, 2014, http://tinyurl.com/ndvwsbz.

2. Tina Rosenberg, "The Family Doctor, Minus the M.D.," *New York Times* (October 24, 2012), http://tinyurl.com/9cjwrvj; TAN, "Fixes" (October 24, 2012), http://tinyurl.com/ke7dmo8.
3. WBUR, "Nursing a Shortage: Inside Out" (January 19, 2007), http://tinyurl.com/ljolky2; CFNA, "Our Favourite Worst Nightmare," TAN (January 19, 2007), http://tinyurl.com/putwtfs.
4. Tony Kushner, writer, Mike Nichols, director, *Angels in America*, HBO Films (2003); CFNA, "Angels in America," TAN (April 4, 2004), http://tinyurl.com/mqcbd3l.
5. The University of Rochester School of Nursing, "Woodhull Study on Nursing and the Media: Health Care's Invisible Partner," Sigma Theta Tau International (1997), http://tinyurl.com/kwgguga; Bernice Buresh, Suzanne Gordon, and Nica Bell, "Who Counts in News Coverage of Health Care?," *Nursing Outlook* 39, no. 5 (September/October 1991): 204–208.
6. Pedro Alcântara da Silva, "A Saúde nos Media. Representações do Sistema de Saúde e das Políticas Públicas na Imprensa Escrita Portuguesa," *Mundos Sociais* (Lisboa, 2011), http://tinyurl.com/l28ltk7.
7. Rodrigo José Martins Cardoso, João Manuel Garcia de Nascimento Graveto, and Ana Maria Correia Albuquerque Queiroz, "The Exposure of the Nursing Profession in Online and Print Media," *Revista Latino-Americana de Enfermagem* 22, no. 1 (Jan-Feb 2014): 144, doi:10.1590/0104-1169.3144.2394, http://tinyurl.com/lr3yo88.
8. Maria Aparecida Baggio and Alacoque Lorenzini Erdmann, "The (In)visibility of Caring and of the Profession of Nursing in the Relations Space," *Acta Paulista de Enfermagem* 23, no. 6 (2010): 745–750, http://tinyurl.com/k6wr62f.
9. TAN, "*Grey's Anatomy* Analyses and Action," accessed January 29, 2014, http://tinyurl.com/pgayg7h.
10. TAN, "*House* Single Episode Reviews" (2011), http://tinyurl.com/py4b5ug.
11. TAN, "*Private Practice* Individual Episode Analyses" (2013), http://tinyurl.com/lecehka.
12. CFNA, "Nurses Are about 100 Times More Likely to Attend Graduate Nursing School than Medical School," TAN (2002), http://tinyurl.com/p7orchc.
13. TAN, "Letting the Exiles Bleed on Main Street" (April 2010), http://tinyurl.com/kunazup.
14. TAN, "Commander" (September 2011), http://tinyurl.com/n8z5zum.
15. TAN, "*A Gifted Man*: The Lionel Messi of Surgeon Glorification" (March 2, 2012), http://tinyurl.com/kr88jes.
16. TAN, "Admiring Their Credentials" (January 12, 2011), http://tinyurl.com/oe9eox7.
17. CFNA, "Cinema Faux," TAN (June 26, 2008), http://tinyurl.com/m48c3bx.
18. TAN, "Physicians Are Awesome" (July 22, 2010), http://tinyurl.com/o7m9olh.

19. TAN, "Scrubbing Out" (October 24, 2013), http://tinyurl.com/nwb8zn9.
20. Jo Brand, Vicki Pepperdine, Joanna Scanlan, Mark V. Olsen, and Will Scheffer, creators, *Getting On*, HBO, accessed March 24, 2014, http://www.hbo.com/getting-on.
21. TAN, "*ER* Episode Analyses" (2009), http://tinyurl.com/odsbmqw.
22. TAN, "*Scrubs* Episode Analyses" (2009), http://tinyurl.com/p9n8e58.
23. TAN, "*Nurse Jackie* Episode Reviews," accessed March 24, 2014, http://tinyurl.com/kqm3k6b.
24. TAN, "*Mercy* Episode Reviews" (2010), http://tinyurl.com/kj3t63s.
25. TAN, "*HawthoRNe* Episode Reviews" (2011), http://tinyurl.com/jwd7neg.
26. TAN, "*Call the Midwife* Episode Reviews," accessed March 24, 2014, http://tinyurl.com/m3bf4lw.
27. Cathryn Domrose, "Mending Our Image," *NurseWeek* (June 26, 2002), http://tinyurl.com/l6j486c.
28. Beatrice J. Kalisch and Philip A. Kalisch, "Anatomy of the Image of the Nurse: Dissonant and Ideal Models," *American Nurses Association Publications* G-161 (1983): 3–23. See generally "The Work of Beatrice Kalisch and Philip Kalisch on Nursing's Public Image and the Nursing Shortage," TAN, accessed January 29, 2014, http://tinyurl.com/lq3ebxh.
29. CFNA, "*A Farewell to Arms*," TAN (2003), http://tinyurl.com/mj7hyo2.
30. CFNA, "*Rear Window*," TAN (2003), http://tinyurl.com/oyre8hy.
31. CFNA, "*One Flew Over the Cuckoo's Nest*," TAN (2003), http://tinyurl.com/pvz3267.
32. CFNA, "*M*A*S*H*" (film review), TAN (2003), http://tinyurl.com/qc58j2k.
33. CFNA, "*M*A*S*H*" (television review), TAN (2003), http://tinyurl.com/opyqegz.
34. TAN, "*ER* Episode Analyses" (2009), http://tinyurl.com/odsbmqw.
35. TAN, "*Strong Medicine* Single Episode Analyses" (2006), http://tinyurl.com/o5q2awp.
36. TAN, "*Scrubs* Episode Analyses" (2009), http://tinyurl.com/p9n8e58.
37. TAN, "*Off the Map* Single Episode Analyses" (2011), http://tinyurl.com/oc5vaqg.
38. Kantar Media, "Kantar Media Reports U.S. Advertising Expenditures Increased 3 Percent in 2012" (March 11, 2013), http://tinyurl.com/lspr69o.
39. Robert Jensen and Emily Oster, "The Power of TV: Cable Television and Women's Status in India" (September 23, 2008), http://tinyurl.com/q4bzpfp.
40. Rajiv N. Rimal and Maria K. Lapinski, "Why Health Communication Is Important in Public Health," *Bulletin of the World Health Organization* 87 (2009): 247, http://tinyurl.com/da6dg3.
41. Jerry C. Parker and Esther Thorson, *Health Communication in the New Media Landscape* (New York: Springer Publishing, 2009), http://tinyurl.com/l2qwnme.

42. Deborah Glik, "Health Communication in Popular Media Formats" (paper presented at the 131st annual meeting of the American Public Health Association, San Francisco, California, November 15–19, 2003), http://tinyurl.com/ohx64ds.
43. Joseph Turow and Rachel Gans, "As Seen on TV: Health Policy Issues in TV's Medical Dramas," Kaiser Family Foundation (2002), http://tinyurl.com/lfpy9jz. See generally Joseph Turow, *Playing Doctor: Television, Storytelling, and Medical Power* (Ann Arbor: University of Michigan Press, 2010), http://tinyurl.com/nmdyvjv.
44. DaimlerChrysler, "It Doesn't Take a Brain Surgeon," Dodge Caravan commercial (2003), http://tinyurl.com/k3qp2n9.
45. Turow and Gans, "As Seen on TV," http://tinyurl.com/lfpy9jz.
46. Bill D. Herman, The *Fight Over Digital Rights: The Politics of Copyright and Technology* (New York: Cambridge University Press, 2013): xv, http://tinyurl.com/mvy2vkp.
47. Kaiser Family Foundation, "Entertainment Education and Health in the United States" (2004), http://tinyurl.com/n33q8uf.
48. Dartmouth College, "Both Good and Bad Movie Characters Who Smoke Influence Teens to Do the Same," *Science Daily* 3 (July 2009), http://tinyurl.com/n2vuea; Susanne E. Tanski, Mike Stoolmiller, Sonya Dal Cin, Keilah Worth, Jennifer Gibson, and James D. Sargent, "Adolescent Smoking: Who Matters More, Good Guys or Bad Guys?," *Pediatrics* 124, no. 1 (July 2009): 135–143, http://tinyurl.com/kwaxbx3.
49. Turow and Gans, "As Seen on TV," http://tinyurl.com/lfpy9jz.
50. Kaiser Family Foundation and Norman Lear Center, "How Healthy Is Prime Time?," Hollywood, Health and Society (September 2008): 1, http://tinyurl.com/ky6x4pk.
51. Matea Gold and Maria Elena Fernandez, "Community Service as a TV Theme," *Los Angeles Times* (October 19, 2009), http://tinyurl.com/pgdqdps.
52. Marc Malkin, "Sarah Chalke's Very Personal *Grey's Anatomy*," *TV Scoop* (March 28, 2013), http://tinyurl.com/qf778kv.
53. Adriene Hill, "Hollywood Writes a New Storyline for Obamacare," Marketplace (October 20, 2013), http://tinyurl.com/lsw66fx.
54. Elena Lesley, "New Soap Helps Battle AIDS," *Phnom Penh Post* (December 3, 2004), http://tinyurl.com/m27couh.
55. Allison Van Dusen, "TV's Medical Missteps," *Forbes* (September 19, 2007), http://tinyurl.com/lg2adh3.
56. Writers Guild of America, West, "Neal Baer to Receive Valentine Davies Award from Writers Guild of America, West," press release (December 1, 2003), http://tinyurl.com/kwgx3wb.
57. Mary Murphy, "The Women Who Revived *ER*," *TV Guide* (February 14, 2014), http://tinyurl.com/lvtmaqh.

58. Ed Gordon, "An Ethnically Diverse 'Grey's Anatomy,'" National Public Radio (March 25, 2005), http://tinyurl.com/phpkpw2.
59. Suzanne Gordon, "Doc Hollywood," *The American Prospect* (November 5, 2001), http://tinyurl.com/kz58hcc.
60. Lisa Liddane, "Paging Dr. Nielsen: TV Medical Shows," *Orange County Register* (October 8, 2006), http://tinyurl.com/lyx3nsx.
61. Mary A. Fischer, "Docs in the Box," *Reader's Digest* (March 2007), reprinted January 15, 2010, http://tinyurl.com/krp7upc.
62. Carol Ann Campbell, "Nurses Urge TV Dramas: Get Real," *The Star-Ledger* (January 28, 2007), http://tinyurl.com/k5ofcbl.
63. Allison Van Dusen, "Playing Doctor: Medical TV Isn't Always Right," *Forbes* (September 20, 2007), http://tinyurl.com/n5jvn7x.
64. Kelly Brewington, "TV Nurses—The Good and the Bad," *Baltimore Sun* (January 7, 2010), http://tinyurl.com/pn7ncku.
65. Faiza Elmasry, "Nurse, I Need a Reality Check," Voice of America (April 13, 2010), http://tinyurl.com/qj6f5do.
66. Jessica Testa, "A Real Nurse Rates the TV Fakes," *More* (March 26, 2012), http://tinyurl.com/qxluqod.
67. Turow and Gans, "As Seen on TV," http://tinyurl.com/lfpy9jz.
68. Kaiser and Norman Lear, "How Healthy" (September 2008): 14, http://tinyurl.com/ky6x4pk.
69. Brian L. Quick, "The Effects of Viewing *Grey's Anatomy* on Perceptions of Doctors and Patient Satisfaction," *Journal of Broadcasting and Electronic Media* 53, no. 1 (March 12, 2009): 38–55, http://tinyurl.com/leogd7d.
70. JWT Communications, "Memo to Nurses for a Healthier Tomorrow Coalition Members on a Focus Group Study of 1800 School Children in 10 US Cities," TAN (2000), http://tinyurl.com/l2q5mma.
71. Gavin R. Neilson and William Lauder, "What Do High Academic Achieving School Pupils Really Think about a Career in Nursing: Analysis of the Narrative from Paradigmatic Case Interviews," *Nurse Education Today* 28 (2008): 680–690, http://tinyurl.com/m8ewewz.
72. Roslyn Weaver, Yenna Salamonson, Jane Koch, and Debra Jackson, "Nursing on Television: Student Perceptions of Television's Role in Public Image, Recruitment and Education," *Journal of Advanced Nursing* 69, no. 12 (December 2013): 2635–2643, http://tinyurl.com/oy6o2or.
73. Jacinta Kelly, Gerard M. Fealy, and Roger Watson, "The Image of You: Constructing Nursing Identities in YouTube," *Journal of Advanced Nursing* 68, no. 8 (2012): 1804–1813, http://tinyurl.com/k5carcm.
74. Karen Donelan, Peter Buerhaus, Catherine Desroches, Robert Dittus, and David Dutwin, "Public Perceptions of Nursing Careers: The Influence of the Media and Nursing Shortages," *Nursing Economics* 26, no. 3 (2008), http://tinyurl.com/mram6xl.

75. Centers for Disease Control (CDC), "Entertainment Education: 2000 Porter Novelli Healthstyles Survey" (2000), http://tinyurl.com/k9qastz.
76. Kaiser Family Foundation, "Entertainment Education and Health in the United States" (2004), http://tinyurl.com/n33q8uf.
77. Susan E. Morgan, Tyler R. Harrison, Lisa Chewning, LaShara Davis, and Mark DiCorcia, "Entertainment (Mis)Education: The Framing of Organ Donation in Entertainment Television," *Health Communication* 22, no. 2 (August 2007): 143–151, http://tinyurl.com/nmde27r.
78. Susan Morgan, Tyler Harrison, Shawn Long, Walid Afifi, Michael Stephenson, and Tom Reichert, "Family Discussions about Organ Donation: How the Media Influences Opinions about Donation Decisions," *Clinical Transplantation* 19, no. 5 (2005): 674–682, http://tinyurl.com/kck563a.
79. Richard J. Crockett, Thomas Pruzinsky, and John A. Persing, "The Influence of Plastic Surgery 'Reality TV' on Cosmetic Surgery Patient Expectations and Decision Making," *Plastic & Reconstructive Surgery* 120, no. 1 (July 2007): 316–324, http://tinyurl.com/6y97d3; Kathleen Doheny, "Cosmetic Surgery TV Shows Get Viewers Pondering," *HealthDay* (August 9, 2007), http://tinyurl.com/l8fae62.
80. Melissa S. Kearney and Phillip B. Levine, "Media Influences on Social Outcomes: The Impact of MTV's *16 and Pregnant* on Teen Childbearing" (January 2014), http://tinyurl.com/nnb8ufu; Nicholas Kristof, "TV Lowers Birthrate (Seriously)," *New York Times* (March 19, 2014), http://tinyurl.com/nnb8ufu.
81. Roslyn Weaver and Ian Wilson, "Australian Medical Students' Perceptions of Professionalism and Ethics in Medical Television Programs," *BMC Medical Education* 11 (2011): 50, http://tinyurl.com/l3z8ss2.
82. Weaver and Wilson, "Australian Medical Students," http://tinyurl.com/l3z8ss2.
83. Victoria Rideout, "Television as a Health Educator: A Case Study of *Grey's Anatomy*," Kaiser Family Foundation (September 16, 2008), http://tinyurl.com/ld27y4s.
84. Henry J. Kaiser Foundation, "Unique Experiment Finds Health Content Placed in *Grey's Anatomy* Episode Quadrupled Awareness Among Audience," press release (September 16, 2008), http://tinyurl.com/lp6krre.
85. P. G. Brindley and C. Needham, "Positioning Prior to Endotracheal Intubation on a Television Medical Drama: Perhaps Life Mimics Art," *Resuscitation* 80, no. 5 (May 2009): 604, http://tinyurl.com/kdwd2sw.
86. Michael M. O'Connor, "The Role of the Television Drama *ER* in Medical Student Life: Entertainment or Socialization?," *Journal of the American Medical Association* 280, no. 9 (September 2, 1998): 854–855, http://tinyurl.com/qdf8ymn.
87. Mollyann Brodie, Ursula Foehr, Vicky Rideout, Neal Baer, Carolyn Miller, Rebecca Flournoy, and Drew Altman, "Communicating Health Information through the Entertainment Media," *Health Affairs* 20, no. 1 (January/February 2001): 192–199, http://tinyurl.com/lutka8m.

88. Kaiser Family Foundation, "Entertainment Education and Health in the United States" (2004), http://tinyurl.com/n33q8uf; Kaiser Family Foundation, "The Impact of TV's Health Content: A Case Study of *ER* Viewers" (2002), http://tinyurl.com/orpdwtm.
89. Thomas Valente, Sheila Murphy, Grace Huang, Jodi Gusek, Jennie Greene, and Vicki Beck, "Evaluating a Minor Storyline on *ER* about Teen Obesity, Hypertension, and 5 a Day," *Journal of Health Communication* 12, no. 6 (September 2007): 551–566, http://tinyurl.com/o3c8kzn.
90. Harvard School of Public Health, "After 'ER' Smallpox Episode, Fewer 'ER' Viewers Report They Would Go to Emergency Room if They Had Symptoms of the Disease," press release (June 13, 2002), http://tinyurl.com/oapocqj.
91. RAND Health, "Entertainment TV Can Help Teach Teens Responsible Sex Messages" (November 3, 2003), http://tinyurl.com/lln6eg7, citing Rebecca Collins, Marc Elliott, Sandra Berry, David Kanouse, and Sarah Hunter, "Entertainment Television as a Healthy Sex Educator: The Impact of Condom Efficacy Information in an Episode of Friends," *Pediatrics* 112, no. 5 (November 2003): 1115–1121, http://tinyurl.com/tku8.
92. Kaiser Family Foundation, "Entertainment Education" (2004), http://tinyurl.com/n33q8uf; CDC, "Soap Opera," http://tinyurl.com/qa5mewv.
93. May G. Kennedy, Ann O'Leary, Vicki Beck, Katrina Pollard, and Penny Simpson, "Increases in Calls to the CDC's National STD and AIDS Hotline Following AIDS-Related Episodes in a Soap Opera," *Journal of Communication* 54, no. 2 (June 2004): 287–301, http://tinyurl.com/lqe3ra7.
94. Sandra G. Boodman, "Anger Management Courses Are a New Tool for Dealing with Out-of-Control Doctors," *Washington Post* (March 4, 2013), http://tinyurl.com/bxcyt3f; TAN, "The Weather in My Head" (March 16, 2013), http://tinyurl.com/q6h6fmx.
95. Alison Gendar, "Nurse Fired for Trying to Expose Roosevelt Hospital's Neglect in Death of Homeless Man: Lawsuit," *New York Daily News* (March 28, 2011), http://tinyurl.com/mwau98t; TAN, "Patients Unattended" (March 28, 2011), http://tinyurl.com/pwyshqr.
96. Michelle Smith, "Brain Surgery Goes Awry in R.I.," *USA Today*/Associated Press (November 27, 2011), http://tinyurl.com/nxgd73e.
97. Amy Turner, "Used Needles are Causing a Health Crisis in India," *Sunday Times* (March 22, 2009), http://tinyurl.com/l7hz8mf; TAN, "Against Everything She Has Been Taught" (March 22, 2009), http://tinyurl.com/mqcqx7v.
98. Rose Chapman, I. Styles, L. Perry, and Shane Combs, "Examining the Characteristics of Workplace Violence in One Non-Tertiary Hospital," *Journal of Clinical Nursing* 19 (2010): 479–488, press release, http://tinyurl.com/m77bhcx;Fran Lowry, "Nurses Are Frequent Targets of Workplace Violence," *Medscape* (February 4, 2010), http://tinyurl.com/ksfow8d.

99. Deborah D. May and Laurie M. Grubbs, "The Extent, Nature, and Precipitating Factors of Nurse Assault among Three Groups of Registered Nurses in a Regional Medical Center," *Journal of Emergency Nursing* 28, no. 1 (2002): 11–17, http://tinyurl.com/ks7cdj9.
100. Chapman, et al., "Examining," http://tinyurl.com/m77bhcx; Lowry, "Workplace," http://tinyurl.com/ksfow8d.
101. May and Grubbs, "The Extent," http://tinyurl.com/ks7cdj9.
102. May and Grubbs, "The Extent," http://tinyurl.com/ks7cdj9.
103. Heather K. Spence Laschinger, Michael Leiter, Arla Day, and Debra Gilin-Oore, "Workplace Empowerment, Incivility, and Burnout: Impact on Staff Nurse Recruitment and Retention Outcomes," *Journal of Nursing Management* 17, no. 3 (April 2009): 302–311, http://tinyurl.com/mby29r4.
104. Dianne Felblinger, "Incivility and Bullying in the Workplace and Nurses' Shame Responses," *Journal of Obstetric, Gynecologic, & Neonatal Nursing* 37, no. 2 (March/April 2008): 234–242, http://tinyurl.com/6s28ut, summary available at http://tinyurl.com/6kyzkq.

II THE GREAT DIVIDE: THE MEDIA VERSUS REAL NURSING

3 COULD MONKEYS BE NURSES?

NBC's campy daytime drama *Passions* offered a very special solution to the nursing shortage: an orangutan. From 2003 until 2005, the monkey played the role of Precious, a private duty nurse. Character Beth Wallace hired Precious to replace her invalid mother's previous nurse, who had blabbed Beth's evil secrets.[1]

The NBC website told us the "dutiful caretaker" changed Mrs. Wallace's diapers, wore "a modern version of a nurse's uniform, complete with cap," adored "handsome Latino men, bananas, fruit smoothies, shopping, food fights, gin and tonics," and wanted "to do the best job possible as Mrs. Wallace's nurse . . . and to have some fun at the same time!"

While *Passions* was known for being somewhat surreal, the role of Precious reflects public sentiment about the work of nurses. There are those who believe nursing requires so little skill that a monkey *could* do it. In fact, in the 1990s, representatives of a California hospital group told top-level union negotiators that nursing was so simple that the union's nurses could be replaced with monkeys.

This chapter explores how recent media has portrayed nursing skill. A number of media items, particularly in print news, have communicated some sense of the advanced scientific skills that nurses use to improve patient outcomes. Unfortunately, much of the most influential media, particularly television, regularly sends the message that nursing is low-skilled loser work unworthy of serious consideration by anyone with a brain.

In addition, countless media items portray important nursing work as being performed by others, particularly physicians, thus robbing nurses of credit they need to save their profession. Others ignore nursing work and expertise, even when nursing actually plays a central role in the relevant subject, such as patient education, managing healthcare errors, or mass casualty events. Still other items suggest that any helpful person or machine is a "nurse," consistent with the broad use of the term "nursing" to include unskilled tending.

The prevailing view of nursing as inferior grunt work undermines nurses' claims to respect and resources. In a May 2008 *Arab News* article, Taqwa Omer Yahia, a nursing dean at Saudi Arabia's King Saud University, described what happened when she gave a lecture at a local university. She was introduced as "Dr. Yahia" and "treated with respect and admiration" until, after her talk, a student asked "what kind of doctor" she was. Dr. Yahia said that her PhD was in nursing. The students' disappointment was palpable, and she felt she had "lost all credibility as a trusted speaker."

The stories of Dr. Yahia and Nurse Precious remind us of research on inattentional blindness. In one famous Harvard study, participants watching a small circle of people throw basketballs to each other were asked to count the passes. As the balls went back and forth, a person dressed in a gorilla costume walked into the middle of the circle, stopped to beat her chest, and left the circle. But most observers later reported seeing no gorilla.[2] In a 2013 variation of this experiment, when white female subjects were first told they would later have to select a coworker or neighbor from online profiles, they were equally likely to notice white and African-American men walk into the circle. But when the subjects were instead told they would later be looking for a friend or mate, goals that were "closer to self," they were more than twice as likely to notice the white man. Even their "unconscious screeners" were biased.[3] Similarly, most of us fail to see what *nurses* really do because we have been conditioned to focus—consciously or unconsciously—on what *physicians* do.

Media Portrayals of Nurses as Serious Professionals

Portrayals of nurses as skilled professionals do exist. They tend to appear in the print news media, but they can be found even on entertainment television and in feature films. Nurses have been depicted as skilled clinicians, vital public health workers, researchers and innovators, healthcare experts and leaders.

"Might Be a Genius": Nursing Skill on Television and in Film

The nurse-focused television dramas that have appeared since 2009 have all shown nurses to have healthcare skills that may surprise viewers, although there has been a little physician nursing on the US shows. For instance, even on those shows, physicians have often done the defibrillation.

Perhaps the strongest examples of nursing skill have appeared on *Nurse Jackie*. Although Jackie Peyton is a "world class liar" who struggles with drug addiction and occasionally disregards ethical obligations, she is also probably the best nurse in television history, a tough clinical virtuoso who excels at physical and psychosocial care, patient advocacy, and mentoring. She regularly saves lives. In the first season, Jackie casually saved a choking restaurant patron with the Heimlich maneuver and taught a precocious 10-year-old girl how to manage her mother's debilitating lupus. Jackie takes innovative, effective approaches to troublesome colleagues, violent patients, and agitated family members. In one July 2009 episode, she used index cards to give a mute stroke victim some pointed options to show his skeptical, obnoxious family that he was still "in there" and in need of their support. Jackie's style of holistic care includes masterfully manipulating an insurance company into covering an expensive surgery for a deaf woman who has had several fingers shot off[4] and blackmailing a wealthy athlete into donating a much-needed $400,000 computed tomography [CT] scanner to the emergency department (ED) in exchange for not revealing his drug possession.[5] Like many real nurses, Jackie has fought to give dying patients the endings they wanted, helping them avoid being tortured with unwanted procedures.[6] Jackie has trained not only her quirky protégée Zoey Barkow, who now displays Jackie-like life-saving skill, but also the somewhat bogus young physician Cooper, who initially struggled with Jackie's blunt critiques. June 2012 episodes found Jackie expertly running the ED during a staffing crisis, leading fellow nurse Sam to marvel that she "might be a genius."[7]

Call the Midwife offers a dramatic look at the exploits of Anglican and lay nurse-midwives caring for poor women and babies in London's East End in the late 1950s. The show can be sentimental, but the nurses are vital health workers, with tough, expert senior midwives guiding the nervous newer ones. The nurses visit pregnant women to monitor their progress, deliver babies under awful conditions, and advise new mothers and their communities, all in an environment without birth control where women seem to function as baby factories and one-person day care centers.[8] In one April 2013 episode, the midwives expertly managed the difficult delivery of an older woman whose twin was extremely hostile to modern health care. Meanwhile, lead character Jenny, temporarily practicing in a hospital, proved a quick study in the operating room (OR) while effectively diagnosing and informing her nurse superior of an abusive surgeon's dangerous neurological problems.[9] In a May 2013 episode, nurse Chummy expertly diagnosed preeclampsia in a pregnant acquaintance, taking a urine sample after swollen ankles aroused her suspicions.[10]

During its one season on the air, *Mercy* also included powerful portrayals of nursing skill. Like Jackie, lead character Veronica Callahan was an assertive clinical leader who had some trouble with rules. In the September 2009 series premiere, after Veronica saw a car crash cause a motorist to suffer a tension pneumothorax, she quickly saved his life by decompressing the collapsed lung with a knife and a coffee straw. Veronica counseled and advocated for a dying older patient, empowering her to tell her adult children that she wanted to stop treatment, even though this same bitter patient had at one point asked what nurses were good for, prompting Veronica to respond: "Well, we do try to keep the doctors from killing you." In another September 2009 episode, the smart novice nurse Chloe Payne (who had a masters degree from Penn!) persuaded a skeptical physician that a patient actually was hearing the sound he said was driving him to seek drugs. In the May 2010 series finale, Chloe diagnosed airport malaria despite resistance from another physician. Too bad the finale also had Chloe vowing to attend medical school following a romantic rejection from a cardiologist. That'll show him! That nursing really is inferior.[11]

HawthoRNe also featured good examples of nurses' health expertise, particularly the authority of nurse managers—who barely exist on other shows—although its portrayals were wildly inconsistent and weaker toward the end of its run. Christina Hawthorne was a commanding chief nursing officer, and ultimately chief operating officer, who also had time to dispense expert clinical care when a crisis arose and to fight for patients with resistant physicians and family members. In one July 2009 episode, Hawthorne went around a powerful surgeon to offer a patient the option of treatment from another surgeon who had more experience in doing a difficult operation. She also determined that the mysterious cause of a teenager's Adderall overdose was a prescription from his pushy physician father. Like the other nurse shows, *HawthoRNe* even included some promising saves by a novice nurse character. Nurse Kelly Epson was often embarrassingly timid, but in an August 2009 episode, her advocacy and alertness to the shifting story of a stroke victim's daughter about when symptoms began saved the victim from a dangerous treatment. In a July 2011 episode, Kelly identified and acted courageously to counter the outbreak of an antibiotic-resistant organism (methicillin-resistant *Staphylococcus aureus* [MRSA]). She even built an isolation ward, alerted the Centers for Disease Control and Prevention, and defibrillated a patient.[12]

Although *ER* featured rampant physician nursing and occasionally denigrated the nursing profession, the show also included some impressive portrayals of nursing skill. Typically these involved the lone major nurse character, who in the show's final years was Samantha (Sam) Taggart, a tough nurse who displayed confidence and skill in performing or advocating for critical care procedures. An October 2008 episode found her fighting back against condescending physician attitudes, at one point successfully taking over an urgent intubation from a flailing intern. In a February 2007 episode, the physicians had trouble intubating another critical patient. Taggart pushed the sides of the patient's chest to force air back up through the trachea, explaining that "the bubbles will show you where to place the tube."

A handful of late 2005 *ER* episodes featured the expert, hard-core nurse manager Eve Peyton. In one scene, busy attending Luka Kovac repeatedly brushed off Peyton's requests that he come help a flailing resident physician with a fiberoptic intubation for a hypoxic accident victim with severe head trauma. When Kovac finally arrived, the resident and the rest of the code team were watching Peyton insert a laryngeal mask airway. The patient quickly improved. Peyton suggested that Kovac consider educating his residents about using the laryngeal mask airway and told him, "Take it from here, Doctor. I'm going to go find a bedpan that needs emptying."[13]

The irreverent sitcom *Scrubs* was similarly dominated by physician characters, but it too included some passing indications of nursing knowledge. Most involved the show's one major nurse character, Carla Espinosa, who at times was presented as a nurse manager. An April 2006 episode showed Espinosa catching intern errors and teaching the interns how to avoid them. In one scene, she even expertly took charge of handling a patient's seizure. A March 2006 episode featured a brief but aggressive defense of nurses' technical expertise, as Espinosa demonstrated her encyclopedic knowledge of the conditions and care plans of specific patients.[14]

Portrayals of nursing skill on shows that are not hospital-focused are rare. From 2009 to 2014 NBC's sitcom *Parks & Recreation* included nurse Ann Perkins, who occasionally displayed knowledge and skill both in the clinical setting and as a local public health official. In an April 2013 episode, Ann not only acted to treat her reluctant city colleague Ron's streptococcal infection by pushing him to go to the hospital, but she also insisted on addressing his overall health, getting him to eat bananas to raise his potassium levels. The physician who saw Ron at the hospital was eager to write him a prescription and move on.[15] The global hit *Downton Abbey* (ITV/

PBS) mostly portrayed World War I–era nursing as very low-skilled, but the first season, broadcast in 2011 in the United States, did include brief depictions of nurse Isobel Crawley, the Downton heir's mother, as a formidable health system organizer with skills that in some ways rivaled those of the local physician.[16] And in an August 2008 episode of TNT's *Saving Grace*, a tough but sensitive veteran nurse played the central role in the care of a badly burned boy, displaying advanced clinical knowledge and interpersonal skills.[17]

A few documentaries have given viewers a good sense of nursing. *24 Hours in A&E* has shown emergency nurses at London's King's College Hospital, like the charismatic senior sister Jen Du-Prat, to be bright, articulate professionals who play a central role in patient care, using very good psychosocial and managerial skills. A couple documentaries on Discovery Health Channel also showcased nursing knowledge, although their audience was limited. *Lifeline: The Nursing Diaries*, a three-part documentary from 2004, followed nurses at Massachusetts General and New York-Presbyterian hospitals. The first part, "The Rookies," produced by master documentary maker Richard Kahn and Linda Martin, may be the best single hour of a nursing documentary that we've seen. It shows highly skilled nurses saving lives, educating patients, and supporting families in intensive care units (ICUs).[18] Helen Holt's *Nurses*, from 2002, was an engaging five-part documentary about Johns Hopkins nurses in oncology, critical care, psychiatric care, pediatrics, and the neonatal intensive care unit (NICU).[19]

A few recent feature-length films have conveyed something of nursing skill. Mike Nichols's *Angels in America*, based on Tony Kushner's play, included one of the best depictions of nursing in feature film history, placing the profession at the center of AIDS care. Shown on HBO in 2003, the six-hour exploration of faith, politics, and sexuality was set at the start of the AIDS era. Nurse Belize used skill, cynical wit, and tough love to keep his stricken friend Prior alive and sane. Meanwhile, at the hospital, Belize provided the AIDS-stricken power broker Roy Cohn with a measure of comfort, dignity, and expert advice, even as they traded invective across a chasm of mutual loathing.[20]

The 2004 overhaul of George Romero's zombie classic *Dawn of the Dead*, by director Zack Snyder and screenwriter James Gunn, was a funny post-9/11 vision of radical fundamentalism overrunning bourgeois society. Character Ana Clark, a smart, tough, resourceful nurse, helped lead some survivors trapped in a suburban mall. She cared for the group's wounds and used her nursing skill to discover vital zombie information.[21] Neill Blomkamp's dystopian 2013 film *Elysium* also included a nurse, lead character Max's childhood sweetheart Frey. She displayed some skill and strength, patching up Max after a knife wound, although her overall role in the plot was far more passive than Ana's in *Dawn of the Dead*.[22]

Although the popular *Meet the Parents* films were not exactly advertisements for nursing, the 2010 installment, *Little Fockers*, included clear signs of nursing expertise along with the frat-boy overtones. In that film, main character Gaylord (Greg) Focker was an articulate nursing manager who directed a medical-surgical unit, wrote scholarly articles, and showed some clinical expertise, mainly helping his father-in-law Jack with the effects of a heart condition.[23]

"Startling Discoveries": Nursing Skill in the News Media

Most of the effective recent portrayals of nursing skill have appeared in the print press. These do not generally have the broad impact of television or movies, although they may reach influential demographics.

Experts, Life Savers, and Leaders

Occasionally the news media presents nurses as healthcare leaders. In December 2012 the *New York Times* ran Daniel Slotnick's strong obituary for Vernice Ferguson, who supervised more than 60,000 nurses and "fought for greater opportunities, higher wages and more respect for nurses as a longtime chief nursing officer" at what became the US Department of Veterans Affairs. Slotnick noted that when the African-American Ferguson graduated from the nursing program at New York University in 1950 with an academic prize, the director of nursing reportedly refused to shake her hand.[24]

In June 2012, the *Baltimore Sun* published a detailed obituary by Frederick Rasmussen for Elizabeth Scanlon Trump, the driven cofounder and longtime nursing director of the University of Maryland's Shock Trauma Center, arguably the finest trauma center in the world. The piece portrayed Trump as "the first trauma nurse."[25]

In March 2012 the *San Francisco Chronicle* printed a remarkably good profile of new University of California San Francisco nursing dean David Vlahov—*on the front page*. Julian Guthrie's piece traced Vlahov's development as a nurse, including his work as a prison clinician and a nursing professor, his time at the Centers for Disease Control and Prevention, his founding of an AIDS clinic in East Baltimore, and his years on the New York City Board of Health.[26]

Other pieces have highlighted the expertise of direct care nurses. A September 2012 tribute to the nurses at the University of Southern California's Keck Hospital by *Los Angeles Times* columnist Steve Lopez had some of that old-time help 'n' comfort imagery. But it also stressed that an alert nurse had saved Lopez's life by performing cardiopulmonary resuscitation (CPR) after his heart stopped following knee-replacement surgery. Lopez gave readers a sense of nurses' professional training and skills, including counseling patients and "translating doctor-speak."[27]

In April 2007 the *Wall Street Journal* published a piece by editor John Blanton, who had gone back to school and become a nurse in a post-9/11 search for meaning. Focused on the crushing workload and fear of error Blanton faced as a new burn unit nurse, the article described what he did for patients and why it mattered:

> With easily shattered confidence, I could start an IV, administer medications, bathe a bed-bound patient and change linens, change dressings, insert all sorts of catheters and tubes, read lab results and electrocardiograms. I knew to be vigilant against infection, pneumonia, pressure ulcers, medication errors and the many other lurking threats to hospital patients. On the burn unit, pain control loomed large. I also knew, as both executor of treatment plans and patient advocate, to keep a close eye on what doctors ordered. They make mistakes, too.[28]

In October 2005 the *Boston Globe* ran Scott Allen's four-part special report about the intense eight-month ICU training of new nurse Julia Zelixon by veteran nurse M. J. Pender. Readers got a vivid sense of the complexity and importance of nursing. Pender's analysis of the patients' conditions and needs was relentless, as the nurses worked to manage different medications, tubes, and monitors. Each patient reportedly needed twenty hours of nursing care daily, the vast majority of it provided by nurses on their own. At one point Pender stopped a physician from speeding a transfusion to an especially critical patient, fearing that it would dilute the medication dripping through the same intravenous line. An anesthesiologist noted that he often feels "we're here more as consultants to the nurses."[29]

Perhaps most rare are items about what nurses, as skilled professionals, do *not* do. In 2004, Garry Trudeau's widely distributed comic strip *Doonesbury* introduced tough Walter Reed character Nurse Jewel, who cared for Lt. B.D. after he lost part of his leg in the Iraq war. In a June strip, Jewel told B.D. that the hospital's nurses "love our soldiers" but that "because we're so good at all the things we do here . . . occasionally a patient is tempted to think of us as his personal concierge service. This is a mistake." B.D. responds, "I can tell." Jewel: "Then let the fun begin! Drain your wound?"[30]

What We're Missing: Reporting on the Shortage

Although many media pieces about the nursing shortage have focused on numbers, some items show why it matters that patients don't have enough nurses. A May 2012 report by Patti Neighmond on National Public Radio's *Morning Edition* described a poll of patients showing widespread nurse understaffing in US hospitals. After twelve hours of trying to care for too many patients nonstop, one nurse said she drove home exhausted but white-knuckled, worrying about the danger to patients. A nurse explained that if she was too busy to detect subtle condition changes, such as that a patient's "jugular vein is just slightly distended, or you check their nail beds and they're a little bit dusky," a patient could decline quickly.[31]

Will Moredock's March 2007 cover story on the shortage in the *Charleston City Paper* included an admirably detailed look at what Medical University of South Carolina Hospital ICU nurse Misty Deason actually did for patients. Moredock seemed surprised by how much nursing mattered; he described studies showing that nurse staffing and education levels affect patient outcomes as "startling discoveries." He marveled at the credentials of his expert sources, nursing leaders with PhDs.[32]

A cover story by John Pekkanen in the September 2003 *Reader's Digest* revealed a system of US hospitals on the verge of breakdown, as angry family members struggled to get the attention of overwhelmed nurses and patients died needlessly because there simply weren't enough nurses.

> Every time a nurse enters a patient's room, she observes his or her color, demeanor, state of mind and speech. Any subtle change can signal trouble. [Deceased liver donor] Mike Hurewitz failed to get this sort of assessment—and none of the devices he was hooked up to could perform that job.[33]

Of course, things are worse in some settings. In July 2004 the *New York Times* ran a powerful report by Celia W. Dugger about the catastrophic effects of the emigration of nurses from AIDS-ravaged Malawi to developed nations. At the labor and delivery ward at Lilongwe Central Hospital, she noted, "a single nurse often looks after 50 or more desperately ill people." One nurse found a baby on his mother's breast, desperate to breathe; she reached him in time to suction his tiny mouth until he was able to breathe on his own. But one night, after the dayshift nurse had "steadfastly" tried to keep the premature babies in the nursery alive, "a tiny baby girl, blue and dead, lay next to her sister, eyes open, tiny fists clenched, mouth yawning."[34]

Some reports have focused on the shortage of nursing in schools. In October 2013, *Salon* posted a strong piece by Jeff Bryant questioning US schools' recent tendency to balance security and budget concerns by hiring more guards but continuing to cut nurses and other health workers.[35] He focused on the tragic case of Philadelphia sixth grader Laporshia Massey, who died of an asthma attack when her school had no nurse. Likewise, in February 2004, *Salon* posted a powerful piece by nurse Elisabeth Ochs, who detailed her efforts to care for 800 elementary school students, an increasing number of whom suffered chronic conditions, such as asthma and obesity.[36] In a June 2013 op-ed in the *Seattle Times*, nurse Kathleen Bartholomew argued strongly that Washington schools need more nurses; the state had only one nurse for every 2,031 students. Bartholomew cited the case of a ten year old who had died because no one in her school knew CPR or that her EpiPen was nearby. Bartholomew also described nurses' skills in addressing substance abuse and mental health issues, serious concerns in schools today.[37]

A Nurse Did What? Public Health Nurses in the News

Even apart from shortage pieces, the media sometimes takes an interest in the work of public health nurses outside clinical settings. Perhaps the work of these nurses is striking because many don't expect to see nurses improve outcomes using *real skill by themselves.*

The school-nurse-as-one-time hero article has become its own minor genre. In December 2007 the *Dallas Morning News* ran a piece by Chris Coats about a tenacious school nurse who had pushed through physician skepticism until an eight-year-old student was correctly diagnosed with leukemia in time to benefit from life-saving treatment.[38] In October 2006, the Kansas City ABC television affiliate KMBC reported that a local high school nurse had been "credited with saving a student's life" by diagnosing a brain aneurysm.[39] New York City school nurse Mary Pappas drew media acclaim for setting in motion the April 2009 government response to the H1N1 flu epidemic, identifying and managing hundreds of students' symptoms at her Queens school. But Pappas also gave a "riveting" account of her experiences and plans to contain H1N1 at a federal summit on the issue, as Lauran Neergaard reported in an excellent July 2009 Associated Press item.[40]

Other public health nurses have also gained some attention. In November 2011 the *Harrow Times* (UK) ran Suruchi Sharma's piece about hospital nurses who had organized a "mouth cancer exhibition" to help the local Asian community get "clued up" about the health risks posed by tobacco products.[41] And there have been stories about the Nurse-Family Partnership (NFP), a cost-effective US program in which nurses make home visits to poor first-time mothers and their children. A February 2006 issue of *The New Yorker* included Katherine Boo's lengthy and powerful "Swamp Nurse," which told how, despite huge obstacles, rural Louisiana nurse Luwana Marts and her NFP colleagues question, teach, and cajole their patients toward better lives.[42]

Ninety Pounds and the Truth: Nursing Research and Innovation

Some recent press items have highlighted the work of nurses on the cutting edge. In April 2010 the *Manchester Evening News* (UK) reported that nurses at Stepping Hill Hospital had won a national award from *The Nursing Times* for showing that using a particular skin wash greatly reduced the risk of developing the virulent staphylococcal infection MRSA from hospital devices, such as intravenous catheters.[43] A January 2006 item by Alan McEwen on the *Scotsman* site described a life-saving initiative by Edinburgh nurse Scott McLean to enable paramedics to treat heart attack victims with "clot-busting" thrombolytic drugs.[44]

Nurse researchers occasionally make news. A June 2010 *New York Times* piece by Milt Freudenheim on geriatric care discussed the work of nursing scholars Mary Naylor and Terry Fulmer, who design new systems to provide cost-effective care for the growing elderly population.[45] A March 2009 *BBC News* story by Jane Elliott described the achievements of pioneering 1950s nurse researcher Doreen Norton, who showed how to properly treat deadly bedsores.[46] In March 2006 Geoffrey Cowley's long *Newsweek* piece about UNAIDS director physician Peter Piot briefly told how, two decades earlier, "ebullient, 90-pound" Kenyan nurse Elizabeth Ngugi pioneered programs that empowered poor Nairobi sex workers to adopt safer sex practices. Ngugi's methods prevent thousands of HIV infections each year.[47] A March 2004 *Parade* magazine cover story profiled six "superstars" of health research, including Loretta Sweet Jemmott, a professor at the University of Pennsylvania and "the nation's leading expert on HIV prevention in teens."[48]

Some articles have highlighted the emerging practice at urban trauma centers to have specially trained forensic nurses take the lead in caring for sexual assault victims and gathering evidence for criminal prosecutions. In

October 2006 *Newsweek* posted "'CSI' Nursing," a Web exclusive by Anne Underwood that introduced readers to forensic nursing, including an interview with New Jersey sexual assault forensic examiner nurse Beryl Skog.[49]

"No One Wants to Hear from a Nurse": The Nurse as Media Health Expert

In a November 2006 *ER* episode, nurse character Sam Taggart declined a chance to speak to a local television news crew about the ED's work because "no one wants to hear from a nurse."[50] This attitude is sadly common among real nurses, who often seem determined to keep their heads down. One reporter from the *New York Times* responded to our critique of her physician-centric coverage of the January 2011 shooting of Congresswoman Gabrielle Giffords by lamenting that although the reporter had tried, she could not get the nurses involved to talk to her.[51]

Even so, nurses have on occasion appeared as experts. In the *New York Times*, a lengthy July 2013 "Ask an Expert" piece featured York College nursing professor and advanced practice nurse Julia Bucher, who gave articulate and sensitive advice to those whose relatives have cancer.[52] Surgeon Pauline Chen, who writes the paper's "Doctor and Patient" column, sometimes relies on nurse experts, as she did in a July 2012 column about threats to nurses' physical and mental health.[53] The *Times* has also published oncology nurse Theresa Brown's pieces on health care and nursing, starting in 2008 on the "Well" blog and more recently in Brown's "Bedside" columns.[54]

There are other isolated examples. In January 2014 the CNN website ran an opinion piece by Johns Hopkins nursing professor and ethics expert Cynda Rushton about issues surrounding a pregnant Texas woman who was reportedly brain dead but being kept alive against her family's wishes because she was pregnant.[55] A December 2010 *Ghana News* website item relied entirely on expert comment from senior nurse midwives, who described the importance of prenatal care and the threat of unsafe abortions.[56] In November 2006 the *New Zealand Herald* ran a story by Cherie Taylor that relied mainly on "diabetes nurse and educator" Shona Tolley in discussing efforts to address diabetes among the Maori and other indigenous peoples.[57]

"Is This All Nurses Do?" Media Contempt for Nursing Skill

Direct expressions of contempt for nursing expertise remain common in some of the most popular and influential media products of our time.

Hollywood Tells the World Nursing Is for Losers

Grey's Anatomy and *House* have attacked nursing more aggressively than any US television shows in decades, although the newer sitcom *The Mindy Project* is in the running. *ER* and *Scrubs* were far less likely to disparage nursing skill directly, but they did so, as have many non-healthcare shows.

Grey's Anatomy: **"You're the Pig Who Called Meredith a Nurse"**

Although most clinical scenes in *Grey's Anatomy* have no nurses, the few that do generally present nursing as a matter of fetching physicians, or holding or moving things for physicians, usually at the edge of the frame. So the "nurses" tend to consist of forearms and background blurs. The few nurse characters who do speak tend to be bitter or fawning lackeys.[58]

The show's March 2005 premiere stressed that smart, tough, attractive women like its surgeon stars do *not* become nurses. In one scene, physician intern Alex diagnosed a postoperative patient as having pneumonia. He told the older, far less attractive nurse to start antibiotics. The nurse bleated, "Are you sure that's the right diagnosis?" He responded, "Well, I don't know, I'm only an intern. Here's an idea, why don't you go spend four years in med school and let me know if it's the right diagnosis. She's short of breath, she's got a fever, she's post-op. Start the antibiotics."

Alex then told intern Meredith Grey, "God, I hate nurses." Meredith noted that it might not be pneumonia. Alex: "Like I said, I hate nurses." Meredith: "What did you just say? Did you just call me a nurse?" Alex: "Well, if the white cap fits." Meredith stalked off. Later Alex responded to a page from this same nurse, who argued that the patient was still short of breath. He blew her off: "Don't page me again." The pathetic nurse watched in silence as he left. Later the chief of surgery endorsed Meredith's views. The nurse had sensed vaguely that something was wrong, but it took a real professional—Meredith—to do anything about it.[59]

The show's second episode, in April 2005, offered more explicit contempt. Meredith's friend, hotshot intern Cristina, told Alex, "You're the pig who called Meredith a nurse . . . I hate you on principle."[60]

In an October 2009 episode, the show returned to the same theme. Star neurosurgeon Derek "McDreamy" Shepherd assigned Meredith's younger sister Lexie, an intern, the job of safeguarding McDreamy's own health during an upcoming marathon surgery. A male physician mocked Lexie: "Have fun playing nurse. It sounds . . . neat!"[61]

The female physicians' reactions to these slurs effectively endorse the assumptions that underlie them. Of course, it would not occur to Meredith, Cristina, or Lexie to say anything in defense of nurses. What they care most about is that they not be regarded as nurses themselves.

Grey's has presented nurses as lost in the face of serious care problems and nursing as disgusting work that the interns get as a punishment. In a November 2005 episode, Cristina dismissed a nurse from a patient's room, saying that the physicians would let her know if a bedpan needed changing. Rather than responding directly, the nurse paged Cristina to do a series of grotesque bodily fluid tasks.[62] This plotline suggested that the problem with antinurse slurs is not that they're inaccurate, but just that, as the chief resident noted, it's "stupid" to "piss off the nurses"—the petty, vindictive cleanup crew of health care. A November 2006 plotline likewise used the "nurse's job" of "digging through crap" as a symbol of professional disaster. Cristina's chief resident punished her by making her sift through the stool of a boy who had swallowed Monopoly pieces. Later the boy started vomiting. Nurse Tyler paged Cristina, who quickly diagnosed a perforated bowel and directed the clueless Tyler to page the chief resident.[63] A January 2007 episode portrayed attending physician Mark Sloane inflicting seemingly grotesque, trivial nursing tasks on interns Meredith and Alex as a punishment. As always, there was no hint that the tasks might be important to patient outcomes.[64]

Grey's has made a few efforts to address concerns that it portrays nurses as unskilled drones, but these have been isolated or deeply flawed. A January 2006 *Grey's* episode with a minor plotline about a nursing strike had a few good lines about short-staffing, but on the whole it suggested that the lack of nurses mostly created burdens in administration and trivial bedside care.[65] In the January 2007 *Grey's* in which Sloane inflicted icky nursing tasks on the interns, the attending also vaguely praised nurses as "smart," "helpful," and "already good at their jobs"—which is a lot easier, of course, when there isn't much to your job.[66]

Late 2007 episodes of *Grey's* introduced OR nurse Rose, temporary love interest of McDreamy. Rose was actually capable of light banter *and* basic OR computer repair, an achievement that the show promoted as helping McDreamy "save a life." So if nurses do help save lives, it must be when they happen to have some *other* useful skill besides nursing. The May 2008 season finale had Rose telling Derek she preferred his usual discussion of "boring science stuff" to his brooding about a clinical trial—"science" sounds like a bewildering subject for those little nurses![67] After McDreamy inevitably resumed his relationship with Meredith, a September 2008 episode showed the upset Rose accidentally cut McDreamy's hand with a scalpel, then flee in embarrassment to a job in pediatrics.[68]

Sadly, none of these plotlines showed how nurses improve outcomes as part of their normal work. Perhaps the show came closest in a couple of episodes airing in late 2010 and early 2011 that included hunky "Nurse Eli" (no last name), the boyfriend/sex toy of star surgeon Miranda Bailey. At a few points Eli played a more robust role in care than any other *Grey's* nurse has, advocating somewhat shrilly for patients and even using his "experience" to stumble upon a practice of removing surgical drains at the right time to reduce postoperative infections. But Eli was more of an intuitive traditional healer than a modern science professional, and the show quickly gave the credit for the drain discovery to Bailey.[69] Ultimately she ended the relationship with Eli—nurses are never more than a temporary dalliance—and went back to her physician ex-boyfriend.

The show carried on as before. In the May 2013 season finale, Bailey struggled to regain surgical confidence after a couple patients died, and she tried to make herself useful by taking blood to the OR. The chief of surgery mistook her for a nurse and had to apologize.[70] That's how far she had fallen!

House: "Clean-Up on Aisle Three!"

As on *Grey's*, nurses appeared occasionally on *House* to perform basic tasks, like moving a gurney. But they were even more likely to be silent, peripheral clerks who scurried out of the way of physicians and even patients, to whom they never spoke. Whereas the direct attacks on nursing in *Grey's* have mostly been delivered by junior physicians, on *House* they usually came from the brilliant lead character, who saw nurses as unskilled morons. None of House's slurs were disproved, so viewers were likely to conclude that they were as ruthlessly correct as his other diagnoses.[71]

A notable May 2005 episode told how House lost partial use of his leg to muscle cell death after a clotted aneurysm led to an infarction. At one point House was in his ICU bed recovering from an operation to restore circulation in his leg. The monitor showed wide-complex tachycardia. House impatiently told the nurse to give him more calcium gluconate. The nurse responded that he had just gotten 5 ml. He insisted. The nurse replied: "I'll talk to your doctor." House told her that would take too long, as he had wide-complex tachycardia and would soon go into cardiac arrest. Her response: "I could get in trouble." House, exasperated and about to lose consciousness, informed the nurse that he was not asking for a narcotic. After House passed out, attending physician Lisa Cuddy rushed in, asking the nurse what happened. The nurse said that House had wide-complex tachycardia. "Who diagnosed it?" Cuddy asked. "He did," the nurse responded. The nurse handed Cuddy the defibrillation paddles, which Cuddy used to save House.[72]

In less than one minute of screen time, the episode did an amazing amount of damage. First, any ICU nurse would have immediately seen from the monitor that House had wide-complex tachycardia. Yet House had to insist that he was having that problem, and Cuddy's question as to who diagnosed the tachycardia assumed it could not have been the nurse. A real ICU nurse would have been the one who told House he needed more calcium gluconate, called the code team, defibrillated, and initiated CPR. House's remark about drug seeking wrongly suggested that nurses are unaware that calcium gluconate is not a narcotic. Without knowledge, initiative, or concern for her patient, all the *House* nurse could do was await the arrival of the almighty Cuddy.

The Greg House character also offered insights on nursing. In one priceless November 2005 scene, House temporarily relieved a patient's thymoma symptoms with a Tensilon injection, then went off on a "playing God" riff. When the drug wore off, as expected, the patient fell to the floor. "This," said House, "is exactly why I created nurses." Then he called out into the hallway, "Clean-up on aisle three!"[73]

In a May 2008 episode, after House sustained a head injury, the show had a home health nurse test his pupils with a penlight while he slept. House woke, and the nurse introduced herself as Nurse Dickerson. House: "I don't need your name. And I got your profession from your supercompetent technique of melting my retinas."[74]

In a telling November 2006 episode, physician Foreman prepared to take a sample of spinal fluid from a patient. When the patient's eleven-year-old sister offered to help, Foreman agreed, noting that it's "quicker than calling a nurse." When Foreman instructed the girl to hold her brother's legs still, she asked, "Is this all nurses do?" Foreman responded, with a wry smile, "My boss [House] doesn't trust 'em to do anything else."[75]

Not every nurse character that appeared on *House* was timid or useless, but the show never really strayed from its basic approach to nursing skills. In a February 2011 episode, a critical patient was coughing up a lot of blood. A nurse was trying to catch the blood in a container, but she said nothing to the patient. Fortunately, an all-physician team arrived to save the day. The agitated nurse gave her report: "I don't know what's wrong. He was stable for a while, and then all of a sudden—!"[76]

The Mindy Project: **"Just a Big Loser"**

The Mindy Project, which focuses on a small obstetrics practice in New York City, is a disaster for nursing. Mindy Kaling's lookin'-for-love character and the show's other obstetrics and gynecology (OB/GYN) physicians are quirky and immature, but there is no doubt that they provide skilled health care, while the three minor nurse characters are inept, bizarre, delusional, and possibly dangerous. (We know—it's just a joke!) As with the female surgeons on *Grey's*, it offends Mindy when others mistake her for a nurse, as was evident in an October 2013 episode in which a male physician did just that.[77]

The practice's first nurse was Beverly, a hostile, drug-abusing, possibly psychotic older woman fired in an October 2012 episode. Recruiting a replacement, Mindy and a physician colleague interviewed one nurse who had good academic and work credentials, which Mindy actually pointed out. The nurse reacted by boasting, without irony, that she "should have been a doctor."[78]

The physicians settled on Morgan Tookers, a well-intentioned ex-convict with lots of kooky ideas but little evident health expertise. Morgan has become the show's main nurse character. Morgan specializes in sincere comments that reveal his idiocy, as in the April 2013 episode in which he noted that he would not be "paying $10 to check a $5 coat" and at another point bragged that his laptop was "the biggest laptop you've ever seen."[79] In an October 2013 episode, Morgan unwittingly ate what were obviously drug-filled cupcakes at a music festival.[80] Then he hurt himself by jumping into what he thought was a pool but was actually a lawn. When Morgan later moaned that he was a drug addict, Mindy reassured him that he was "not cool enough" for that, but instead was "just a big loser." In another episode that month, Morgan consoled a heartbroken Mindy by noting that he himself had been dumped by women 36 times.[81] In a November 2013 episode, when one of the physicians could not continue leading a birthing class, Morgan was unable to rescue the class with any actual health knowledge; instead, he claimed to be there to name the patients' babies—he named two "Grover."[82]

Meanwhile, in a February 2013 episode, Mindy's practice rehired Beverly, this time as an office assistant, although she soon proved to be clueless about even the most basic office technology.[83] In March 2013, Mindy found Beverly moonlighting in a restaurant and guiltily promoted her to some kind of executive assistant position, in which Beverly continued to inject occasional bizarre comments.[84] In one April 2013 episode, Mindy considered converting to Christianity for her boyfriend, and Beverly observed: "I've changed my tune for any number of guys. I've been Jewish, super-Jewish, Buddhist, People's Temple, Heaven's Gate, People's Temple again, normal . . . "[85]

During a period in which Morgan had temporarily left the practice, the OB/GYNs hired a third nurse, Tamra, an African-American woman who has at times functioned as a demented insult comic reminiscent of Perry Cox from *Scrubs*, except without Cox's expertise, authority, or fundamental sanity. In a May 2013 episode, Tamra persisted in calling the macho OB/GYN Danny "girl."[86] In a September 2013 episode, after Mindy returned from a mission in Haiti with a shorter haircut, Tamra failed to recognize her: "Unh-uh, I told you, we don't want no candy bars, little boy." Mindy pointed out that she had worked at the practice for years and had actually hired Tamra.[87] Tamra has been plenty capable of foolish behavior. In a January 2014 episode, she mistakenly ordered 1,000 *boxes* of examination gloves (rather than 1,000 gloves) for the small practice.[88]

Other Hollywood Television Shows: "Any Idiot Can Be a Nurse"

Many other shows have also presented nurses as unskilled. Nurses make easy targets for insults and jokes, because writers can count on much of the audience sharing a sense of nursing as trivial work for dimwits and wannabe physicians.

The *Grey's* spinoff *Private Practice*, set mainly at a Los Angeles "wellness clinic" and a nearby hospital, generally followed the *Grey's* model of brilliant physicians and anonymous wallpaper nurses, but with one twist: the first three seasons included cute surfing receptionist Dell Parker, a nurse who was studying to be a midwife. Despite his good intentions, Dell initially seemed to know little more than a layperson, and it was not clear why any nurse would work as a receptionist, making a fraction of the salary. (Maybe this is what "RN" stands for in Hollywood: Receptionist Nurse.) Dell did become a midwife and occasionally displayed some skill, even delivering a few babies, but he also seemed to retain an office administrator role. When the show killed him off in May 2010, it added drama by highlighting his elation at having just been admitted to medical school. Toward the very end of its run, the show also included a few clinical scenes with physician Sam Bennett's girlfriend, the strong, smart labor and delivery nurse Stephanie. But her skills appeared to consist mainly of anticipating physician needs, and in the January 2013 series finale, Sam dumped Stephanie and returned to his physician ex-wife.[89]

ER always had one competent major nurse character, but it also denigrated nursing skill and professional status. In one September 2006 episode, new physician Abby Lockhart was the mother of a premature infant in the NICU. The NICU nurses were utterly incompetent. One, a lactation consultant, was oblivious to Lockhart's distress. The nurse tried to get Lockhart to breastfeed, proclaiming inanely that "breast is best!" and advising that the breast shield goes "between the boob and the tube!" instead of providing any helpful guidance. The other NICU nurse blithely dismissed the concerns of Lockhart's mother about a critical heart monitor alarm. Mom had to virtually yell at the nurse to go get the physicians—the real life savers.[90]

ER also told viewers that nursing was inferior more directly, by having authoritative physician characters make virulent antinurse comments and by suggesting that smart nurses excel by going to medical school. A May 2004 episode did both. In that one, then-nurse Lockhart passed her medical boards, a fitting end to a season in which the show had exhaustively chronicled her medical school experiences. The episode also included a scene in which new nurse character Sam Taggart asked Lockhart if she could cover a nursing shift for Taggart. Attending Kerry Weaver snapped, "Find another nurse. [We] can't have one of our interns changing bedpans during their residency." The nurses had no notable reaction.[91] Abrasive physician characters on such shows often make scathing statements about nursing. When there is no rebuttal, as on *House*, it suggests that the comments are harsh but true.

In fact, data show that nurses are one hundred times more likely to attend graduate school in nursing than in medicine.[92] But *ER* never presented that as an option for its nurse characters until—after we had been making these points to the producers for years—October 2008 episodes indicated that Taggart was starting a nurse anesthetist program. That was a fine idea. But the show still had its characters (particularly nurses) celebrate what it saw as Lockhart's elevation to physician status and, in a May 2008 episode, even celebrate her new attending physician status.[93]

Scrubs also suggested that nursing is low-skilled assistive work. In a notable February 2007 episode, chief of medicine Bob Kelso simply took over as "head nurse" while Carla Espinosa was on maternity leave. Kelso's foray into "nursing" included silly girl talk and trivial scheduling tasks. To mock nurse Kelso, attending Perry Cox ordered Kelso to get him some fresh scrubs from housekeeping.[94] Of course, the idea that Kelso could step directly into any nurse's job is absurd because of nurses' unique knowledge and skills, as explained in Chapters 1 and 4.

In a February 2005 *Scrubs* episode, during a hospital quarantine, Espinosa told her surgeon husband Turk, "We're shorthanded," and asked him to redress a patient's bedsores. Turk said, "That's nurse stuff," and added that he did not "have the expertise." Espinosa responded that "any idiot can be a nurse." Turk: "I know." Espinosa shoved him, saying, "I knew you thought that. I knew it."[95] We see that Espinosa objects to Turk's rudeness, but that does not disprove what he said.

The HBO sitcom *Getting On*, which follows the hapless staff at a geriatric care facility, makes a serious effort to show how challenging that setting is for the nurses and of course for the patients. Nurse Dawn Forchette does know something about health care, at times displaying an understanding of patient conditions; in the first season finale, she had a better sense of when a patient would die than did physician Jenna James. But Dawn also seems to have problems with infection control, and she is such a weak, pitiful character that it's hard to imagine that viewers see her as a serious professional.[96] In another December 2013 episode, when James was berating Dawn for not understanding the importance of the physician's fecal studies, James accused the nurse of never even having heard of the *New England Journal of Medicine*. Dawn's response, a blank stare, seemed to confirm her ignorance.[97] "Nurse" Didi Ortley appears to be a licensed vocational nurse (with one year of training), although she once called herself an "orderly" (six to eight weeks of training).[98] Didi has common sense and a good rapport with patients, but she seems to know very little about health care.

Many other health-oriented shows have suggested that it doesn't take much to be a nurse. In a December 2013 episode of MTV's nurse reality show *Scrubbing In*, one cast member failed to get her dream job at a Beverly Hills plastic surgery practice after showing up at the interview with a resume that misspelled her title as registered "nuse."[99] School nurses are a popular target. In the January 2011 series premiere of *Off the Map*, a hot young US physician who had recently arrived at a remote South American clinic staffed mainly by hot young US physicians complained that a colleague was lucky to have a critical patient to care for, because the first physician just "handed out Band-Aids today . . . like a school nurse!"[100] Nurses have virtually never appeared on USA Network's *Royal Pains* (2009–); when one did briefly in an August 2013 episode, she was a patient's romantic interest named Daisy who was nice but none too skilled.[101] In the June 2009 series premiere of that show, after brilliant physician and lead character Hank Lawson was blackballed by a New York hospital, he lamented, "No institution will touch me. I can't even get a job as a school nurse!"[102]

Popular shows that do not focus on health care are no better. In an October 2009 episode of Fox's *Glee*, character Terri applied for a school nurse job in order to keep an eye on her teacher husband Will, even though her healthcare training consisted of a CPR course. The principal and the ensuing plotline suggested that a school nurse ought to have more training, but Terri still got the job and put the students at risk.[103] *Glee* returned to the same basic theme four years later when an October 2013 episode had a college student named Penny, who had not yet begun nursing school, giving vaccinations and other school nurse care as "an internship." The show made clear that Penny was dangerously incompetent and it implied that a real nurse would be better, but she was still identified as "Nurse Penny" and the effect was again to make a joke of school nursing.[104] A December 2013 episode of the ABC sitcom *Modern Family* revealed that Dylan, the sweet but notoriously clueless sometime boyfriend of main character Haley Dunphy, was attending nursing school.[105] And in a May 2004 episode of ABC's sitcom *8 Simple Rules*, hospital nurse Cate tried to extricate herself from a meeting with a school principal. When she said patients would die if she was not at work, the principal gave her a skeptical look. Cate admitted patients would not die, but said they might wet the bed. The laugh track encouraged viewers to find this remark hilarious.[106]

In Hollywood's view, any type of nursing is worth leaving. NBC's drama *Heroes* featured hospice nurse Peter Petrelli, but the fall 2006 series premiere presented hospice nursing as a dead-end job for dreamy, unduly self-sacrificing losers, stressing the contempt of Peter's successful family, who saw the work as just sitting with the dying. Peter soon dropped nursing.[107] On *The Glades*, hospital nurse Callie occasionally displayed real knowledge, but she was always a part-time medical student, and 2013 episodes stressed how eager she was to continue with medical school, so it was not clear that any of her skill could be attributed to nursing. What seemed to matter to the show was that physicians held her in high esteem.[108]

"More Than a Nurse": How the News Media Disrespects Nurses

Even the most respected news media sources belittle nursing. In October 2006 the *Boston Globe* website posted a poll in its business section after a successful nurses' strike at a local hospital. The item said that the strike was about a plan to reduce what were, according to the hospital, "excessively generous" contracts under which the "average nurse . . . working a 40-hour week makes $107,000 a year." The site then asked if the nurses "deserve this six-figure salary for what they do."[109] We doubt the paper would have questioned a "six-figure salary" for lawyers, advertising executives, or newspaper editors. But for *nurses* to make such a salary evidently suggested to the editors that our society has its priorities wrong, because "what they do" is pretty simple.

In November 2005, National Public Radio's *Morning Edition* ran a report by science correspondent Brenda Wilson about developing world physicians migrating to wealthier nations. At one point Wilson, reporting from a community health center in a Kenyan village, said that "because there are not enough doctors, the center is run by a clinical officer." To explain the expertise of these officers, Wilson said they are "not quite a doctor but more than a nurse."[110]

Also in November 2005, *Good Housekeeping* included seventy-five "surprising" health tips from "doctors" nationwide. One "Dr. X" offered hot ED tips, like telling patients to lie to the triage nurse about when symptoms began—never to say it was more than four hours earlier—in order to be seen faster. However, he advised, "tell the doctor exactly when symptoms began."[111] But in fact, effective triage requires accurate information, which can mean the difference between life and death. And saying that symptoms began more recently will not necessarily indicate greater severity or get you seen faster.

Many people get news from *The Daily Show with Jon Stewart*. In October 2012 the show ran a segment about reintegrating veterans into the civilian workforce that featured two former US military medics, who appeared to have significant experience stabilizing wounded soldiers, following EMT Basic training. To show that the medics' experience was not being adequately recognized, Stewart insisted that they were vastly overqualified to be school nurses. Even though he noted that one school nurse position he had found for the medics required a bachelor of science in nursing, Stewart mocked school nurses as being all about "kickball" and "tummy aches."[112]

News media diversions can also undermine nursing. In February 2007, one *New York Times* Crossword Puzzle included the following as one of its clues: "I.C.U. helpers." The "correct" answer was "RNs."[113] *Helpers*? Nurses let Puzzle Master Will Shortz know this was wrong, but the Puzzle nevertheless returned to the theme in April 2009, seeking "nurse" with the clue "hospital attendant."[114] The references may seem trivial, but when the premier crossword in the world says that the nurses who play the central role in high-tech ICU care are just peripheral bit players, it has a real effect.

A subtle problem is the news media's tendency to suggest that nurses who are not providing direct care at the bedside are not nurses. In other words, nursing is not a science profession that confers enduring status or that one might pursue through health management, research, advocacy, or policy-making. John Colapinto's generally strong December 2010 *New Yorker* profile of Duchenne muscular dystrophy advocate Pat Furlong portrays her as a smart, ruthlessly effective health leader fighting the disease that claimed her sons, but it also calls her a "former nurse."[115] In April 2006 the *Long Beach Press Telegram* ran a piece about Judy Fix, who had saved the life of an injured motorist at the roadside. The headline: "Ex-Nurse Didn't Forget." Fix was referred to as an "administrator" at Memorial Medical Center and a "former nurse."[116] In fact, Judy Fix was the hospital's *chief nursing officer* and senior vice president of patient care services, managing 1,800 RNs. The media would not refer to Memorial's chief of medicine as an "ex-physician." What's the difference? The view that nursing involves simple physical labor and not education, leadership, or professional expertise.

"Don't Forget to Pack a Nurse": Even Good Intentions Can Go Wrong

In recent years many media items have tried to pay tribute to nurses. Unfortunately, even these efforts can suggest that nurses are not so much skilled professionals as they are durable, hardworking, and useful in the way of a handy tool.

In a May 2005 edition of the *Mercury* (South Africa), Xoliswa Zulu's "Have You Thanked a Nurse Today?" marveled at nurses' endurance and ability to tolerate foul-smelling wounds and bedpans. But readers did not get a sense that nurses are educated professionals.[117]

Even efforts to highlight nursing knowledge do not always show much respect for it. A November 2011 segment of *The Dr. Oz Show* called "NURSES' SECRETS That Can Save Your Life,"[118] like the *Reader's Digest* cover story "50 Secrets Nurses Won't Tell You"[119] from that same month, had some good information. But both items were marred somewhat by the condescending focus on "secrets." That approach presented nurses less as college-educated professionals than as a group of employees who had hung around healthcare settings long enough to have picked up basic tips 'n' tricks, some of which might strike people as pretty minor and hardly "life-saving."

The *New York Times* has, in trying to convey the value of nursing, compared nurses to inanimate objects. In a basically helpful November 2002 "Cases" piece in the *Times,* physician Abigail Zuger suggested that an elderly patient of hers who had died might have survived if not for the nursing shortage. The headline was "Prescription, Quite Simply, Was a Nurse."[120] In September 2005 the *Times* ran a piece by Alina Tugend about the trend toward hiring private nurses to compensate for hospital short-staffing. The headline: "Going to the Hospital? Don't Forget to Pack a Nurse."[121]

If It's Important Work, Credit Anyone but a Nurse

In many entertainment and news media products, nursing work is seen to have real value. It saves patients' lives and improves outcomes. That would be great—except that the work is presented as having been done by someone other than a nurse.

Physician Nursing: Prime-Time Physicians Do Nursing Work

Aside from the 2009 nurse shows, every recent US hospital drama has featured rampant physician nursing: the shows' structure makes it inevitable. Virtually every major character is a physician, and the prevailing practice is that the drama must run through these characters. But because the real physician role is actually somewhat limited, physician characters are often shown doing dramatic work in which real-life nurses take the lead. Thus, physician characters handle bedside surveillance and interventions, psychosocial care, patient advocacy and education—and all decision-making.

Grey's Anatomy may have more physician nursing than any other recent Hollywood drama. In the May 2013 season finale, after a big storm knocked out the hospital's power, guess who gave all the skilled care to twelve critically ill infants in the NICU? Supposedly, just two nurses managed to make it to the hospital in the storm—evidently the six NICU nurses who would have been on duty at the time of the storm just abandoned their tiny patients—so the surgeon characters and the worried parents ventilated and otherwise cared for the babies. The impression was that physicians provide all meaningful NICU care, disinformation that was especially ironic because the episode seemed to be based in part on the heroic real-life evacuation of New York University hospital's NICU during Hurricane Sandy—which was conducted, of course, by the nurses who actually play the primary role in NICU care.[122]

Physician nursing was also abundant in several November 2010 episodes of *Grey's*.[123] One actually included a limited portrayal of a nurse as a strong, knowledgeable advocate—for her own critically ill son. But residents Meredith Grey and Alex Karev seemed to be the only hospital workers who gave any significant physical or psychosocial care to the boy. *No practicing nurse appeared.* The plotline was a good example of the show's occasional practice, seen a couple of times on *House* as well, to have nurses briefly display health knowledge when appearing as patients or family members in isolated episodes, perhaps as a token effort to mollify critics without upsetting the natural all-physician order. In another *Grey's* episode that same month, senior surgeon Miranda Bailey ordered resident Jackson Avery to closely monitor a postoperative patient with a pancreatic fistula. Avery complained that Bailey had him "watching a post-op for fluid into a bag every two minutes." In real life, nurses monitor patients for fluid loss and other subtle signs of decline, and they initiate rescue measures if needed.

In one May 2008 episode, cardiac surgeon Erica Hahn provided emotional care to a distraught transplant candidate in isolation. Alex Karev gave the patient intravenous medication. When the patient's lung collapsed, Alex alone intervened to save her, issuing a command to the ether to get Hahn. A nurse-blur responded, "Right away, Dr. Karev!"[124] Meredith Grey provided all psychosocial care to a soldier with a brain tumor. She managed the tension between this soldier's father and his male lover. After the surgery, Meredith monitored the patient's intracranial pressure. Later the patient coded, and a nurse handed Meredith the paddles so she could defibrillate. Alex even got the transplant patient's family into protective gear so they could enter the isolation bubble with her. In real life, every one of these actions would be performed primarily or completely by a nurse. Finally, resident Cristina Yang gave a bitter speech about another surgeon's winning a medical award without crediting her help. She complained that she was "the unseen hand to his brilliance," an astonishing echo of the episode's own crediting of physicians for work nurses really do.

In a December 2005 *Grey's* episode, hours after a quintuplet birth, each of the five major intern characters sat in the NICU keeping watch over his or her own quint, with no nurses in sight. The physician characters also provided cobedding for the quints and emotional support for the quints' distressed mother. Another subplot involved a patient Alex "killed" when he "told a nurse" to administer an incorrect dosage of hypertonic saline, thus dehydrating the patient's brain.[125] No one suggested that the nurse had a duty to scrutinize prescriptions to prevent dangerous errors, which Alex's prescription clearly was.

House also generally had physicians do everything important in the hospital. In fact, like the *Grey's* surgeons, House's team did the meaningful work of many other types of health workers—not just nurses—including the work of physicians with other specialties.[126]

In the May 2008 *House* season finale, when a patient had multiple organ failure, House's team of diagnosticians did a typical range of critical nursing tasks. They infused solutions and intravenous medications. They set up and maintained a cardiac bypass without nurses. They did ambu-bagging, which nurses, respiratory therapists, or anesthesia professionals usually do. They provided all monitoring and psychosocial care. They performed nurse-free surgeries. They induced hypothermia with cooling blankets. They alone performed resuscitation and effected an interhospital transfer of the critical patient. All of these actions are unthinkable without nursing involvement.[127]

In a May 2006 *House* episode, the physicians did virtually all monitoring, psychosocial care, and therapeutic care. The most amusing part was a nurse-free scene in which physician Robert Chase walked a patient with major facial swelling around after his surgery and even took him to the toilet! Perhaps a physician has done this, but we've never heard of it.[128]

TNT's *Monday Mornings*, which only lasted one season in early 2013, is a good example of the many television dramas that come and go quickly but still leave millions of viewers with the idea that physicians provide all the hospital care that matters. The show, based on a novel by CNN medical reporter and physician Sanjay Gupta, focused on the tense morbidity and mortality conferences held at a Portland, Oregon hospital. All major characters were physicians. Nurse characters were rarely seen, much less heard, and health care seemed to consist of smart physicians interacting with patients, families, and each other. Junior physicians, not nurses, advocated for patients and woke attendings in the middle of the night. In the April 2013 finale, a man waiting in the ED stopped a nearby surgeon, complaining that he'd been waiting more than two hours. The surgeon, acting as triage nurse, assured the man that they'd be with him as soon as they could![129]

On *ER,* where nurse characters had far more realistic roles than their counterparts on most other dramas, there was still plenty of physician nursing, and wallpaper nurses often watched physicians do work that nurses really do. In a May 2007 episode, nurse Sam Taggart generally came off as a tough, skilled patient advocate, but the care of a physicist with septic shock featured relentless physician nursing. In the ED, Taggart called for the hospital's rapid response team to help this unstable patient. The team was composed solely of physicians and medical students. In fact, rapid response teams generally consist mainly of nurses and respiratory therapists.[130] An anonymous nurse helped OR resident Neela Rasgotra push the physicist's gurney from the surgical ward to the ICU. But the nurse did not seem to be managing the patient's second-to-second care, as real nurses do during these trips. When ICU attending Kevin Moretti approached, the nurse departed without a word. The patient crashed, and while Moretti, Rasgotra, and a medical student resuscitated her, a bit of a nurse did appear at the edge of the frame a couple of times. The episode also included an intern taking a patient to CT scan alone, a serious ambulance admit with no nurse involvement, and physician medication administration.[131]

Physician nursing infects nonhospital shows as well. Episodes of NBC's *Law and Order: Special Victims Unit* broadcast in November 2004 and September 2010 featured a special spin on physician nursing. In these episodes, commendably, a sexual assault forensic examiner nurse actually cared for a rape victim. Those specially trained nurses, not physicians, do typically take the lead in providing critical care and forensic work for sexual assault victims at major trauma centers. Sadly, the 2004 episode depicted one of the show's two main *detective* characters directing and doing the key work. In real life, the police probably would not even have been present. But here, the nurse character came off as an awkward and insensitive assistant, as the detective explained what was going on, took photographs, and provided the only real emotional support the patient received.[132] In the 2010 episode, the nurse seemed more autonomous, but she was a callous evidence collector who *did not say a word* to the distraught rape victim, even when she caused the victim pain. The detective provided all psychosocial care.[133]

Physician Nursing: The News Media Knows Who Saves Lives

Physicians Get the Credit

Many news accounts, particularly those written by physicians, assign credit for nursing work to physicians. In May 2007 the *New York Times* ran a long piece by reporter Lawrence K. Altman, MD, about New Jersey Governor Jon Corzine's recovery from a serious automobile crash: "In Corzine's Recovery, Doctors Cite Grit and Luck." Corzine spent eighteen days in Cooper University Hospital, eleven of those in the ICU—where elite nurses take the lead 24/7, running high-tech machinery, managing a complex regimen of treatments, and monitoring patients for the slightest changes in condition. Yet in the midst of many statements about what physicians thought and did, the only specific credit any nurse got in this article was for lip-reading Corzine's requests for medication and water while he was on the ventilator. The article noted, "At Cooper, doctors typically take turns caring for trauma patients every day."[134] The writer must have meant that different physicians are assigned to such patients on different days, but for most readers, this statement would likely confirm the prevailing misconception: physicians do all the important "caring" at the bedside for critical patients like Corzine.

Later that same month, the US Department of Transportation sponsored a public service announcement featuring Governor Corzine urging television viewers to use seat belts. Corzine credited "a remarkable team of doctors and a series of miracles" with saving his life. The public service announcement was a good public health effort, but it ignored the nurses and other "team" members who likely provided most of the skilled care that saved his life.[135] Of course, the public service announcement creators are not alone in their limited view of what saves lives. The title of physician Sanjay Gupta's 2009 book is *Cheating Death: The Doctors and Medical Miracles That Are Saving Lives Against All Odds*.

In October 2004 a long, unsigned article in the *Wall Street Journal* on allowing family presence during major hospital procedures recognized that nurses had been most active on that issue and even featured quotes from nursing experts. Unfortunately, even that article repeatedly suggested that physicians perform major procedures alone, so the nurses are largely observers who have time to worry about how the family may react. The piece referred to steps to alleviate "one of medicine's most trying ordeals: That wait in the hall while doctors are working on a loved one." Later, the report noted that a Boston hospital had begun allowing family members to stay during codes when "doctors may need to shock the patient or open up the chest to massage the heart." And one of the reported benefits of family presence? "Families can give on-the-spot medical information to trauma doctors."[136]

A March 2012 piece in *Haaretz* (Tel Aviv, Israel) included a special spin on physician nursing: reporting that does not tell readers which type of health professional is responsible for important healthcare work, but that is likely to leave the impression that it's a physician or other nonnurse. In this piece, Dan Even reported that a new study by scholar Sigal Shafran-Tikva examined the factors that can lead to violence by Israeli hospital patients. Unfortunately, the report failed to mention that Shafran-Tikva is a nurse, leaving readers to guess her profession based on their understanding of health care.[137] Perhaps those publicizing the study themselves downplayed the nursing element so the research would be taken more seriously, but the net effect was to bury nursing expertise.

Physicians Get the Blame

The media commonly assigns all blame for clinical healthcare problems to physicians. It would be natural for nurses not to object. But they should, because this practice signals that the media regards physicians as the ones who provide all important care and decision-making. Being seen as an integral part of the healthcare picture means receiving credit when things go well and being held responsible when things do not.

A September 2008 *New York Times* article by Laurie Tarkan discussed emergency patients' poor understanding of their care. Patient education is a key nursing responsibility, and nurses generally spend far more time on it than physicians do, if staffing allows. But this piece gave no hint of that fact, instead relying on multiple statements from five named physicians. Not one nurse was consulted, although nurses did get a mention—in discussion of a "dual discharge" approach in which a physician discusses care with patients and a nurse "follows up with computerized discharge instructions."[138]

In June 2004 the *New York Times* published a column by Bob Herbert about malpractice claims against an OB/GYN physician. The piece suggested that a critical problem for one baby born with severe brain damage was improper checking of a fetal monitoring strip while the physician was absent. Herbert stated, with unmistakable contempt, that the physician "blamed the ensuing tragedy on the nurse."[139] In fact, the apparent monitoring and assessment error described *would* generally be a nurse's job.

In December 2005 the *Baltimore Sun* ran Fred Schulte's massive series "Masking Malpractice Cases." The gist was that Maryland's system for overseeing physician practice was failing to protect patients. The article focused on the small number of physicians who have had unusually high numbers of malpractice claims or payments. Readers would plainly see the *Sun's* report as addressing the full universe of healthcare errors. Yet there are four times as many registered nurses as physicians,[140] and although nurses are not seen as the litigation targets physicians are, there is no reason to think nurse errors are any less numerous or consequential. Healthcare errors are the third leading cause of death in the United States,[141] and nurses are deeply involved in the care in which such errors occur. In fact, research shows that nurses prevent the majority of potential hospital errors.[142] But in this entire *Sun* report, whose text exceeded 9,500 words, neither the word "nurse" nor the word "nursing" appeared even once.[143]

A couple of thoughtful reports on hospital errors in early 2010 did use fatal nursing mistakes as examples, although the pieces still consulted physicians to a greater extent than nurses, and so they were likely to leave the impression that physicians had more responsibility. Liz Kowalczyk's February *Boston Globe* report described events surrounding the tragic death of a Massachusetts General Hospital patient whose heart monitor alarm had been left off. The reporter included a few helpful quotes from the hospital's chief nurse, but none from national nurse experts or direct care nurses who deal with those monitors constantly. Instead, the piece relied on physician safety experts and engineers involved in improving the safety of such technologies.[144] Laura Landro's piece in a March edition of the *Wall Street Journal* discussed efforts to treat the health workers involved in errors fairly, focusing on the well-known case of Wisconsin nurse Julie Thao, who mistakenly gave a pregnant patient a fatal dose of a painkiller. The piece included a little indirect commentary from Thao, but all the expert quotes were from physicians and non-nurse safety experts, rather than the nurses who have more direct knowledge of medication errors.[145] Perhaps as a result of inadequate input from nurses, neither piece mentioned the extent to which nurse-related errors are due to inadequate staffing or nurses' relatively low level of power, which discourages nurses from speaking up about problems.

Nursing Just Happens

Many press pieces effectively suggest that important nursing care has been done by hospitals or machines, or else that it has simply occurred, with no actor named. A December 2012 Associated Press report did not just say that "doctors" were assessing the condition of then-Secretary of State Hillary Clinton following her hospitalization for a blood clot. Rather, the piece also passively stated that Clinton was "under observation" and "was being treated with anti-coagulants."[146] In fact, nurses take the lead in "observing" patients, and nurses give medications and carefully monitor their effects.

An October 2011 issue of *The New Yorker* included a piece by Ken Auletta about Jill Abramson's ascendancy to the editorship of the *New York Times*. Auletta described injuries Abramson suffered after a truck knocked her down and rolled over her, breaking bones and causing "extensive internal injuries." Physicians were the only health workers mentioned; supposedly, "surgeons administered blood transfusions," although of course nurses would have done that, and later surgeons "told [Abramson] that she needed to spend six weeks in bed." But Auletta also said that "an ambulance rushed" Abramson to Bellevue Hospital's trauma center, and "many months of painkillers, excruciating rehab, and physical therapy followed, as she progressed from wheelchair to crutches to cane."[147] Note the lack of nurses, first responders, and physical therapists. The ambulance must have driven itself and taken care of Abramson on the way! No one conducted the physical therapy; it just "followed." And Abramson apparently had only painkillers for professional company during her weeks in bed. But in reality, nurses provide hundreds of hours of skilled, life-saving care to patients with severe injuries like these.

In February 2006 National Public Radio's *Morning Edition* ran a report by Richard Knox about the lack of intensive care resources that would be needed to handle a bird flu pandemic: US hospitals would not have enough ventilators or "hospital beds."[148] The report wrongly implied that care for patients would revolve mainly around whether physicians granted access to the ventilators or beds, and it quoted only physicians—as if either the physicians provide all the associated care, or the ventilators and hospital beds do it themselves. In fact, nurses and respiratory therapists carefully monitor patients' tolerance to ventilators, wean them off the machines, and teach them how to breathe afterward. Without nurses, ventilators and beds save no one.

Innovation: Which Nonnurse Thought of That?

Some recent reports discuss the work nurses do on innovative health projects, often outside the usual clinical settings. But even these pieces may present the nurses as carrying out work engineered by others. Of course, it may be that a specific project *was* designed by someone else. But nurses are not empty vessels into which others have poured expertise. Nurses have long been expert in community health and holistic preventative care, as explained in Chapter 1. It often seems that the nursing care model gains attention only when it is embraced by physicians or others with more social status.

Consider recent reports on the work of the Nurse-Family Partnership (NFP) to improve the health of poor mothers and children, such as an August 2007 *CBS Evening News* report by Katie Couric.[149] We have seen no major mainstream article that cites the NFP program's debt to the long tradition of home-based nursing care, so the whole idea that "nurse-visitors" can improve maternal–child health may seem to have originated with NFP founder David Olds, a developmental psychologist. The pieces have also failed to convey how much of the nurses' success is due to their nursing skill, not just to Olds's program design or the nurses' personal attributes, trusted image, or on-the-job experience.

In October 2006 an Associated Press piece by Alicia Chang reported that insurers increasingly rely on "health coaches" to help patients manage chronic conditions at home, thereby cutting costs and improving outcomes.[150] The report barely managed to note that most of the coaches are nurses, so it failed to discuss why nurses are uniquely qualified to play such roles. Instead, it credited a Colorado physician for the specific care "model" it discussed, which may imply that this kind of work is a recent physician innovation.

Ghosts in the Machine: Nurses Go Missing in the Media

The media often simply ignores nursing, even when reporting on skilled work in which nurses play a central role, such as hospital care or foreign aid work. Nurses are not generally recognized as career health care "heroes," and they are rarely consulted as health experts.

Lost in Hollywood

Popular Hollywood products often ignore the role nursing would really play in their area of interest. For example, *Grey's Anatomy* includes many clinical scenes in which no nurses appear, even though the patients are in critical condition and would require a great deal of skilled nursing.[151]

Ignoring nursing also results in a failure to portray recent nurse-led advances in care that television producers would almost certainly take great interest in if the developments had originated with physicians. For instance, in hospital dramas, family members are forever freaking out to see their loved ones in distress, then causing disruption. Physician characters often command nurses to remove the family. We have never seen a nurse character advocate for family to stay, or discuss the trend toward allowing family presence, which nursing research has shown to have real benefits.[152] Likewise, although recent episodes of *Grey's* and other shows have focused on NICUs, they have largely failed to reflect recent nurse-led developments in kangaroo care (keeping the infant at its mom's or dad's chest for certain periods), cobedding for multiples, or breastfeeding. A November 2009 *Grey's* episode did finally portray kangaroo care, but no nurses were involved; surgeon Miranda Bailey initiated the care, and it was actually provided by junior physician Alex Karev.[153]

Most documentaries, reality shows, and daytime shows about health care have taken a similar physician-centric approach. Since 2008, the popular daily syndicated daytime talk show *The Doctors* has generally lived up to its name. Airing in nations around the world, this *Dr. Phil* spin-off features a "dream team" of four physicians dispensing advice and opinions on topics ranging from cosmetic plastic surgery to various practical health issues, including many in which the physician hosts seem to have little expertise, such as home birth and midwifery. Although nurses are expert in patient education, they have so far had no significant role on *The Doctors*.[154]

Terence Wrong's multipart *ABC News* documentaries *Hopkins 24/7* (2000),[155] *Hopkins* (2008),[156] *Boston Med* (2010),[157] and *NY Med* (2012 and 2014)[158] have been mainly about glorifying surgeons. The *Hopkins* documentaries ignored nursing almost completely, and although the more recent series did occasionally feature emergency nurses, those segments were really just diversions. For the most part, the focus was not on the nurses' skill but on their personal lives and the difficult behavior of the patients they confront.

The 2008 documentary feature *Living in Emergency: Stories of Doctors Without Borders* profiled four developed world physicians who worked on Médecins Sans Frontières/Doctors Without Borders aid missions in war-torn Congo and Liberia. The film offered some valuable insights on foreign aid work, but it ignored Médecins Sans Frontières' nurses and logistics officers, all of whom play key roles in the Nobel Prize–winning group's work. Indeed, nurses are the most numerous Médecins Sans Frontières health professionals,[159] but this film was almost entirely about physicians, who did virtually all of the talking and acting.[160] In the end, the film's distorted treatment of emergency aid mirrored that of Médecins Sans Frontières' name.

Lost in the News

News items often ignore nurses or nursing, even when covering areas in which nurses play key roles. An October 2011 issue of *The New Yorker* included "A Child in Time: New Frontiers in Treating Premature Babies," by Harvard physician Jerome Groopman. In this "medical dispatch," physician work was dominant and only physicians were consulted as NICU experts (along with one social worker, briefly). *No nurses were even named.*[161] Granted, one key focus was physician research, but nurses also perform key research on the care of premature babies and they spend much more time providing skilled care to those babies than does anyone else. NICU nurses did appear here and there in Groopman's account, but he described them doing assistive things that lay people could also do: swaddling babies, sitting with families, handing things to people, and placing candles.

In a June 2004 "Cases" item in the *New York Times*, Richard A. Friedman, MD, discussed whether July is a perilous time to visit US hospitals because of the influx of recent medical school graduates with little experience. Friedman admitted that it was rational to be concerned about "July syndrome" but argued that there is little basis to think care suffers, because of "vigilant supervision" by attending physicians. In fact, a great deal of the "vigilance" is supplied by nurses, who also play a key role in teaching the interns how to practice safely. But the word *nurse* did not appear in this piece.[162]

When nurses spearhead groundbreaking research or policy proposals, they are often ignored by elite media sources. In September 2009, John Hopkins University issued a press release about the pain management research of its nursing scholars Gayle Page and Sharon Kozachik. United Press International ran a short item in response, noting that the nurses have "determined through research that pain management is not only a matter of compassion, but a medical necessity for patients to heal."[163] It was a rare example of press coverage of nursing research. Indeed, although the United Press International item was noted on a few health-oriented websites, we saw no other mainstream press coverage.

In October 2004 the Columbia University School of Nursing issued a press release about its striking plan, published in *Nursing Economics*, to provide universal health coverage in the United States at an annual cost of about $2,000 per person. Despite the obvious link to the impending general election, more than a week later the only major press coverage appeared to be a short item by Laura Gilchrest on the *CBS Marketwatch* website.[164] It is hard to avoid the conclusion that the Columbia plan was ignored because of the professional status of those who created and published the plan.

Nurses Evacuated from Disaster Areas

It's remarkable how invisible nursing often is in news accounts about responses to mass casualty events, considering the central role nurses actually play.

One notable exception was Elizabeth Cohen's short April 2013 piece on the CNN website about the experience of nurses Stephen Segatore and Jim Asaiante, who provided emergency care on-site after the Boston Marathon bombing. Although there were few specifics on the nurses' skills beyond tourniquets and intravenous lines, the piece did quote them and make clear that their trauma experience had been critical to their work as members of a *team* of event health workers who saved lives that day.[165] Of course, other CNN reports, like a July 2013 follow-up piece about a victim who lost her leg, focused only on physicians as experts and care providers.[166]

An extensive April 2013 *New York Times* report on the bombing response was a tour de force of elite news physician-centrism. "Doctors Saved Lives, If Not Legs, in Boston," by Gina Kolata, Jeré Longman, and Mary Pilon, focused on the care given on-site and initially at local hospitals. In a 1,500-word piece that aimed to describe the full range of care given that day, the word "nurses" appeared twice; once, notably, in the statement that "at least eight doctors and what seemed to be 20 or more nurses were stationed in the tent." Yet despite all those nurses, the piece did not name or quote any. Instead, it quoted six physicians and a chaplain (briefly), repeatedly telling readers what "doctors" alone did and said, as if only that mattered. The reporters were not short on space; at one point, they noted that a surgeon was so tired he took a nap. This same surgeon woke up to explain that "surgeons were notified, emergency-room physicians were notified, operating-room personnel were notified, everyone was notified."[167] Yeah, guess that about covers it, dude.

In early 2007 NPR's *Morning Edition* aired interviews with disaster health experts. In February it ran an interview with a former US Coast Guard officer, who said at one point that a community had to ask whether it could handle hundreds of thousands of casualties, "all requiring triage and other kinds of life-and-death care." Show host Steve Inskeep asked if that meant asking whether such a place had "hundreds of vacant beds . . . hundreds of idle doctors?" In a March interview, when the chief of medical affairs at a New Orleans hospital noted that a lack of "health care providers" was hampering efforts to restore area hospitals to full capacity after Hurricane Katrina, Inskeep wondered whether even hospitals that had remained open "don't have enough doctors available." In fact, most of the critical care in such emergencies, such as triage, is provided by nurses. At least the guest experts in both stories sooner or later worked nurses into the conversation.[168]

In September 2005 many outlets ran an Associated Press piece by Marilynn Marchione about hospital care immediately after Katrina. The *Yahoo!* headline was typical: "Doctors Emerging as Heroes of Katrina." The Associated Press report portrayed physicians as having done virtually everything of note for patients at New Orleans hospitals after the storm. Apart from a passing reference to RNs and EMTs, and one sentence about a Pennsylvania paramedic, the piece was all physicians all the time, with many references to what "doctors" did, as well as multiple quotes and descriptions of no fewer than eight named physicians and a medical student. Not one nurse was mentioned, although nurses played a central role in keeping patients alive under the extreme conditions during and after Katrina.[169]

Can We Be "Heroes"?

The media often salutes the careers of healthcare "heroes." Nurses are rarely recognized in that way, consistent with the view that life-saving is not a regular feature of nursing, although nurses may be honored for saving lives outside of their usual practice settings.

In November 2005, *Time* magazine published a massive report on global health. Slightly more than half of the total report was devoted to profiles of eighteen "heroes" whose "energy and passion are making a difference" in the fight against disease worldwide. Of the fifteen healthcare professionals profiled, twelve were physicians. Not one "hero" was recognized for her nursing, although a profile of a nutritionist noted that she had a nursing degree. Only one brief mention in the whole report could be considered a tribute to the work of the world's estimated 16 million nurses to stem disease. That was in the concluding essay by rock star Bono.[170]

In July 2004 Discovery Health Channel aired the *Discovery Health Channel Medical Honors*. The star-studded special saluted thirteen "medical heroes" for "bringing awareness to many challenging health and medical issues of our time." The thirteen honorees consisted of eight physicians, a biosciences researcher, a nonprofit leader, a political science professor, a health system CEO, and an advertising executive. No nurses made the cut, but nurses were represented—by actress Yvette Freeman, who played nurse Haleh Adams on *ER* and who appeared at the ceremony as a presenter.[171] You go, nurses!

When nurses do appear as "heroes," it's often because they have surprised people by saving lives in unexpected ways. In November 2012, the ABC current affairs show *20/20* included a segment about the New York University NICU nurses who transported their fragile patients to safety after power failed at their flooded hospital during Hurricane Sandy. The segment, part of a feature about dramatic rescues during the storm entitled "The Heroes Among Us," did include references to the nurses' knowledge and skill, although the nurses were generally treated more like bystanders who stepped up in a tragedy rather than highly trained health professionals.[172]

It also seems to be amazing when nurses save lives by themselves on plane flights. In January 2014 the Southern California NBC affiliate Channel 4 reported that nurses Linda Alweiss and Amy Sorenson had recently provided "cardiac life support" to a pilot having a serious heart attack on a cross-country flight.[173] Similarly, Nicole Brodeur's helpful May 2005 *Seattle Times* column told how ED nurse Joanne Endres saved a man having a heart attack on a plane flight. The theme of that column, "Flying Solo, Nurse Is Enough," was that the public does not understand what nurses do. Brodeur proved it by quoting a passenger who said of Endres, "She just knew what to do. . . . And there wasn't even a doctor there!"[174]

Nurses? Healthcare Experts?

The media regularly fails to consult nurses in healthcare items, even on topics about which nurses are expert. A January 2009 article by Gina Kolata in the *New York Times* described a supposedly radical physician innovation: getting ICU patients up and walking around as a way to improve recovery. The piece featured extensive commentary by five physicians. Kolata noted in passing that this new "tactic" required the help of nurses and therapists. In fact, nurses have been walking patients around to improve recovery in ICUs for decades without the need of any physician request. But the *Times* piece failed to quote a single nurse.[175]

In May 2006 a huge *Time* cover story by Nancy Gibbs and Amanda Bower stressed that not even health workers are safe from the health threats posed by . . . hospitals. The story, "Q: What Scares Doctors? A: Being the Patient," presented an all-physician vision of hospital care, based on expert comment by twelve physicians. It excluded nurses. At one point, the writers wondered who the "sentinels" and "advocates" in hospitals would be now that family physicians have supposedly been excluded from the role. Hint: that's what the nurses who make up the majority of professional hospital staff do, or *would* do if they had the staffing and other resources.[176]

In 2007, Google formed a Health Advisory Council, a group of eminent health "experts" that would help the dominant media company consider how to "contribute to the health care industry." The council of more than twenty prominent health figures included thirteen physicians and many members without any formal health care training. No nurses.[177]

Can Any Helpful Person or Thing Be a Nurse?

The media uses the term *nurse* broadly. It often refers to female caregivers as "nurses" no matter how little health training they have. For example, the Hollywood films *The Skeleton Key*[178] (2005) and *The Grudge*[179] (2004) were widely promoted as having "nurse" characters, but the characters were actually nonnurse caregivers. A nursing assistant who played a key role in the powerful 2012 documentary *The Waiting Room* was described as a "nurse" not only by some reviewers, but also by the film's *director* Peter Nicks in an interview.[180]

Of course, the verb form of *nurse* has long been used to describe unskilled tending, especially by females. And as we explained in Chapter 1, the term *nurse* can accurately be applied to professionals with a range of educational backgrounds.

Even so, the media has some obligation to consider the effects of its use of the term. It might start by making sure that those it calls "nurses" actually *are* nurses. Let's try the nouns first, and maybe we can work our way up to the verbs!

I, Robot, Will Be Your Nurse

Sometimes the media refers to new healthcare technology as a "nurse," as in "robot nurse" and "electronic nurse." In some cases, developers or marketers themselves call their products "nurse." These products may assist with nursing tasks, but equating machines with college-educated health professionals is unhelpful.

The press often suggests that "robot nurses" may be critical to the future of health care. A March 2011 Associated Press item reported that Purdue University researchers were developing a "robotic scrub nurse" that could *recognize five hand gestures*![181] In March 2009 Agence France-Presse reported that Japan hoped that "robo-nurses" would soon play a key role in caring for its aging population.[182] In January 2007 the *Scotsman* ran Angus Howarth's "Robot Nurses Could Be on the Wards in Three Years, Say Scientists." The piece reported on a project by European Union–funded scientists to develop machines to "perform basic tasks" at hospitals. These include cleaning up spills, guiding visitors around, and perhaps distributing medicines and taking temperatures. The article proposed other imaginative names for the machines, such as "nursebots" and "mechanised 'angels.'"[183]

Other assistive health technology may also receive the title "nurse." Tim Bajarin's March 2009 column "Meet Nurse iPhone" in *PC Magazine* extolled the virtues of new applications that turn Apple's popular phone into a "surprisingly competent medical assistant," enabling timely transmission of health information.[184] Similarly, in March 2006 the website of Wis10 (the Columbia, SC, NBC affiliate) posted an item by Chantelle Janelle, "Health Alert: Electronic Nurse." It described a $70 machine used to help real nurses do home health monitoring by asking patients basic questions.[185]

You Just Haven't Earned It Yet, Baby Nurse

Many in-home newborn nannies market themselves as "baby nurses," regardless of whether they have any health training. The media has repeated the term, even shortening it to "nurse." This practice continues even though some jurisdictions have made "nurse" a restricted title, in order to protect the public from unlicensed practitioners.

In an April 2010 episode of the CBS sitcom *Accidentally on Purpose*, the pregnant main character Billie hired an attractive "baby nurse" named Nicole. Characters twice referred to Nicole simply as a "nurse," and at one point we heard that she had a "nursing degree from Cal." But few if any "baby nurses" are registered nurses, and there was no suggestion that Billie's baby would need the advanced skills a real neonatal nurse would provide. At first Nicole did seem professional, but she turned out to be a manipulative nymphomaniac, seducing two friends of the baby's father for a three some practically on sight. So, she was less a real nurse than a real naughty nurse.[186]

In February 2007 Vickie Elmer's item in the "Jobs" section of the *Washington Post* repeatedly referred to the infant caregiver it profiled as a "baby nurse," even though the provider had virtually no health care training. In response to criticism, the *Post* pointed out that there is a historic association between infant caregiving and the word "nurse," as in "nursemaid."[187]

But to use "nurse" this way today sends a dangerous message about professional nursing. Indeed, in August 2005 the *New York Daily News* ran a piece about the lack of regulation and awareness of the minimal training "baby nurses" have, focusing on the case of Noella Allick, who reportedly "confessed to violently shaking and seriously injuring two babies in her care." The article rightly suggested that a key problem is that anyone can call herself a "nurse."[188] New York State later made "nurse" a protected title.[189] But the term "baby nurse" remains common.

I Say You're a Nurse, and the Shortage Is Over

In clinical settings, many people—including some physicians—refer to any female who is not a physician as a "nurse." Such "nurses" may include technicians, medical assistants, nurses' aides, and clerks. Hospitals may see no reason to clarify matters, because most have placed unlicensed assistive personnel into nursing roles to save money. But when a patient asks an apparent "nurse" with only a few weeks' training to explain his condition, and the "nurse" cannot do so, the patient may conclude that nurses as a group are not highly skilled.

The media reflects and reinforces this tendency to equate "nurse" with "female health worker." For instance, in a 2005 episode of the popular *Dr. Phil* television show, the host—a psychologist—repeatedly referred to a nurse's aide as a "nurse."[190] In a January 2006 CVS drugstore company television advertisement, a pharmacist explained that he had spent several hours teaching a patient's husband to administer her twenty different medications. The pharmacist twice said that the husband was now "a nurse."[191] Modern drug regimens are complex, and the health financing system has left many families with the impossible task of trying to nurse themselves. But this advertisement wrongly suggested that pharmacists could train nurses and that training a nurse might take only a few hours.

Or none. In November 2011 posters appeared in the Washington, DC Metro system as part of an extensive "Care Not Cuts" campaign, a lobbying effort by the US long-term care industry to prevent federal reimbursement cutbacks. One advertisement featured text reading: "Today, you're an accountant. Tomorrow, you're dad's nurse."[192] An August 2009 article in the *Philippine Daily Inquirer*, headlined "Daughter Kris Was Aquino's Nurse," suggested that one of the daughters of former President Corazon Aquino had cared for her dying mother so faithfully that one friend said she had "attended to her mother's bedside needs like a professional nurse." But there was no indication that Kris, a television host, had any actual health care training.[193]

This sense that anyone can be a nurse goes hand in hand with ideas to resolve the shortage by recruiting those with few other options. In March 2006 the news magazine *Der Spiegel* ran a piece by Guido Kleinhubbert about a new German government program to train prostitutes to become "care workers for the elderly," including "nurses."[194] It is possible they were to be nurse's aides. But policymakers and press pieces have also suggested that solutions to the developed world's nursing shortage lie in recruiting those on public assistance,[195] desperate nurses from poor nations,[196] or foreign physicians who can't pass their physician licensing examinations.[197] Excellent nurses may come from any of these categories, but the sense we get from many of these press stories is that these ideas make sense because being a "nurse" requires little critical thinking or knowledge.

Media creators have also presented plans to address the shortage or achieve other policy goals by "streamlining" educational requirements to get more nurses into practice faster. For example, in an October 2012 presidential debate, President Obama stated that former military medics who wanted to become nurses had to "start from scratch," so we should "change those certifications."[198] Of course veterans and others should receive appropriate credit for prior education, but ideas that effectively result in less education for nurses are not in the interests of nurses or their patients. A June 2005 article by Joel Dresang in the *Milwaukee Journal-Sentinel* approvingly described a large Wisconsin program to address the nursing shortage that included ideas to "streamline" nursing coursework.[199]

Simply finding new groups of people to plug the holes in the nursing workforce does nothing to fix the reasons those holes exist, which include poor working conditions and a lack of real understanding of nursing skills. Would media creators uncritically discuss plans to address a physician shortage by "streamlining" medical school or recruiting those with few other options?

Notes

1. CFNA, "NBC's 'Passions' Solves Nursing Shortage: Monkeys Can Do the Job!," TAN (September 12, 2003), http://tinyurl.com/jww254k.
2. Daniel Simons and Christopher Chabris, "Gorillas in Our Midst: Sustained Inattentional Blindness for Dynamic Events," *Perception* 28 (1999): 1059–1074, http://tinyurl.com/ykg833m; video available at http://tinyurl.com/2pl5d.
3. Keith Payne, "Your Hidden Censor: What Your Mind Will Not Let You See," *Scientific American* (June 11, 2013), http://tinyurl.com/kzf9t6b.
4. Liz Brixius and Linda Wallem, writers, Paul Feig, director, "Comfort Food," *Nurse Jackie*, Showtime (March 22, 2010); TAN, "Blade Runner" (March 22, 2010), http://tinyurl.com/mapznaw.
5. Clyde Phillips, writer, Randall Einhorn, director, "Happy F**king Birthday," *Nurse Jackie*, Showtime (April 14, 2013); TAN, "Cunning, Baffling, Powerful" (April 14, 2013), http://tinyurl.com/kgrdrne.
6. Rick Cleveland, writer, Craig Zisk, director, "Tiny Bubbles," *Nurse Jackie*, Showtime (July 13, 2009); TAN, "Who Must Do the Hard Things?" (July 13, 2009), http://tinyurl.com/k3n88ug.
7. TAN, "*Nurse Jackie* Episode Reviews" (2013), http://tinyurl.com/kqm3k6b.
8. TAN, "*Call the Midwife* Episode Reviews" (2012), http://tinyurl.com/m3bf4lw.
9. John Martin, Heidi Thomas, and Jennifer Worth, writers, Roger Goldby, director, "Season 2, Episode 3," *Call the Midwife*, BBC/PBS (February 3, 2013), http://tinyurl.com/cm8tpvg.
10. Heidi Thomas, writer, Minkie Spiro, director, "Season 2, Episode 8," *Call the Midwife*, BBC/PBS (March 19, 2013).
11. TAN, "*Mercy* Episode Reviews" (2010), http://tinyurl.com/kj3t63s.
12. TAN, "*HawthoRNe* Episode Reviews" (2011), http://tinyurl.com/jwd7neg.
13. TAN, "*ER* Episode Analyses" (2009), http://tinyurl.com/odsbmqw.
14. TAN, "*Scrubs* Episode Analyses" (2009), http://tinyurl.com/p9n8e58.
15. Megan Amram, writer, Craig Zisk, director, "Animal Control," *Parks & Recreation*, NBC (April 11, 2013), http://tinyurl.com/kjqo6ve.
16. TAN, "A Tale of Two Nurses" (January 27, 2013), http://tinyurl.com/pzv2juv.
17. TAN, "I Just Do" (2008), http://tinyurl.com/nqk9f2t.
18. CFNA, "Lifeline: The Nursing Diaries," TAN (2004), http://tinyurl.com/ob9df8c.

19. Greg Rienzi, "TV Documentary Explores Nursing," *The Gazette Online* 29, no. 42 (July 31, 2000), http://tinyurl.com/q8kqald; CFNA, "Nurses," TAN (2002), http://tinyurl.com/qzjaldh.
20. Tony Kushner, writer, Mike Nichols, director, *Angels in America*, HBO Films (2003); CFNA, "Angels in America," TAN (April 4, 2004), http://tinyurl.com/mqcbd3l.
21. George Romero and James Gunn, writers, Zack Snyder, director, *Dawn of the Dead,* Universal Pictures (2004); CFNA, "Dawn of the Dead," TAN (2004), http://tinyurl.com/py9holr.
22. Neill Blomkamp, writer and director, *Elysium*, TriStar Pictures (2013); TAN, "Elysium" (October 17, 2013), http://tinyurl.com/olqoxef.
23. John Hamburg and Larry Stuckey, writers, Paul Weitz, director, *Little Fockers*, Tribeca/Everyman Pictures (2010); TAN, "Little Fockers" (August 4, 2011), http://tinyurl.com/oko5yzw.
24. Daniel Slotnik, "Vernice D. Ferguson, Leader and Advocate of Nurses, Dies at 84," *New York Times* (December 21, 2012); TAN, "Fear No Evil: Whatever the Boys Have" (December 21, 2012), http://tinyurl.com/qhfr7vy.
25. Frederick Rasmussen, "Elizabeth S. Trump: Longtime Director of Nurses at Maryland Shock Trauma Center Worked Closely with Founder Dr. R Adams Cowley," *Baltimore Sun* (June 9, 2012); TAN, "Fear No Evil: The First Trauma Nurse" (December 21, 2012), http://tinyurl.com/pohupcn.
26. Julian Guthrie, "David Vlahov Is New UCSF Nursing School Dean," *San Francisco Chronicle* (March 11, 2012); TAN, "You Just Have to Listen" (March 11, 2012), http://tinyurl.com/ncsmen2.
27. Steve Lopez, "A Note of Gratitude to Nurses: An Alert Nurse's Quick Action Saves the Columnist's Life and Opens His Eyes to His Medical Team's Dedication and Compassion," *Los Angeles Times* (September 1, 2012); TAN, "All Pros" (September 1, 2012), http://tinyurl.com/9h56qwm.
28. John Blanton, "Care and Chaos on the Night Nursing Shift; In a Search for Purpose, an Editor Changes Careers; 'He's Asking for You Again,'" *Wall Street Journal* (April 24, 2007); CFNA, "There and Back Again," TAN (April 24, 2007), http://tinyurl.com/ndu5dx8.
29. Scott Allen, "A Crash Course in Saving Lives," *Boston Globe* (October 23–26, 2007), http://tinyurl.com/axoun4o; CFNA, "As I Lay Dying," TAN (October 23–26, 2007), http://tinyurl.com/mnm2zkh.
30. Gary Trudeau, "Doonesbury" (June 25 and 28, 2004), http://tinyurl.com/pqdkekm and http://tinyurl.com/mx4jtzg; CFNA, "Nurse Jewel Shows B.D. the Tough Love," TAN (July 3, 2004), http://tinyurl.com/ndmswyl.
31. Patti Neighmond, "Need a Nurse? You May Have to Wait," *National Public Radio* (May 25, 2012), http://tinyurl.com/7kf9eab; TAN, "Are Your Knuckles White?" (May 25, 2012), http://tinyurl.com/nhdpoas.
32. Will Moredock, "Critical Condition: S.C.'s Nursing Shortage Could Use Some Intensive Care," *Charleston City Paper* (March 14, 2007), http://tinyurl.com/

mpdgzfv; CFNA, "Startling Discoveries," TAN (March 14, 2007), http://tinyurl.com/pko6wuj.

33. John Pekkanen, "Condition Critical: With Nurses Leaving in Droves, a Stay at the Hospital Gets Scarier Every Day," *Reader's Digest* (September 2003): 84–93, http://tinyurl.com/keeggj9; CFNA, "Reader's Digest: Nursing Shortage Is 'America's Biggest Health Care Crisis,'" TAN (September 2003), http://tinyurl.com/m6ouj9e.
34. CFNA, "Exodus," TAN (June 29, 2006), http://tinyurl.com/oalpeeg.
35. Jeff Bryant, "'School Nurse Cuts Killed My Daughter': Laporshia Massey Died Because Our Priorities Are Wrong," *Salon* (October 18, 2013), http://tinyurl.com/n7df67t.
36. Elisabeth Ochs, "Help Us," *Salon* (February 5, 2004), http://tinyurl.com/pr4duqv; CFNA, "Homeland Security," TAN (February 5, 2004), http://tinyurl.com/ocq23cd.
37. Kathleen Bartholomew, "Students in Washington Schools Need Nurses," *Seattle Times* (June 11, 2013), http://tinyurl.com/lj54b79.
38. Chris Coats, "Christmas Angel Saves 8-Year-Old Boy," *Dallas Morning News* (December 21, 2007), http://tinyurl.com/ow8o2fj.
39. Jim Flink, "School Nurse Helps Save Student With Aneurysm," KMBC, Kansas City (October 20, 2006); CFNA, "Assessment," TAN (October 20, 2006), http://tinyurl.com/pgwro3t.
40. Lauran Neergaard, "NYC School Nurse Recounts Swine Flu Triage," Associated Press (July 9, 2009), http://tinyurl.com/mql8kud; TAN, "Post-Its and Other Priorities: Every School Needs a Nurse" (July 9, 2009), http://tinyurl.com/nqdpj2g.
41. Suruchi Sharma, "Nurse Tells Asian Community to Get 'Clued Up' about Tobacco at Northwick Park Hospital," *Harrow Times* (November 25, 2011), http://tinyurl.com/mev326u; TAN, "Wicked Local Public Health Advocates: Getting Clued Up" (December 2011), http://tinyurl.com/q5xqvaq.
42. Katherine Boo, "Swamp Nurse," *The New Yorker* (February 6, 2006), http://tinyurl.com/mvs5fe; CFNA, "The Overcomer: Nurse-Family Partnerships in the Louisiana Bayou," TAN (February 6, 2006), http://tinyurl.com/pcmov73.
43. Amanda Crook, "MRSA Award for Nurses," *Manchester Evening News* (April 17, 2010), http://tinyurl.com/ou736nv.
44. Alan McEwen, "Pioneer Nurse Wins Award for Life-Saving Heart Scheme," *Scotsman* (January 3, 2006), http://tinyurl.com/o46fumn; CFNA, "Pioneer Nurse Wins Award for Life-Saving Heart Scheme," TAN (January 3, 2006), http://tinyurl.com/o8ezbrm.
45. Milt Freudenheim, "Preparing More Care of Elderly," *New York Times* (June 28, 2010), http://tinyurl.com/qf5q677; TAN, "Nurse and Patient: How to Survive" (October 21, 2010), http://tinyurl.com/oezjzs3.

46. Jane Elliott, "How One Nurse Helped Stop Killer Bedsores," *BBC News* (March 21, 2009), http://tinyurl.com/cq935f; TAN, "Think Different: BBC News Article by Jane Elliott, March 21" (March 2009), http://tinyurl.com/yh997r4.
47. *Newsweek*, "The Life of a Virus Hunter" (May 14, 2010), http://www.newsweek.com/life-virus-hunter-110499; CFNA, "90 Pounds and the Truth," TAN (May 15, 2006), http://tinyurl.com/put3fg6.
48. Dianne Hales, "The Quiet Heroes," *Parade* (March 21, 2004), http://tinyurl.com/pz4m986; CFNA, "Parade Profiles Leading Nursing Scholar," TAN (March 21, 2004), http://tinyurl.com/pmf87hu.
49. Anne Underwood, "Inside Forensic Nursing: Crime and Care," *Newsweek* (October 6, 2006), http://tinyurl.com/n7f3eeg; CFNA, "Who Are You?," TAN (October 6, 2006), http://tinyurl.com/o6h99p2.
50. CFNA, "We Want to Hear from a Nurse," TAN (November 2, 2006), http://tinyurl.com/nvyaow3.
51. TAN, "Sung and Unsung: Nurses Won't Talk" (January 25, 2011), http://tinyurl.com/puvslg5.
52. Julia Bucher, "Advice for Caregivers of Relatives with Cancer," *New York Times* (July 3, 2013), http://tinyurl.com/nxce4y6; TAN, "Diplomacy: This Message is Important to Share" (July 3, 2013), http://tinyurl.com/o6rcwda.
53. Pauline Chen, "When It's the Nurse Who Needs Looking After," *New York Times* (July 5, 2012), http://tinyurl.com/7w2dd2p; TAN, "Oh, Inverted World" (July 5, 2012), http://tinyurl.com/lm3q8nl.
54. Theresa Brown, accessed March 23, 2014, http://www.theresabrownrn.com.
55. Cynda Hylton Rushton, "Take Pregnant Woman off Ventilator?," *CNN Opinion* (January 8, 2014), http://tinyurl.com/pv5fzwu.
56. Ghana News Agency, "Unsafe Abortion Leading Cause of Birth Complications - Nurse" (December 31, 2010), http://tinyurl.com/mwos7kn; TAN, "Ask the Senior Midwife" (December 31, 2010), http://tinyurl.com/o9pe37a.
57. Cherie Taylor, "Diabetes about Lifestyle - Not Race: Rotorua Nurse," *New Zealand Herald/Rotorua Daily Post* (November 14–15, 2006), http://tinyurl.com/jw92vwv; CFNA, "Lifestyle," TAN (November 14, 2006), http://tinyurl.com/p3tlwug.
58. TAN, "*Grey's Anatomy* Analyses and Action," accessed March 26, 2014, http://tinyurl.com/pgayg7h.
59. Shonda Rhimes, writer, Peter Horton, director, "A Hard Day's Night," *Grey's Anatomy*, ABC (March 27, 2005); CFNA, "ABC's *Grey's Anatomy*: So Chunky with Hollywood's Contempt for Nursing, You'll Be Tempted to Use a Fork. But Use a Scalpel!," TAN (March 27, 2005), http://tinyurl.com/nay5lvy.
60. Shonda Rhimes, writer, Peter Horton, director, "The First Cut is the Deepest," *Grey's Anatomy*, ABC (April 3, 2005); CFNA, "You're the Pig Who Called Meredith a Nurse . . . I Hate You on Principle," TAN (April 3, 2005), http://tinyurl.com/nk7jvm2.

61. William Harper, writer, Allison Liddi, director, "I Saw What I Saw," *Grey's Anatomy*, ABC (October 22, 2009); TAN, "*Grey's Anatomy*: Have Fun Playing Nurse!: Complaining of Pain" (August 2010), http://tinyurl.com/k8r85ea.
62. Stacy McKee, writer, Adam Davidson, director, "Something to Talk About," *Grey's Anatomy*, ABC (November 6, 2005); CFNA, "The Drunk and the Ugly," TAN (November 6, 2005), http://tinyurl.com/o7ob6nt.
63. Mark Wilding, writer, Dan Minahan, director, "Where the Boys Are," *Grey's Anatomy*, ABC (November 9, 2006); CFNA, "Digging through Crap," TAN (November 9, 2006), http://tinyurl.com/q5oxkmr.
64. Eric Buchman, writer, Michael Grossman, director, "Great Expectations," *Grey's Anatomy*, ABC (January 25, 2007); CFNA, "The Soft Bigotry of Low Expectations," TAN (January 25, 2007),http://tinyurl.com/ptkrlyy.
65. Tony Phelan and Joan Rater, writers, Adam Davidson, director, "Tell Me Sweet Little Lies," *Grey's Anatomy*, ABC (January 22, 2006); CFNA, "Sweet Little Lies," TAN (January 22, 2006),http://tinyurl.com/pbauv6b.
66. Eric Buchman, writer, Michael Grossman, director, "Great Expectations," *Grey's Anatomy*, ABC (January 25, 2007); CFNA, "The Soft Bigotry of Low Expectations," TAN (January 25, 2007), http://tinyurl.com/ptkrlyy.
67. Shonda Rhimes, writer, Rob Corn, director, "Freedom 2," *Grey's Anatomy*, ABC (May 22, 2008), http://tinyurl.com/pkaomsr.
68. Shonda Rhimes, writer, Rob Corn, director, "Dream a Little Dream of Me (1)," *Grey's Anatomy*, ABC (September 25, 2008).
69. TAN, "Who's the Man?" (October 13, 2011), http://tinyurl.com/onha8uc.
70. Stacy McKee, writer, Rob Corn, director, "Perfect Storm," *Grey's Anatomy*, ABC (May 16, 2013), http://tinyurl.com/lcuw6y6.
71. TAN, "*House* Single Episode Reviews" (2011), http://tinyurl.com/py4b5ug.
72. CFNA, "What's the Differential Diagnosis for Chronic Handmaiden-itis with Persistent Physician Nursing? Quick! The Patient is Dying!," TAN (May 24, 2005), http://tinyurl.com/o5ejlfq.
73. CFNA, "And on the Eighth Day, the Lord Physician Created Nurses, to Clean up the Mess," TAN (November 15, 2005), http://tinyurl.com/o4qdogh.
74. David Foster, Peter Blake, Garrett Lerner, and Russel Friend, writers, Greg Yaitanes, director, "House's Head (Part 1)," *House*, Fox (May 12, 2008).
75. CFNA, "Is This All Nurses Do?," TAN (November 21, 2006), http://tinyurl.com/p4mw8yw.
76. TAN, "Helpful and Caring and the Whole Sponge Bath Thing" (February 22, 2011), http://tinyurl.com/nlasf6l.
77. Mindy Kaling and Matt Warburton, writers, Michael Weaver, director, "Music Festival," *The Mindy Project*, Fox (October 1, 2013).
78. Mindy Kaling, Ike Barinholtz, and David Stassen, writers, Michael Spiller, director, "Hiring and Firing," *The Mindy Project*, Fox (October 2, 2012).

79. Mindy Kaling and Tucker Cawley, writers, Rob Schrab, director, "Pretty Man," *The Mindy Project*, Fox (April 4, 2013); TAN, "Clicking and Clacking" (May 14, 2014), http://tinyurl.com/oj3w76y.
80. Kaling and Warburton, "Music Festival."
81. Mindy Kaling and Tracey Wigfield, writers, Neal Brennan, director, "Magic Morgan," *The Mindy Project*, Fox (October 8, 2013).
82. Mindy Kaling and Charlie Grandy, writers, Beth McCarthy-Miller, director, "Sk8er Man," *The Mindy Project*, Fox (November 5, 2013).
83. Mindy Kaling, Ike Barinholtz, and David Stassen, writers, BJ Novak, director, "Mindy's Minute," *The Mindy Project*, Fox (February 19, 2013).
84. Mindy Kaling and Adam Countee, writers, Claire Scanlon, director, "Mindy's Birthday," *The Mindy Project*, Fox (March 19, 2013).
85. Mindy Kaling and Jack Burditt, writers, Wendey Stanzler, director, "Triathlon," *The Mindy Project*, Fox (April 30, 2013).
86. Mindy Kaling and Tracey Wigfield, writers, Michael Weaver, director, "Frat Party," *The Mindy Project*, Fox (May 7, 2013).
87. Mindy Kaling, writer, Michael Spiller, director, "All My Problems Solved Forever . . . ," *The Mindy Project*, Fox (September 17, 2013).
88. Mindy Kaling and Charlie Grandy, writers, Rob Schrab, director, "Danny Castellano Is My Personal Trainer," *The Mindy Project*, Fox (January 7, 2014).
89. TAN, "*Private Practice* Episode Analyses" (2013), http://tinyurl.com/lecehka.
90. CFNA, "Between the Boob and the Tube," TAN (September 28, 2006), http://tinyurl.com/lk84eaf.
91. CFNA, "The Swan, M.D.," TAN (May 13, 2004), http://tinyurl.com/qd9vfn7.
92. CFNA, "Nurses Are About 100 Times More Likely to Attend Graduate Nursing School than Medical School," TAN (2002), http://tinyurl.com/p7orchc.
93. Virgil Williams, writer, Anthony Hemingway, director, "Tandem Repeats," *ER*, NBC (May 8, 2008).
94. Bill Lawrence and Mike Schwartz, writers, Linda Mendoza, director, "His Story IV," *Scrubs*, NBC (February 1, 2007); CFNA, "'Scrubs,' Lift Us up Where We Belong," TAN (February 1, 2007), http://tinyurl.com/nh2t6a5.
95. Bill Lawrence and Ted Quill, writers, Michael Spiller, director, "My Quarantine," *Scrubs*, NBC (February 8, 2005); CFNA, "Can Any Idiot Be a Nurse? Don't Forget the Sponge Baths and Happy Endings!" (February 8, 2005),http://tinyurl.com/qaanymw.
96. Jo Brand, Joanna Scanlan, Vicki Pepperdine, Mark V. Olsen, and Will Scheffer, creators, *Getting On*, HBO (2013-).
97. Mark V. Olsen, writer, Howard Deutch, director, "If You're Going to San Francisco," *Getting On*, HBO (December 1, 2013).
98. Mark V. Olsen, writer, Miguel Arteta, director, "Born on the Fourth of July," *Getting On*, HBO (November 24, 2013).

99. Dave Caplan, Mark Cronin, and Shannon Fitzgerald, executive producers, "The Surprise Visit," *Scrubbing In*, MTV (December 26, 2013), http://tinyurl.com/mtd4vx9.
100. TAN, "Admiring Their Credentials" (January 12, 2011), http://tinyurl.com/oe9eox7.
101. Andrew Lenchewski, John P. Rogers, and Jessica Ball, writers, Ed Fraiman, director, "Pins and Needles," *Royal Pains*, USA Network (August 14, 2013).
102. Andrew Lenchewski and John P. Rogers, writers, Jace Alexander, director, "Pilot," *Royal Pains*, USA Network (June 4, 2009); TAN, "Post-Its and Other Priorities" (July 9, 2009), http://tinyurl.com/nqdpj2g.
103. Ryan Murphy, writer, Elodie Keene, director, "Vitamin D," *Glee*, Fox (October 7, 2009); TAN, "Vitamin F" (October 7, 2009), http://tinyurl.com/p4xzp2z.
104. Ian Brennan, writer and director, "Tina in the Sky with Diamonds," *Glee*, Fox (October 3, 2013).
105. Megan Ganz, writer, Beth McCarthy-Miller, director, "The Big Game," *Modern Family*, ABC (December 4, 2013); TAN, "Problems with Nursing" (December 4, 2013), http://tinyurl.com/kz43lrn.
106. Seth Kurland, writer, Lynn M. McCracken, director, "The Principal," *8 Simple Rules for Dating My Teenage Daughter*, ABC (May 11, 2004); CFNA, "8 Simple Rules for Portraying Nurses in Your Hollywood Sitcom," TAN (September 3, 2004), http://tinyurl.com/ohkbuwm.
107. CFNA, "Falling without Style," TAN (October 9, 2006), http://tinyurl.com/nhjg6cv.
108. Marlene Bokholdt, "Working as a Nurse," TAN (September 2011), http://tinyurl.com/np8qoe4; TAN, "Hell of a Doctor" (August 2013), http://tinyurl.com/l2gfpxd.
109. Christopher Rowland, "Chaotic but Brief UMass Strike," *Boston Globe* (October 27, 2006) http://tinyurl.com/l67d6hm; CFNA, "'Do They Deserve This Six-Figure Salary for What They Do?,'" TAN (October 26, 2006), http://tinyurl.com/p5y7bml.
110. Brenda Wilson, "Developing Countries See Health Care 'Brain Drain,'" *National Public Radio* (November 3, 2005); CFNA, "NPR Science Correspondent Explains It All for You: Kenyan Clinical Officers Are 'Not Quite a Doctor, but More than a Nurse,'" TAN (November 3, 2005), http://tinyurl.com/klcav6o.
111. CFNA, "Tip No. 76: For Even Quicker Attention, Drive Your Hummer Straight into the ER. Then Offer the Triage Nurse a Chocolate if He'll Let You See the Physician Before All Those Little Pedestrians!," TAN (November 2005), http://tinyurl.com/q4r8r9n.
112. TAN, "You Will Be Required to Deal with Bruising" (October 24, 2012), http://tinyurl.com/kj78oom.
113. CFNA, "4. Crossword Helper (3 Letters)," TAN (February 27, 2007), http://tinyurl.com/mbf6za.

114. TAN, "Hospital Attendant" (April 27, 2009), http://tinyurl.com/nfabnfr.
115. John Colapinto, "Mother Courage," *New Yorker* (December 20, 2010), http://tinyurl.com/d79aa7n; TAN, "The Talk of the Town" (December 2011), http://tinyurl.com/mu88h9u.
116. CFNA, "Nurse or Leader: Pick One," TAN (April 1, 2006), http://tinyurl.com/q2luguv.
117. CFNA, "Serenading the Unsung Heroines in South Africa," TAN (May 12, 2005), http://tinyurl.com/qfcfzbr.
118. TAN, "Ridiculously Easy Tricks Help Local Nurses Save Lives!" (November 21, 2011), http://tinyurl.com/q7xcm5k.
119. TAN, "The Experts" (November 2011), http://tinyurl.com/p3wjkdc.
120. Abigail Zuger, "CASES: Prescription, Quite Simply, Was a Nurse," *New York Times*, November 19, 2002, accessed March 21, 2014, http://tinyurl.com/pwt5c2j.
121. CFNA, "In Juggling Your Hectic Business Schedule Prior to Your Stay Here at Ritz Memorial, Did You Forget to Pack One of Those Little Essentials, Like Toothpaste, Shampoo, or a Nurse? If So, Our Concierge Is Pleased to Provide Them with Our Compliments," TAN (September 17, 2005), http://tinyurl.com/q3ng6hy.
122. Stacy McKee, writer, Rob Corn, director, "Perfect Storm," *Grey's Anatomy*, ABC (May 16, 2013); TAN, "Heroes Among Us" (November 3, 2012), http://tinyurl.com/nzbknp4.
123. TAN, "Right Away, Doctor!" (November 2010), http://tinyurl.com/q982g5q.
124. CFNA, "Looking for Mr. McSteamy," TAN (May 8, 2008), http://tinyurl.com/oj3ybyy.
125. CFNA, "Plot Devices in Scrubs," TAN (December 11, 2005), http://tinyurl.com/nhlj8nd.
126. TAN, "*House* Single Episode Reviews" (2011), http://tinyurl.com/py4b5ug.
127. Peter Blake, David Foster, Russel Friend, and Garrett Lerner, writers, Katie Jacobs, director, "Wilson's Heart," *House*, Fox (May 19, 2008).
128. CFNA, "Golem," TAN (May 23, 2006), http://tinyurl.com/o9ydmvo.
129. Amanda Johns, David E. Kelley, Karen Struck, writers, based on the novel of Sanjay Gupta, Bill D'Elia, director, "Family Ties," *Monday Mornings*, TNT (April 8, 2013); TAN, "Picking Battles" (April 2013), http://tinyurl.com/n65ovcn.
130. Carol C. Scholle and Nicolette C. Mininni, "How a Rapid Response Team Saves Lives" *Nursing2006* 36, no. 1 (January 2006): 36–40; Laurel Tyler, Diane Sanders, Nancy Dahlberg, and Carol Wagner, "Rapid Response Teams" (slide presentation), Washington State Hospital Association (2006), http://tinyurl.com/kuu4rlo.
131. Lisa Zwerling, writer, Laura Innes, director, "Sea Change," *ER*, NBC (May 10, 2007); CFNA, "Nothing More than a Persistent Illusion," TAN (September 13, 2007).

132. Margorie David, writer, Ted Kotcheff, director, "Doubt," *Law and Order: Special Victims Unit*, NBC (November 23, 2004); CFNA, "Take Care of Yourself!," TAN (November 23, 2004), http://tinyurl.com/oe4d32x.
133. Jonathan Greene, writer, Helen Shaver, director, "Behave," *Law and Order: Special Victims Unit*, NBC (September 29, 2010); TAN, "The Sexual Assault Nurse" (September 29, 2010), http://tinyurl.com/ovl3cje.
134. CFNA, "Physicians Save Corzine; Other Work Occurs," TAN (May 13, 2007), http://tinyurl.com/oenh2by.
135. CFNA, "Living with His Mistake," TAN (May 2007), http://tinyurl.com/otzqc4b.
136. *Wall Street Journal*, "Hospitals Let Families Witness Procedures: Staying with Patient in ER or ICU Can Have Benefits, but Some Doctors Object" (October 12, 2004); CFNA, "Family Presence and Nursing Presence," TAN (October 12, 2004), http://tinyurl.com/pnnzjhv.
137. Dan Even, "Medical Staff Partly to Blame for Patients' Violence, Israeli Study Finds," *Haaretz* (March 13, 2012), http://tinyurl.com/lctyj82; TAN, "A Seemingly Innocuous Incident" (March 13, 2012), http://tinyurl.com/o2rxnxg.
138. Laurie Tarkan, "E.R. Patients Often Left Confused After Visits," *New York Times* (September 15, 2008), http://tinyurl.com/pdrba7f.
139. CFNA, "I Can't Even Say I Made My Own Mistakes. Really—One Has to Ask Oneself—What Dignity Is There in That?," TAN (June 20, 2004), http://tinyurl.com/nd578gk.
140. US Department of Labor, Bureau of Labor Statistics, "Occupational Employment Statistics: May 2012 National Occupational Employment and Wage Estimates," http://tinyurl.com/q2ywzuv, and "Physicians and Surgeons," accessed January 15, 2014, http://tinyurl.com/77ghlzk.
141. Leah Binder, "Stunning News on Preventable Deaths in Hospitals," *Forbes* (September 23, 2013), http://tinyurl.com/mk4zraj.
142. Lucian L. Leape, David W. Bates, David J. Cullen, Jeffrey Cooper, Harold J. Demonaco, Theresa Gallivan, and Robert Hallisey, "Systems Analysis of Adverse Drug Events," *Journal of the American Medical Association* 274, no. 1 (1995): 35–43, http://tinyurl.com/m7dwymb; Geri L. Dickson and Linda Flynn, "Nurses' Clinical Reasoning: Processes and Practices of Medication Safety," *Qualitative Health Research* 22, no. 1 (2011): 3–16, http://tinyurl.com/qe7ywza.
143. Fred Schulte, "Masking Malpractice Cases," *Baltimore Sun* (December 20, 2005), http://tinyurl.com/kee5txa; CFNA, "If Only We Could Find a 10,000-Word Major Metropolitan Newspaper Article on Nursing Malpractice, That Would Be So Great!," TAN (December 20, 2005), http://tinyurl.com/o8pl6cs.
144. Liz Kowalczyk, "MGH Death Spurs Review of Patient Monitors," *Boston Globe* (February 21, 2010), http://tinyurl.com/y99fbua; TAN, "Background Noise" (March 16, 2010), http://tinyurl.com/ns95szd.

145. Laura Landro, “New Focus on Averting Errors: Hospital Culture,” *Wall Street Journal* (March 16, 2010), http://tinyurl.com/mtuflpe; TAN, “Disabling the Off Switch” (March 16, 2010), http://tinyurl.com/ney7lwq.
146. Matthew Lee and Marilynn Marchione, “Hillary Clinton Hospitalized with Blood Clot,” Associated Press/*BusinessWeek* (December 31, 2012), http://tinyurl.com/myzoy4m; TAN, “I’m Not There” (January 2013), http://tinyurl.com/p396p7h.
147. Ken Auletta, “Changing Times,” *New Yorker* (October 24, 2011), http://tinyurl.com/3lb6nuh; TAN, “The Talk of the Town: Times Not Changing Enough” (December 2011), http://tinyurl.com/nhyfu7v.
148. Richard Knox, “Health Officials Consider Strategy for Possible Bird Flu Pandemic,” *National Public Radio* (February 10, 2006), http://tinyurl.com/9ccbb; CFNA, “The Ventilated Elite,” TAN (March 12, 2006), http://tinyurl.com/pkw39u5.
149. Christine Lagorio, “The Nurse-Family Partnership,” *CBS Evening News with Katie Couric* (July 11, 2007), http://tinyurl.com/k86lz4v.
150. Alicia Chang, “Health Coaches Helping Patients Avoid Return Trips to Hospital,” Associated Press/*Union Tribune* (October 12, 2006), http://tinyurl.com/l3pz3z4; CFNA, “Put Me In, Health Coach!,” TAN (October 12, 2006), http://tinyurl.com/leobqq2.
151. Stacy McKee, writer, Rob Corn, director, “Perfect Storm,” *Grey’s Anatomy*, ABC (May 16, 2013), http://tinyurl.com/lcuw6y6.
152. Janice Mangurten, Shari Scott, Cathie Guzzetta, Jenny Sperry, Lori Vinson, Barry Hicks, Douglas Watts, and Susan Scott, “Family Presence: Making Room,” *American Journal of Nursing* 105, no. 5 (May 2005): 40–48.
153. Stacy McKee, writer, Jessica Yu, director, “Invest in Love,” *Grey’s Anatomy*, ABC (November 5, 2009).
154. Andrew Scher, Carla Pennington, Jay McGraw, Jeff Hudson, executive producers, *The Doctors*, syndicated television show, accessed March 26, 2014, http://www.thedoctorstv.com.
155. Terence Wrong, executive producer, *Hopkins 24/7*, ABC (2000).
156. Terence Wrong, executive producer, *Hopkins*, ABC (2008); CFNA, “Cinema Faux,” TAN (June 26, 2008).
157. Terence Wrong, executive producer, *Boston Med*, ABC (2010); TAN, “Physicians Are Awesome” (July 22, 2010), http://tinyurl.com/o7m9olh.
158. Terence Wrong, executive producer, *NY Med*, ABC (2012, 2014).
159. CFNA, “Infirmieres Sans Frontières,” TAN (December 3, 2006), http://tinyurl.com/jwa9goe.
160. Mark Kaplan, director, Mark Kaplan, Naisola Grimwood, and Daniel Holton-Roth, producers, *Living in Emergency: Stories of Doctors Without Borders*, Red Floor Pictures (2009); TAN, “Living in Emergency: Stories of Doctors Without Borders” (March 23, 2010), http://tinyurl.com/qdf64yr.

161. Jerome Groopman, "A Child in Time: New Frontiers in Treating Premature Babies," *The New Yorker* (October 24, 2011), http://tinyurl.com/mv7rwhk; TAN, "The Talk of the Town" (December 2011), http://tinyurl.com/mu88h9u.
162. Richard Friedman, "Their Coats Are White, but Their Hands Are Green," *New York Times* (June 29, 2004), http://tinyurl.com/lo49wt5; CFNA, "The 'July Syndrome:' Who's Minding the Interns?," TAN (June 29, 2004), http://tinyurl.com/nmcpd6n.
163. United Press International, "Nurses: Pain Affects Everything Else" (September 14, 2009), http://tinyurl.com/m6rswre; TAN, "Nurses: Pain Affects Everything Else" (September 14, 2009), http://tinyurl.com/ov2n282.
164. CFNA, "Maybe I Wrote in Invisible Ink," TAN (October 29, 2004), http://tinyurl.com/o68u9pm.
165. Elizabeth Cohen, "Nurses Relied on Trauma Experience to Help Bombing Wounded," CNN (April 16, 2013), http://tinyurl.com/kxy4wns; TAN, "Everyone Worked in Tandem" (April 17, 2013), http://tinyurl.com/k4mun2n.
166. Poppy Harlow and Sheila Steffen, "Woman Gets New Leg—and New Life—After Boston Bombings," CNN (July 17, 2013), http://tinyurl.com/mhmqht7.
167. Gina Kolata, Jeré Longman, and Mary Pilon, "Doctors Saved Lives, if Not Legs, in Boston," *New York Times* (April 16, 2013), http://tinyurl.com/lslx8hd.
168. Steve Inskeep, "Disaster Would Overwhelm Hospitals, Author Warns," *National Public Radio* (February 22, 2007), http://tinyurl.com/msgs6ea; CFNA, "Mourning Edition," TAN (March 1, 2007), http://tinyurl.com/p5ncv6m.
169. Marilyn Marchionne, "Doctors Weathered the Storm and Became Heroes," Associated Press/*USA Today* (September 9, 2005), http://tinyurl.com/k4johsc; CFNA, "Nurses Evacuated from AP Report on Katrina," TAN (September 9, 2005), http://tinyurl.com/oxf73du.
170. Nancy Gibbs, "Saving One Life at a Time," *Time* (October 30, 2005), http://tinyurl.com/oubx8sn; CFNA, "We Can Be 'Heroes,'" TAN (November 7, 2005), http://tinyurl.com/odkbjbq.
171. Mark Poertner, executive producer, David Stern, producer and director, *Discovery Health Channel Medical Honors*, Discovery Health Channel (2004); CFNA, "Nation's Elite Honors 13 'Medical Heroes'; Heroic Nurses' Invitations Lost in Mail?", TAN (July 8, 2004), http://tinyurl.com/pst2gny.
172. Gail Deutsch, Mark Dorian, and Adam Sechrist, producers, "Heroes Among Us," *20/20*, ABC (November 2, 2012), http://tinyurl.com/mqk3wfm.
173. Patrick Healy, "'Heroic Actions' by SoCal Nurse Save Pilot Mid-Flight," NBC4 News (January 10, 2014), http://tinyurl.com/mmkllwa.
174. Nicole Brodeur, "Flying Solo, Nurse Is Enough," *Seattle Times* (May 3, 2005), http://tinyurl.com/lqygpob; CFNA, "'And There Wasn't Even a Doctor There!,'" TAN (May 3, 2005), http://tinyurl.com/3qdez2a.
175. Gina Kolata, "A Tactic to Cut I.C.U. Trauma: Get Patients Up," *New York Times* (January 12, 2009), http://tinyurl.com/khnz56j.

176. Nancy Gibbs and Amanda Bower, "Q: What Scares Doctors? A: Being the Patient," *Time* (April 23, 2006), http://tinyurl.com/kzlccsd; CFNA, "Q: What Scares Nurses? A: Who Cares?," TAN (May 14, 2006), http://tinyurl.com/on2ldfq.
177. Google, "New Advisory Group on Health" (June 27, 2007), http://tinyurl.com/29ptre.
178. Ehren Kruger, writer, Iain Softley, director, *The Skeleton Key*, Universal Studios (2005).
179. Stephen Susco, writer, Takashi Shimizu, director, *The Grudge*, Columbia Pictures (2004).
180. Craig Phillips, "*The Waiting Room*: Interview with Filmmaker Peter Nicks," PBS (October 17, 2013), http://tinyurl.com/ma3vfz9.
181. *TechNewsDaily*, "Toyota Debuts 'Robot Nurses' to Aid the Disabled" (November 3, 2011), http://tinyurl.com/mp46wr8; TAN, "That Leg Brace Graduated First in Its Nursing School Class!" (November 3, 2011), http://tinyurl.com/qfkulnl.
182. Agence France-Presse, "Japan Plans Robo-Nurses in Five Years: Govt." (March 25, 2009), http://tinyurl.com/ckc84m.
183. Angus Howarth, "Robot Nurses Could Be on the Wards in Three Years, Say Scientists," *The Scotsman* (January 22, 2007), http://tinyurl.com/lrxd4rg; CFNA, "Interaction and Intelligence," TAN (January 22, 2007), http://tinyurl.com/mln6lp6.
184. Tim Bajarin, "Meet Nurse iPhone," *PC Mag* (March 23, 2009), http://tinyurl.com/d5qgjn.
185. WisTV, "Health Alert: Electronic Nurse" (March 31, 2006), http://tinyurl.com/mkkcv4f; CFNA, "$70 Machine Claims to Be 'Nurse'; Background Check Underway," TAN (March 31, 2006), http://tinyurl.com/o24wk28.
186. Kevin Bonani and Jenn Lloyd, writers, Ted Wass, director, "Face Off," *Accidentally on Purpose* (April 7, 2010); TAN, "Nympho Nurse #3" (April 7, 2010), http://tinyurl.com/oglwt4u.
187. Vickie Elmer, "Bringing Balance to Life with New Babies," *Washington Post* (February 25, 2007), http://tinyurl.com/mq9c73d; CFNA, "The Nursemaid Who Wouldn't Disappear," TAN (February 25, 2007), http://tinyurl.com/mdnju89.
188. Pete Donohue and Caitlin Kelly, "Scandal of 'Baby Nurses,'" *New York Daily News* (August 28, 2005), http://tinyurl.com/mnk5ms4; CFNA, "Nursing the Baby Nurses," TAN (August 28, 2005), http://tinyurl.com/ku4gekk.
189. American Nurses Association, "Title 'Nurse' Protection: Summary of Language by State," accessed March 25, 2014, http://tinyurl.com/kne4ko3.
190. CFNA, "Feel Good, Inc.," TAN (July 14, 2005), http://tinyurl.com/n6opthx.
191. CFNA, "CVS Pharmacist Returns from Matrix; Can Now Download Entire Nursing Curriculum into Your Brain in Four Hours!," TAN (January 24, 2006), http://tinyurl.com/mwvx9bj.

192. St. John & Partners, "Today You're An Accountant. Tomorrow You're Dad's Nurse" (November 2011), http://tinyurl.com/pnp75zl.
193. Fe Zamora, "Daughter Kris was Aquino's Nurse," *Philippine Daily Inquirer* (August 1, 2009), http://tinyurl.com/mseq8j.
194. Guido Kleinhubber, "Prostitute Retraining Program: From Johns to Geriatrics," *der Spiegel* (March 14, 2006), http://tinyurl.com/c92bhjp; CFNA, "*Der Spiegel*: 'From Johns to Geriatrics,'" TAN (March 14, 2006), http://tinyurl.com/mrngpkn.
195. Nancy Pindus, Jane Tilly, and Stephanie Weinstein, "Skill Shortages and Mismatches in Nursing Related Health Care Employment," Urban Institute (April 2002), http://tinyurl.com/kv82hjr; VHA Health Foundation, "Welfare to Work" (March 2001), http://tinyurl.com/kz8kt6n. *See also* Eric Westervelt, "One Approach to Head Start: To Help Kids, Help Their Parents," *National Public Radio* (April 23, 2014), http://tinyurl.com/mohaqeh.
196. Yu Xu, "Are Chinese Nurses a Viable Source to Relieve the US Nursing Shortage?," *Nursing Economics* 21, no. 6 (2003): 269–274, http://tinyurl.com/lbjgvfb.
197. Alan Tomlinson, "Foreign Doctors Fill Florida's Nursing Gap," *National Public Radio* (February 17, 2004), http://tinyurl.com/mdfqd5u; CFNA, "Foreign Physicians as One Answer to the U.S. Nursing Shortage: From 'Giving Orders' to 'Receiving Orders'?," TAN (February 17, 2004), http://tinyurl.com/l7ynnmr; Adam Geller, "Filipino MD Picks Life as Nurse in U.S.," Associated Press/*USA Today* (January 1, 2007), http://tinyurl.com/kkzgpoy; CFNA, "Somebody Changed: AP Article," TAN (March 14, 2007), http://tinyurl.com/qjrb2zl.
198. TAN, "You Are Required to Deal with Bruising" (October 24, 2012), http://tinyurl.com/kj78oom.
199. CFNA, "Dear Applicant: We Are Pleased to Inform You That You Have Been Accepted into Our Nursing Program! Your Diploma Is Enclosed," TAN (June 12, 2005), http://tinyurl.com/mcq28yl.

4 YES, DOCTOR! NO, DOCTOR!

Most of society regards physicians as the captains of the healthcare ship and nurses as their helpful crew. In fact, nursing is an autonomous profession, as we explained in Chapter 1. Some media products reflect this reality, but many, particularly influential television shows like *Grey's Anatomy*, reinforce the damaging myth that physicians manage nurses. The handmaiden stereotype often appears together with the unskilled image discussed in Chapter 3, but they are distinct problems.

Of course, the media has not simply invented the idea that nurses are physician subordinates. Many physicians themselves believe they manage nurses. The May 2008 issue of *California Lawyer* magazine featured a piece by a physician who had attended Stanford, become a lawyer, and worked at a major national law firm.[1] L. Okey Onyejekwe Jr.'s piece described his residency at Columbia, from 2000 to 2003:

> I was a 25-year-old resident trying to establish authority in an emergency room where many of the nurses and staff had been practicing since before I was born. Despite being the least-experienced, lowest paid, and youngest person in the ER, I was responsible for managing the ER staff and for the health and well-being of numerous patients.

In fact, as a new resident, Onyejekwe was not "responsible for managing the ER staff." He was one member of a team, reporting to a physician manager. The nurses and others reported to their respective managers. Actually, one of nurses' most important professional roles is to act as an independent check on physician care plans to protect patients and ensure good care. Another key nursing role is to educate physicians, especially residents, about how to recognize changes in patient conditions and respond with appropriate treatments. These roles are rarely acknowledged by physicians or the media.

So why would a new physician think it was his job to "manage" veteran health staff? We doubt he had a medical school course entitled "The New Physician's Burden: Managing All Other Health Professionals." We assume his thinking was based on professional and cultural assumptions that nurses and other staff are relatively unskilled subordinates—and so physicians do and must manage all of health care. These ideas are deadly. They contribute greatly to healthcare errors and poor outcomes. Nurses are the patient advocates, the last line of defense. If they are viewed as subordinate, they cannot do their jobs effectively.

Of course, physicians still have greater social and economic power, so it is often difficult for nurses to resist their plans. Nurses' input may not be welcome. In December 2004 the *Times of India* reported that, after a nurse pointed out to a physician that he had failed to place a used syringe in the proper receptacle, offended physicians chose to "start a fight" with the nurses. Police were called in to restore order.[2]

An October 2010 cover story in *Reader's Digest* on hospital errors included an essay by nurse Sunnie Bell, who recounted how a patient had died after an esteemed senior physician ignored Bell's repeated warnings that the patient appeared to have a bowel obstruction.[3] Another essay in that issue was by Johns Hopkins physician Peter Pronovost, a healthcare errors expert who promotes the use of checklists and other safety measures. Pronovost stressed that nursing empowerment was a key element of reform, and he argued that some hospital procedures should require nursing agreement.[4]

Sometimes nurses have been able to protect patients despite limited recognition of nursing autonomy. In December 2013, the *Irish Examiner* reported that a nurse had told a panel investigating alleged incompetence by a physician about a 2009 incident in which the nurse had "snatched a scalpel from [the] doctor's hand, moments before he was about to cut into an elderly patient's vein in order to take a blood sample."[5] In March 2006 the Associated Press cited a police report that the chief of neurosurgery at an Oakland hospital had been "arrested after allegedly throwing a drunken fit when a nurse refused to let him operate."[6] Recall our friend Dan Lynch from Chapter 1, the nurse who fought successfully to persuade his heart patient's surgeon that a new heart valve had a potentially fatal problem.

Aside from the direct harm to patient care, the "handmaiden" stereotype sets nurses up as mere assistants. The image contributes to poor relations with patients and physicians, who sense they can abuse nurses with impunity, a major factor in nursing burnout and the nursing shortage. In November 2005 South Africa's *Cape Argus* reported that research in South Africa, the United

Kingdom, and the United States suggested that nurses experience disproportionately high physical and psychological abuse by patients and colleagues, especially physicians. The article noted that 80 percent of nurses surveyed in a recent South African study had said that private sector nurses were leaving the profession because of abuse, largely by male physicians.[7] In June 2009 the *Colorado Springs Gazette* reported that an operating room (OR) nurse had filed a lawsuit against a local hospital after allegedly being demoted for complaining that a senior surgeon had assaulted her, in one instance by throwing and hitting her with a patient's bloody pericardium (the layer of tissue that surrounds the heart).[8] In February 2010, as the *New York Times* reported, a Texas jury acquitted nurse Anne Mitchell after a four-day trial for misusing official information in reporting a physician's allegedly unsafe practices to the state medical board. Mitchell and a nurse colleague had also been fired from their hospital, but evidently that wasn't enough. The *Times* explained that the physician, the local sheriff, and the prosecutor who brought the case had close ties.[9]

The handmaiden stereotype affects who pursues nursing careers. Few ambitious people want to take years of rigorous science courses and endure extraordinary workplace burdens just to be assistants to the professionals who receive all the glory.

Are You Sure Nurses Are Autonomous? It Sure Looks like Physicians Call All the Shots

Well, it sure looks that way on television. That's what we've been heavily conditioned to see. Figure 4.1 shows how most of society views the relationship of nurses and physicians.

Yet nursing is a self-governing profession and a distinct scientific discipline. Nurses have a unique, holistic patient advocacy focus; a unique scope of practice under law; and a unique body of knowledge, including special expertise in such areas as public health, wound care, and pain management. As members of an autonomous profession, nurses are educated by nursing scholars, typically in nursing science degree programs at colleges. They use textbooks authored by those scholars. More than 50,000 US nurses have PhDs or other doctoral degrees, and more than 375,000 US nurses have at least a master's degree in nursing.[10] Highly educated nurses—not physicians—are the theoretical and practical leaders of the nursing profession. The actual relationship of the two disciplines in terms of knowledge is shown in Figure 4.2.

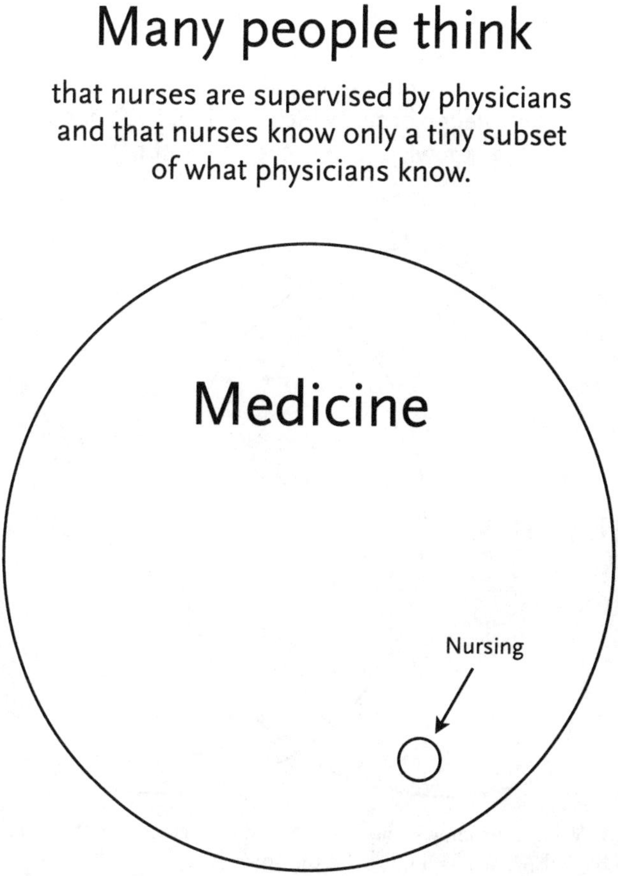
Many people think
that nurses are supervised by physicians
and that nurses know only a tiny subset
of what physicians know.
Medicine
Nursing

FIGURE 4.1 Many people think that nurses are supervised by physicians and that nurses know only a tiny subset of what physicians know.

As Figure 4.2 illustrates, there is a significant overlap with medicine, but nursing is not a subset of the medical profession. In the United States, nurse-controlled state boards administer rigorous nurse licensing examinations, and practicing nurses have independent malpractice liability and codes of ethics. State laws typically describe nursing practice in broad terms that do not depend on physicians. California's Nursing Practice Act defines nursing as care that promotes health and "require[s] a substantial amount of scientific knowledge or technical skill."[11] This Act provides that the profession includes patient care, disease prevention, health assessment and intervention, and the administration of medications and other procedures "ordered" by physicians or other advanced practitioners. These state laws make clear that nursing manages itself. They define nursing practice to include a wide range of critical

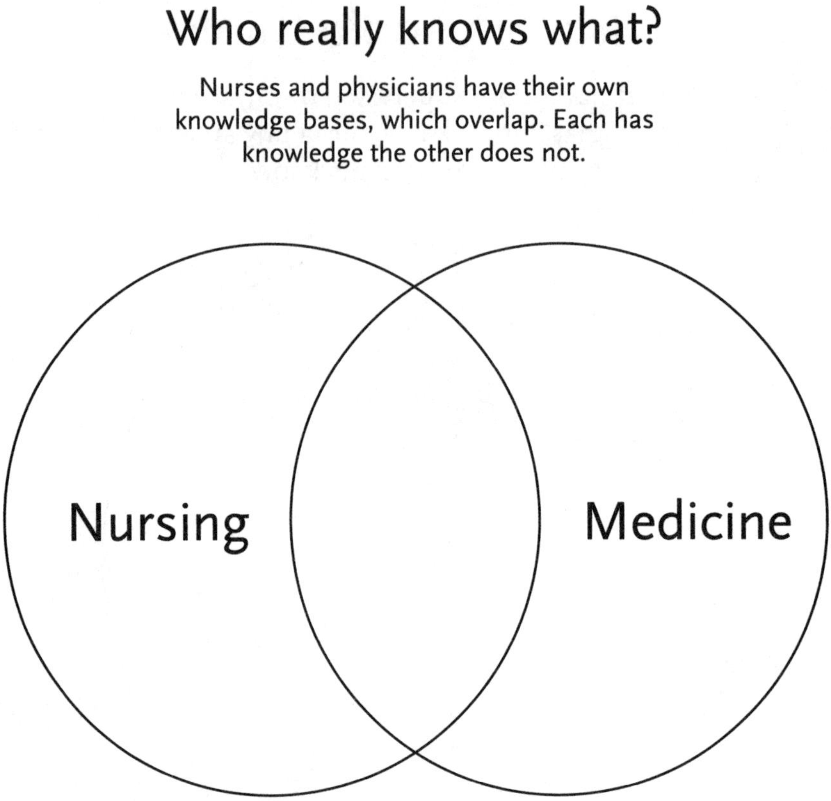
Who really knows what?
Nurses and physicians have their own knowledge bases, which overlap. Each has knowledge the other does not.
Nursing
Medicine

FIGURE 4.2 Who really knows what? Nurses and physicians have their own knowledge bases, which overlap. Each has knowledge the other does not.

prevention and care functions that do not depend on physicians or anyone else. Of course, physicians have more practical power. Reasons include the economic benefits physicians receive in healthcare financing structures, physicians' generally higher levels of education and political clout, long-standing class and gender disparities, and the social esteem physicians enjoy. Figure 4.3 shows the basic relation of nursing to medicine in terms of power.

Nurses administer treatments prescribed by advanced practitioners, and some language in these nursing practice acts (e.g., "ordered" in the California law) may suggest a subordinate relationship as to those tasks. In media portrayals, nurses often follow physician "orders" automatically, as if they were mandatory military orders. But these are really prescriptions or care plans, not orders. The very use of the term "orders" should end, because it does connote subservience, as Chuck Reuter and Virginia Fitzsimons argue in an excellent op-ed in the August 2013 issue of the *American Journal of Nursing*.[12]

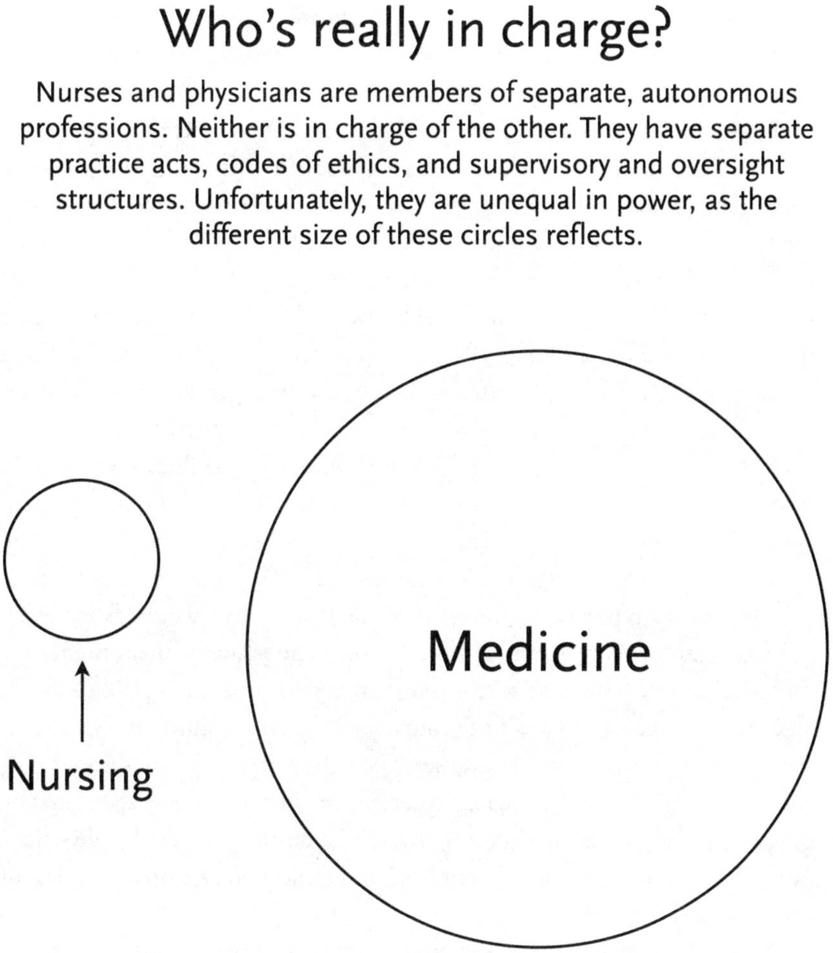
Who's really in charge?
Nurses and physicians are members of separate, autonomous professions. Neither is in charge of the other. They have separate practice acts, codes of ethics, and supervisory and oversight structures. Unfortunately, they are unequal in power, as the different size of these circles reflects.
Medicine
Nursing

FIGURE 4.3 Who's really in charge? Nurses and physicians are members of separate, autonomous professions. Neither is in charge of the other. They have separate practice acts, codes of ethics, and supervisory and oversight structures. Unfortunately, they are unequal in power, as the different size of these circles reflects.

Nurses have ethical and legal obligations to assess all planned care. They are not relieved of malpractice liability simply because they were administering treatment as prescribed. Nurses' patient advocacy may include persistent negotiation with advanced practitioners, refusing to participate in care plans they deem unsafe, and if necessary getting appropriate authorities to stop such actions.

Do nurses find any of that easy to do, given current power structures? No. Speaking up is especially hard for nurses who have recently emigrated from developing nations to wealthier ones. These nurses may have a tenuous immigration status and families who depend greatly on their continued income. Some may not have been trained to assert themselves with physicians.

Does nurses' advocacy sometimes fail because physicians have more power? Of course. Hospitals have fired nurses for advocating for patients, particularly when that advocacy has run counter to the desires of powerful physicians who are seen as revenue generators. Some years ago a Canadian nurse friend of ours was fired from a Caribbean hospital for telling a tourist patient that she should return to the United States for an operation, rather than allow a dangerously inept local surgeon to do it. Physicians pressured nursing managers to fire the nurse, and sadly, the managers gave in to the pressure. But that still does not make nurses subordinate to physicians.

In fact, nurses have significant practical autonomy in clinical settings. In hospitals, where most US nurses practice, nurses are hired, fired, and managed by other nurses. Hospital nurses are typically led by a chief of nursing, who reports to the hospital's chief executive. We have never heard of a chief of nursing who reported to the chief of medicine. Physicians lack expertise in many areas of nursing, and it would make little sense for them to manage nurses. The same basic structure is found in nursing homes. In public schools and other public health positions, nurses are effectively autonomous within the scope of their professional duties. Even the nurses who practice in outpatient offices are operating autonomously within the scope of their nursing practice, although they may be employees of a business owned by physicians or others. Nurses must follow their legal and ethical obligations regardless of their employer's identity.

Courts have begun to awaken to the fact that nursing is a distinct scientific profession with its own standards and scope of care. For decades, US courts tended to wrongly regard nursing as a subset of medicine. Accordingly, physicians were permitted to testify as to the standard of nursing care in malpractice actions, as Ellen K. Murphy noted in a November 2004 article in the *Association of periOperative Registered Nurses Journal*.[13] But in *Sullivan v. Edward Hospital* (2004), the Illinois Supreme Court concluded that a physician was not qualified to testify as to a nursing standard of care because he was not a nurse. This case was specific to the Illinois statutory and judicial context, but Murphy rightly described it as "judicial recognition [of] nurses' long-time assertion that nursing is an independent profession with a unique body of knowledge and not simply a subcategory of medicine."[14] In a later case, *Smith v. Pavlovich* (2009), an Illinois appeals court concluded that a physician was not qualified to testify about the standard of care of an advanced practice nurse.[15]

The American Association of Nurse Attorneys explained why only nurses should be allowed to provide expert testimony as to nursing care in a September 2004 position paper:

> Nursing is a profession, unique, identifiable and autonomous. As a profession, nursing has the authority and responsibility to define its standards of practice.... It is clear that the profession of nursing, though closely related to the practice of medicine, is, indeed, distinct with its own licensing scheme, educational requirements, areas of specialization, Code of Ethics, models, theories and contract with society.... The nurse is not a "junior doctor" nor is the nurse a mere "underling" of the physician. To so hold would negate the existence of nursing as a profession and would render the Nurse Practice Acts of every state, commonwealth and territory meaningless. It is unlikely that any physician, unless he/she has completed a nursing program and has practiced as a nurse, can offer competent, reliable expert opinion on these nursing standards.

The notion that nurses report to physicians has several sources. Historically, nurses deferred to physicians, for reasons that include the disparity of power between the genders. Many nurses remain reluctant to challenge physicians or to assert themselves generally, as Bernice Buresh and Suzanne Gordon showed in their groundbreaking book *From Silence to Voice*.[16] More than 90 percent of nurses are still female, and overall gender equality has not been achieved. At the same time, assertive women do have a wide range of career choices, and many avoid nursing because they want to break gender boundaries, not be confined by them. In addition, physicians' combination of economic power and social status remains unmatched. Physicians have more years of formal education than most (although not all) nurses. Most physicians are not well-informed about nursing, and many believe they are in charge of patient care. Consistent with this authoritarian vision, physician disrespect, disruptive behavior, and even abuse remain issues in many care settings, as Gordon showed in *Nursing Against the Odds* (2005).[17]

Assumptions about physician supervision run so deep that some nursing advocates seem to doubt that nursing is autonomous, including Suzanne Gordon and Dana Beth Weinberg, who wrote *Code Green: Money-Driven Hospitals and the Dismantling of Nursing* (2003).[18] In reaching these flawed conclusions, some of these advocates rely on the views of workplace sociologists rather than nursing leaders. But there is a difference between having less power and being subordinate, which suggests that one party reports to another in a formal sense (i.e., a master-servant relationship). Physicians are no more the conceptual "masters" of nurses than the United States is the master of India. Just as human rights do not cease to exist simply because they are not fully observed, nursing autonomy does not cease to exist simply because it is subject to daunting practical constraints.

Even some prominent nurses do not seem to understand nursing autonomy. In a March 2013 post on the *New York Times* site, oncology nurse Theresa Brown discussed the choices nurses face when they disagree with a physician's care plan. Brown stated that there is a "legal, established hierarchy between doctors and nurses" and that physicians are "ultimately responsible for clinical decisions," apparently because nurses implement physician "orders."[19] In a May 2011 *Times* op-ed about physician bullying, Brown opined that "if doctors are generals, nurses are a combination of infantry and aides-de-camp."[20] Brown's pieces are generally helpful, but her views on autonomy are not.

Career seekers who have the qualities nursing requires value autonomy greatly. It is not hard to see why they would have little interest in the subordinate images they often see in the media. They must understand that nurses can be healthcare leaders and that nurses' autonomous practice has saved countless lives, despite the prevailing belief that it does not exist. Nursing has been a kind of shadowy superhero, saying little and doing much: the Dark Knight Nurse. But that must change if the profession is to meet the health challenges ahead.

Media Portrayals of the Nurse as an Autonomous Professional

The most influential entertainment media regularly presents nurses as physician handmaidens who are peripheral to serious health care. But some news and even entertainment items do convey a sense that nurses operate with autonomy.

Nursing Authority in Television and Film

Bitches and Autonomous Professionals

Very little entertainment television presents nurses as autonomous. It's true that all three of the US nurse shows introduced in 2009, as well as the United Kingdom's *Call the Midwife*, have generally portrayed nurses as operating on their own without the need of direct physician supervision. But only *Call the Midwife* has avoided suggestions that nurses report to physicians.

On *Call the Midwife*, nurse-midwives provide autonomous care and health advice to patients in a poor London neighborhood in the 1950s. Most clinical scenes involve the midwives seeing patients on their own in the community. Physicians do appear occasionally, particularly at a clinic for pregnant women that the midwives open periodically, but overall the focus is on the nurses, in a reversal of the standard Hollywood model. The senior midwives guide the junior ones, and all report to the wise, authoritative yet tactful mother superior, Sister Julienne. In the series premiere, broadcast in the United States in September 2012, local police tried ineffectually to stop a street fight between two women, one of whom was a pregnant patient of the midwives. The commanding Sister Evangelina appeared and brought the proceedings to a halt with one sharp question, then escorted her patient away. It is difficult to imagine this senior midwife uttering an obsequious "right away, doctor!"[21] In an episode broadcast in the United States in April 2013, lead character Jenny encountered an abusive surgeon while working at a local hospital. The episode showed the surgeon's undue power, but it did not suggest that Jenny reported to him. Instead, she took her concerns about his abuse and his dangerous errors to her nurse manager.[22]

Nurses on *Nurse Jackie* also generally follow their own practice model, managing patients' physical and psychosocial care. The emergency department (ED) nurses report to manager Gloria Akalitus, a nurse whose exact role is unclear but who seems to have some supervisory authority over the pharmacy and to some extent even the physicians. Jackie mentors the gifted newer nurse Zoey Barkow, a valuable illustration of nursing autonomy that mirrors the common physician training focus of more conventional hospital shows. Jackie has also helped to train new physicians, particularly Fitch Cooper, arguing against misguided care plans, showing him how to relate to patients, and even, in early 2013 episodes, how to do a better job training a seemingly incompetent junior physician. In June 2012 episodes, Jackie actually took over the ED in the midst of a staffing crisis, running it expertly until the hospital CEO and physician Mike Cruz fired her.[23]

Unfortunately, in recent seasons the show has repeatedly suggested that physicians direct nurse staffing and care. Spring 2011 episodes had physician Eleanor O'Hara removing nurses from cases based on her perceptions of where they fit best,[24] something nurse managers do and physicians have nothing to do with. In 2012, Cruz demoted Akalitus and the show had no nurse managers at all, as if Cruz was playing that role.[25] The 2013 plotlines featured Zoey, who has always deferred too much to physicians, doing various nonnursing tasks for them. A May 2013 episode showed her transcribing Cooper's dictation, a horrendous handmaiden touch.[26] In June 2013 episodes, she spent a lot of time helpfully organizing the office of the chief of ED medicine Ike Prentiss, a symptom of subordination that was not relieved when it was revealed that the two were also having sex.[27]

HawthoRNe addressed nurse-physician power relations more than the other nurse shows, partly through its focus on a chief nursing officer, but also in its frequent portrayals of interactions between staff nurses and physicians. Christina Hawthorne was in command of her nursing staff, and showing viewers the nursing authority structure has great value. Christina also stood up to physicians and the hospital CEO, fighting hard for nurses and patients alike (unrealistically, she often provided direct care). But the show also suggested more than once that she reported to the chief of surgery.[28]

The *HawthoRNe* staff nurses generally followed their own practice model. But those nurses were often weak and submissive. The contemptuous surgeon Brenda Marshall repeatedly argued that the nurses had to do whatever she said, and although the show at times indicated that she was a poor physician, it did not really refute her views of nurse-physician relations. In the June 2009 premiere, nurse Ray Stein knew that Brenda's insulin prescription would endanger a diabetic patient and he challenged it. But faced with her abuse, he wrongly told himself that he had to do what physicians said, and he gave the drug anyway. The patient soon crashed.[29] By the summer 2011 episodes, Brenda had mellowed somewhat. But a long plotline in which the gifted young nurse Kelly Epson moved from pediatrics to the OR reduced Kelly to a silly neophyte begging Brenda to hire and mentor her.[30]

Nurses on *Mercy* also seemed to be engaged in their own health practice in caring and fighting for patients. Veronica Callahan resisted some physician care plans. In the September 2009 series premiere, she advocated successfully to give a dying cancer patient the option to stop treatment.[31] The next month, Chloe Payne pushed relentlessly (with no physician involvement) to locate scarce rabies vaccine for a patient in desperate need.[32] The show also included occasional appearances by Helen Klowden, who was increasingly portrayed as a nurse manager. In a November 2009 episode, nurse Sonia Jimenez urged a high schooler to follow the student's own instincts about whether to have sexual reassignment surgery. The student's parents complained to Helen, who defended Sonia.[33]

But there were also indications that nurses report to physicians. In early episodes, when Veronica lost control, she got in trouble with physician managers. In the premiere, the apparent chief of medicine threatened to "fire" her.[34] In an October 2009 episode, Veronica refused chief of ED medicine Dan Harris's command to discharge a homeless veteran whose hepatitis

Veronica wanted to treat. Harris asked Veronica: "Can you read the letters on my [ID] badge? Mine has an M and a D, yours has an R and an N. I tell *you* what to do." Veronica responded by throwing a cinder block through Harris's car windshield, but that did not prove his statement wrong.[35] In a May 2010 episode, nurse Angel Garcia begged Harris to let him stay on a case, as if physicians controlled nurse staffing.[36]

ER at times showed its nurse characters working with a degree of independence, although the show has also been one of the most persuasive purveyors of the handmaiden image. Nurse manager Eve Peyton, who appeared in some late 2005 episodes, managed the ED nursing staff with authority and resisted physician care plans when necessary, although her management style did cause other characters to see her as a "bitch." Peyton upset chief resident Archie Morris by holding a nursing staff meeting, and she embarrassed him with her superior clinical knowledge when he tried to break it up. Later a chastised Morris told fellow physicians that he could not interfere because nurses are "autonomous professionals."[37] Peyton's departure in December 2005 was deeply flawed, as we will see in Chapter 8, although she was at least fired by the "nursing supervisor."[38] Major nurse character Sam Taggart often operated with some autonomy, advocating strongly for patients with physicians and others. In one December 2006 episode, she took the lead in caring for a homeless patient found on the street in the freezing Chicago winter after another local hospital had dumped the patient. Sam forced that hospital to deliver the grateful patient to her parents' house an hour away.[39]

The sitcom *Parks & Recreation* has included a few good illustrations of nursing autonomy. In recent seasons nurse Ann Perkins, the best friend of the lead character, was the public relations director for the city health department. Ann seemed to operate more or less on her own. Her public health efforts did run up against the dysfunction that surrounded her. In one September 2011 episode, she asked the telegenic city manager Chris to star in a public service announcement about diabetes, although the show audience's main takeaway was likely how Chris acted as if he was making an Oscar contender.[40]

Another show that displayed significant nursing autonomy was the miniseries *RAN: Remote Area Nurse*, which aired on Australia's SBS-TV in early 2006. The drama's public health nurse Helen Tremaine was the only licensed health professional living on a Torres Strait island, and she provided a range of care on her own. Tremaine pushed back against a visiting physician's attempts to tell her what to do with an at-risk pregnant patient—"Since when does a registered nurse outrank a qualified physician?"—though there remained a sense that he was the ultimate health authority.[41]

Some television documentaries have effectively conveyed nursing autonomy. The United Kingdom's *24 Hours in A&E* has shown emergency nurses managing challenging patients at London's King's College Hospital and providing a wide range of care on their own. In an installment broadcast in the United States in November 2011, senior sister Jen seemed to be more or less running the unit. One of her main tasks was trying to keep rival gangs apart while allowing them some access to their wounded comrades.[42] The recent *Showtime* documentary series *Time of Death* included a few good, if limited, portrayals of autonomous hospice and oncology nurses. In the November 2013 series premiere, an oncology nurse gave a patient good advice about helping her children cope with her impending death at the same time as the nurse was expertly administering chemotherapy.[43] The Discovery Health Channel documentaries *Lifeline: The Nursing Diaries*[44] (2004) and *Nurses*[45] (2002), discussed in Chapter 3, showed skilled nurses working autonomously at major US hospitals, suggesting that physicians do not direct nursing care. One 2003 episode of the National Geographic Channel's *Doctors Without Borders: Life in the Field*, a series about the nonprofit organization, actually focused primarily on the independent work of its nurses. The episode included the stories of a veteran nurse running a healthcare system in an Ivory Coast prison, as well as nurses fighting tuberculosis during a refugee crisis in Sierra Leone and in a depressed region of Uzbekistan.[46]

Confronting the Zombies

A few of the recent films discussed in Chapter 3 also suggested nursing autonomy through strong major nurse characters providing vital health care with little or no physician involvement. In the *Meet the Parents* installment *Little Fockers*, lead character Greg Focker had the usual comic misadventures, but he also directed a medical-surgical unit and provided important care on his own, including acting quickly to save his father-in-law after an apparent heart attack.[47] In Zack Snyder's apocalyptic zombie film *Dawn of the Dead*, nurse character Ana was the lone health professional patching up and caring for her band of survivors.[48] In Mike Nichols's HBO adaptation of Tony Kushner's play *Angels in America*, nurse Belize appeared to be the only real health practitioner on his New York AIDS ward. When physician Henry came to have his patient Roy Cohn admitted one night, Henry was annoyed that Belize did not jump to attention. Henry sniffed that nurses were supposed to wear white. Belize responded that physicians were supposed to be home in Westchester, asleep.[49]

Nichols explored some similar territory in his 2001 HBO adaptation of Margaret Edson's play *Wit*. The film portrayed the tough but emotionally homeless scholar Vivian Bearing's confrontation with a life-threatening illness. Nurse Susie Monahan was not an intellectual, but she did want to provide Vivian with professional health care. That brought her into conflict with the self-indulgent research physicians pushing Vivian's chemotherapy and heroic measures to prolong her life. Despite their differences, the two women formed an important bond. Audra McDonald's performance as Susie was a bit too meek, but she displayed a fiery core in stopping the physicians from going against Bearing's wishes.[50] (McDonald moved on to play a heroic physician on *Private Practice*.)

Recent films about World War II have also offered glimpses of nursing autonomy. Joe Wright's 2007 film adaptation of the 2003 novel *Atonement* followed Ian McEwan's characters into the carnage of World War II, and in doing so it included a look at British wartime nursing. The movie added visuals to the book's powerful account of hospital care, showing the formidable authority of the senior nurses and the courage required of all the nurses caring for the horrifically wounded soldiers.[51] Neither the film nor the book conveyed much of the expertise that nursing requires, but both presented nurse-centered visions of care in which physicians played virtually no role.

True Colors in the News Media

Some of the lengthy press accounts of nursing discussed in Chapter 3 are also effective portrayals of nursing autonomy. Julian Guthrie's March 2012 *San Francisco Chronicle* profile of University of California San Francisco nursing dean David Vlahov traced the career path of a healthcare leader with no suggestion that it depended on physicians.[52] John Blanton's April 2007 *Wall Street Journal* piece describing his experience as a new burn unit nurse gave readers a detailed account of nurse-driven care, with the physician role limited to a reference to the need to "keep a close eye on what doctors ordered."[53] The value of these accounts is not that they suggest physicians' work does not matter, but that they show that nursing care is based on nurses' own unique scope of practice.

Likewise, items that consult nurses as experts send the message that they are independent health authorities. For example, although the *New York Times* remains far more likely to consult physicians, in July 2013 the paper ran a long "Ask an Expert" column featuring York College nursing professor and advanced practice nurse Julia Bucher. She gave practical, sensitive advice to readers caring for relatives with cancer.[54] In May 2013, the *Times* had a short "Room for Debate" feature about the ethics of force-feeding inmates on hunger strike at the Guantanamo Bay prison. One of the five "debaters" was Ann Gallagher, director of the International Centre for Nursing Ethics at Surrey University, who argued that it is ethical for nurses to decline to force-feed inmates.

Two December 2004 items presented nurses as the driving force in outpatient clinics. South Africa's *Star* ran a piece by Kerry Cullinan about the challenges faced by nurse managers at the legendary Alexandra Clinic, which handles chronic illnesses and labor and delivery in an overcrowded township.[55] A column by Phillippa Stevenson in the *New Zealand Herald* paid tribute to palliative care nurse Cynthia Ward, founder of True Colours, a health service that "aims to support families at and from the moment their child is diagnosed with a chronic, serious or life-threatening illness."[56]

Some press pieces showcase the autonomous work of public health nurses. Of course, stories about school nurses may do that. An August 2013 Associated Press report by Carolyn Thompson stressed the independent leadership role of modern school nurses in disease prevention and detection, managing chronic conditions, and mental health.[57] An August 2011 United Press International item reported that research to be published in the *Journal of School Health* had shown that a curriculum developed by Cincinnati Children's Hospital nurse and "suicide prevention expert" Cathy Strunk significantly reduced rates of attempted suicide.[58] With regard to older patient populations, in May 2013 *BBC News* published a report by Adam Brimelow about a nurse-run Dutch home care firm that employs thousands of district nurses. Those nurses work in "self-steering teams" to provide holistic, cost-effective care, reducing hospital and nursing home stays; the nurses complement their community-building with a weekly health radio show.[59] Similarly, in July 2007 the *Copenhagen Post* ran a piece about a "mobile nurse task force"—that is, two nurses on bicycles—who diagnose and treat most of their elderly patients' problems at the patients' homes, avoiding traumatic and costly hospital visits.[60] In January 2004 the *Toronto Star* ran Scott Simie's piece about the work of "street nurse" Cathy Crowe, one of Canada's most prominent advocates for the homeless.[61]

Although Hollywood's depictions of military nurses have focused on the past, the news media has offered more current accounts of military nurses practicing with autonomy. In June 2012 PBS aired a segment as part of its "Need to Know" series in which William Brangham profiled three San Diego nurses who provide ongoing outpatient care to veterans who have returned home with posttraumatic stress disorder and other problems. The profile of nurse scientist Jill Bormann, who was investigating the use of mantram therapy to manage posttraumatic stress disorder, was especially impressive.[62] In March 2007 NPR ran a *Leading Ladies* profile, "Clara Adams-Ender: Army Achiever." Cheryl Corley interviewed the retired general, who headed the Army Nurse Corps from 1987 to 1991. General Adams-Ender discussed her career, although the profile had little to say about nursing.[63] In fact, General Adams-Ender had apparently established the first neonatal intensive care unit in Germany, but NPR failed to mention it. Still, the piece did show that nurses can lead at the highest levels.

"Nurse, Hand Me My Laptop": Media Portrayals of the Nurse as Handmaiden

The handmaiden image infects even media directed at children. In Holly Hobbie's 2008 book *Fanny*, an inventive girl made her own "Annabelle" doll after her mother refused to buy her glamorous Barbie-like "Connie" dolls like those her friends had. When the friends all decided to play veterinary hospital, "Dr. Annabelle performed operations on every stuffed animal . . . while the glamorous [Connie] nurses assisted." "Dr. Annabelle" listened to a teddy bear with a stethoscope. The "nurse" dolls looked pretty but useless in skimpy white dresses.[64]

In June 2009 the *Examiner* websites posted a transcript of an interview in which *The View* co-host Whoopi Goldberg explained the professional aspirations of Brenda, the lead character in the *Sugar Plum Ballerinas* children's books Goldberg had written. Goldberg said that Brenda's desire to be a physician is not unusual today, because girls these days have seen "*ER* in reruns" and have not "been told what they couldn't do," in contrast to girls of Goldberg's generation, who "all heard, 'You have to be a nurse first. You have to be a helper. You can't be a doctor. Be a helper.' "

In November 2007 Seattle's Group Health ran Internet advertisements for its "Ask the Doc" service, in which patients communicate with advanced practitioners by email. The tag line: "Nurse, hand me my laptop." Yes, maybe laptops are the new stethoscopes. But get your own laptop, buddy, we're busy saving lives. Of course, nurses do hand physicians things when care requires. However, these advertisements suggested that nurses are gofers whose use of advanced care technology consists mainly of handing it to physicians, the *real* health experts. But in hospital settings and many others, nurses are the main patient educators. Nurses at Group Health itself regularly communicate with patients by email!

Those nurses persuaded Group Health to pull the advertisement. Ms. Goldberg returned our calls and discussed our concerns that her comments presented nurses as handmaidens, indicating that she would bear them in mind going forward. But the popular media sends these same messages every day. Influential entertainment television shows often portray authoritative physicians telling submissive nurses what to do. These scenarios reinforce the prevailing notion that nursing is all about doing physicians' bidding, especially since the great majority of nursing is rarely shown.

Grey's Anatomy: "You're the Man"

No one could possibly think from watching the hundreds of episodes of *Grey's Anatomy* that have aired since 2005 that nurses were anything but physician subordinates. The vast majority of nurses who appear are silent servants. Time and again, the show has told viewers that the nurses report to physicians. Nurses on *Grey's* have occasionally displayed resentment and petty vindictiveness when abused by their physician masters.[65] But that is not the same as being an autonomous professional.

Grey's nurses have, very rarely, questioned physician care plans. In a December 2013 episode, a hospital patient crashed. The weak junior surgeon Leah Murphy rushed in with a nurse and informed the nurse that the patient was having a myocardial infarction, ordering her to get an electrocardiogram and crash cart. The nurse mutely complied. Soon, the bullying junior surgeon Shane Ross insisted on operating. First Murphy and then the nurse urged Ross to wait for a senior surgeon. The nurse caved after Ross barked that he would wait, but then the nurse would have to explain to the attending physician that the patient had died "because you wouldn't let me help him." In the OR, the patient began bleeding heavily. Murphy and then an OR nurse suggested bypass. But Ross insisted on trying to stitch up the perforation, and they allowed him to do so, even as he became desperate and lost control, clearly in over his head. Finally, Murphy found senior surgeon Richard Webber to help; only he could pry Ross away. In terms of nursing advocacy, these two scenes were among the strongest in the show's long run. But these nurses were still just gentle patient safety speedbumps, echoing Murphy's cautious impulses. The physicians were in charge.[66]

Even the episodes with the more assertive nurse Eli, discussed in Chapter 3, reinforced the handmaiden image in the end.[67] Consider a March 2011 episode in which Eli pressed surgeon Miranda Bailey to explain to a patient the risks of participating in a clinical trial—right in front of the patient! Later, Bailey claimed that Eli had violated the hospital's "doctor-nurse protocol." Although the lovebirds made up near the end of the episode, that happened after Eli made this forceful speech:

> Miranda Bailey, we are not inside the hospital. Inside the hospital, you're the man. That's the protocol. But outside, I'm the man. *I . . . am the man*. Me. You can call me Cro-Magnon, or old-fashioned, but that is not gonna stop me from taking you home to my bed tonight and showin' you what kind of man I am. Now, how's that? Does that protocol suit you?

Rather than vomiting, Bailey looks impressed. But having a nurse character endorse the idea that physicians are "the man" inside the hospital is, well, Cro-Magnon.

In an October 2009 episode, the *Grey's* hospital merged with another hospital, and chief of surgery Richard Webber—who also seemed to function as the hospital's chief of medicine and CEO—made staff cuts. With no suggestion that nurse managers exist, Webber let many nurses go, including the pathetic nurse Olivia.[68] Surgeon Derek "McDreamy" Shepherd offered to give Olivia a reference, since he doubtless knew her nursing skills well after years of supervising her! (Of course, not really.)

In a May 2008 episode, Seattle Grace's nurses boycotted all surgeries of plastic surgeon Mark "McSteamy" Sloane because he had loved and left too many of them. The nurses actually complained to their union, and a union representative showed up to get Webber to force all physicians and nurses to submit the names of their sexual contacts. Among other things, that was a clear suggestion that the chief of surgery managed nurses. Finally, chief resident Miranda Bailey called about forty of the nurses together in the hospital atrium to publicly chastise them and get them back to work. Bailey called Sloane a "whore" but stressed that he was a good surgeon and the nurses all knew his reputation, so "let us all close our knees and get back to our jobs." Not a single nurse could reply. Bailey shouted "Disperse!" and the nurse-sheep ambled back to their pastures.[69]

The January 2007 episode in which Sloane praised nurses also had him punishing the interns by dumping nurses' apparently disgusting work—debriding bedsores—on the interns. (Few real nurses would find this disgusting; it is an important professional responsibility.) Presumably, Sloane supervised both the interns and the nurses. His statement that the nurses were "helpful" actually reinforced damaging assumptions. Of course "helpful" is a good thing in general, but this comment in context suggested that nurses are helpful in the physician mission of providing all meaningful health care, rather than in providing autonomous nursing care. "Helpful" is pretty faint praise for life-saving health professionals. Would anyone suggest that physicians, as a class, are "helpful?"

In a September 2006 episode, nurse Tyler smugly informed intern Cristina that he was part of a team that had just saved a life in a code.[70] But Tyler said that only to justify his failure to earn the $20 Cristina had paid him to act as a lookout so she could have sex with her boyfriend in his hospital bed. Tyler seemed to get the last laugh, but he was still a lackey who accepted $20 tips for tasks other than his real job. Later, Tyler paged intern George O'Malley to tell him that a cancer patient had been shoplifting and was planning to leave without having her operation. Then Tyler stepped back to let George handle the important psychosocial issues. Plainly, Tyler worked for George, not the patient.

The January 2006 nurses' strike episodes repeatedly told viewers that the nurses report to the chief of surgery.[71] These episodes made a few points about short-staffing and forced overtime. But the episodes presented the nurses as bitter serfs and suggested that nursing is mostly about paperwork, room assignments, and trivial patient quirks. The chief of surgery's "assistant" Patricia was described as someone who "used to" be a nurse. But now, Patricia managed the nursing crisis. After all, the show has no nurse managers. Patricia lectured some temporary nurses about how the patient charts are organized by room number, then addressed nearby attending surgeons Burke and Shepherd: "You know why I stopped being a nurse? Doctors. Doctors who don't know how to pitch in." These two surgeons told the chief he should resolve the strike, but the chief said it would take $2 million per year to hire the extra nurses needed. Finally, the chief admitted to Patricia that "we" need the nurses, and, at her suggestion, he ended the strike by forgoing the purchase of a surgical robot he had recently ordered.

An April 2005 episode presented a scrub nurse as a loyal subordinate of the surgeons. The nurse, a dying pancreatic cancer patient named Elizabeth Fallon, was formidable and savvy.[72] She had worked for decades with Ellis Grey, the legendary surgeon mother of lead character Meredith. Ellis recalled that Fallon was an "excellent" nurse, but Fallon was also seen as a career physician appendage, focused on gruffly charting the progress of the physicians around her. Fallon's remark that she was "Ellis's scrub nurse for eighteen years" was an insult to perioperative nurses, who are professionals with their own science-based scope of practice. Nurses work *with* surgeons, not for them.

House: Help! Golems Are Loose in the Hospital!

Nurse characters on *House* probably spoke and did even less than nurses on the other major Hollywood hospital shows, and as a result, the show's handmaiden portrayal may have been the most absolute. The vast majority of nurse appearances involved a character popping up out of nowhere to absorb a physician command, like the golems of Jewish folklore—mute, brainless humanoids crafted from inanimate material for basic tasks by the wisest and holiest, notably early rabbis.[73] Recall from Chapter 3 that House himself joked during a "playing God" monologue in a November 2005 episode that cleanup tasks were why he had "created nurses."[74] Nurses could also be timid bureaucrats; from time to time *House* showed a nurse acting as a silent administrative assistant to "dean of medicine" Lisa Cuddy. A very minor exception was Nurse Jeffrey, a snarky, effeminate nurse who appeared in three episodes in the show's final years and made some effort to match House's obnoxious comments. But serious clinical practice was not a focus of Jeffrey's scenes.[75]

In the April 2008 episode with the nurses' strike plotline, House glibly announced that he did not "use nurses."[76] House could have said he doesn't "practice" with nurses, or (translating into House-speak) that he wouldn't let those fools with Daffy Duck on their clothes get near his patients. But "use" suggests that nurses are just physician tools. The show confirmed this attitude in an exchange between House and Cuddy in which both physicians indicated that Cuddy was in charge of the striking nurses. In fact, dealing with the nurses would presumably be the job of the chief nursing officer. But *House* had no nurse managers.

A May 2007 episode showed the main facets of nurses' role on the show. The complete dialogue of the nurse characters in the episode was as follows: "Yes, doctor." "Right away." "I was just trying to get a urine sample, and he went crazy!"[77] These are the words of handmaidens who perform menial assistive tasks but panic in an emergency, relying on physicians to supply all thinking, expertise, and courage. At one point House entered Cuddy's office. She sat at her desk, as a nurse stood beside her. House: "You girls can gossip later." A moment later, when the nurse had not left, House addressed her: "When I said you girls can gossip later, I was throwing you out in a polite way." Cuddy handed some paperwork to the nurse and made a face suggesting, "You know how he is, we'll come back to this later." The nurse left without a word. After Cuddy and House bantered a while, Cuddy sent House away: "Send in Nurse Unger on your way out." Yes, House trashed everyone, but physician characters like Cuddy were smart and able, and they dealt it back to House in spades. The nurses slinked away like wounded mice.

A May 2006 episode offered excellent examples of the show's "golem" portrayal, with nurses effectively conjured into existence to perform unskilled tasks.[78] At one point physician Chase was with a patient and her father. Giving the patient a chelating agent intravenously to help her body dispose of unwanted iron, Chase explained the procedure to the father. The nurse who would actually perform and explain this task was not there. The patient went into respiratory distress, and a monitor beeped. Chase calmly said, "Crash cart." Within five seconds, two nurses were in the room with a crash cart. One of the nurses handed Chase an intubation tool and he saved the patient's life. Throughout, the nurses said nothing. Later House was alone with this patient and her father. No one else was shown in the room. The intubated patient suddenly had a breathing problem. House wanted to eject the father, ostensibly so he could do some scary procedure (actually he just wanted to continue berating the patient). House turned to a nurse, who simply was not there before, and commanded, "Get him out of here." The nurse mutely complied. After all, she served House, and there was but one House.

ER: "I'm the Doctor. This Is My Call."

ER ended its long run several years ago, but it remains one of the most powerful modern sources of the handmaiden image. That's because the series' hundreds of episodes have been shown around the world for so long, because its relatively realistic portrayal of hospital care is so persuasive, and because the skilled handmaiden image is so central to the show's nursing portrayal.[79]

Although *ER*'s nursing depictions improved in the show's final years, the handmaiden image continued to appear. In one December 2008 episode, after nurse Sam Taggart had taken time off to care for her injured son, chief of emergency medicine Cate Banfield offered to give Taggart more time—clearly indicating that nurses report to the chief ED physician.

November 2007 *ER* episodes also suggested that nurses report to physicians. One had chief of ED medicine Kevin Moretti implementing new triage policies and actually telling Taggart, "Sam, you're supposed to be covering triage right now." Taggart complied. In another scene, intern Tony Gates and Taggart led some nurses through the ED explaining new policies, including treating pain at triage and recording the Wong-Baker pain score. Gates:

"Put it in your charts, the docs will be checking."[80] These scenes told viewers that physicians direct nurses and that physicians direct triage. In fact, nurse managers do that. And it is nurses who have led the way in pain management, despite decades of physician resistance.

Another plotline in the November 2007 episodes was about a precocious thirteen year old named Josh, who was dying of an incurable neurological disorder.[81] The boy wanted to avoid the ventilator, and Gates cleared that idea with his attending and the hospital's ethics office—but not the boy's mother or Taggart. When Taggart saw this plan presented to the boy's mother as a foregone conclusion, she objected. Outside, Gates informed the veteran nurse how nasty ventilators are, no doubt based on his superior knowledge of ventilator care and his more holistic approach. (We're kidding.) Gates contemptuously told Taggart that they would not be intubating. Taggart started to call the ethics line, but Gates said he'd already discussed it with ethics, then grabbed the telephone from Taggart and slammed it down, yelling, "Stop! I'm the doctor. This is my call. Now you can either mix this morphine drip or you can take yourself off this case, because we're done here." Taggart stalked off.

Thus, as was usually the case when *ER* physicians dismissed nurses like this, Taggart had no answer, leaving the impression that although Gates was harsh, what he said was correct—major care decisions we indeed "his call." The story showed Taggart as a spirited patient advocate and educator, but also as a somewhat myopic subordinate who could be excluded from key care discussions and who ultimately had to give way to the end-of-life wisdom of the *physicians*. This incident also seemed to be a turning point in Gates's development. Uppity nurse Sam thought she could question Dr. Gates's decisions because he was just a resident, but Gates was growing fast, learning to be a *real* physician.

Even the late 2005 Eve Peyton episodes included handmaiden messages. For example, the December 2005 episode in which Peyton got fired began with new chief of ED medicine Luka Kovac sending three ED nurses home—and calling them "support staff"—because he foresaw a light shift.[82]

In an astonishing October 2003 episode, ED nurses staged a walkout when they learned that the hospital planned to reduce their hours and hire supposedly cheaper traveling nurses and new graduates who would work for "minimum wage" (don't ask). In response to the walkout, chief of ED medicine Robert Romano summarily fired six nurses. Then-nurse Abby Lockhart told Romano that he "can't fire nurses." Romano said he could if they walked off the job. To this Lockhart had no real response. There was no evident involvement from any nursing manager. In another scene, ED physician Susan Lewis forbade Lockhart to tell a teenage girl that she had a fatal heart/lung condition, at the behest of the girl's parents. The girl was panicked because she was getting clues that something serious was wrong, but no one would tell her the truth. Lewis impatiently reminded Lockhart that Lewis was the patient's physician, Lockhart was the patient's nurse, and so Lockhart had to do as Lewis said. Lockhart had—you guessed it—no response except to look hurt.[83]

Shut Up and Follow Orders: Nursing on Other Healthcare Shows

Other healthcare shows have done no better than the major ones in portraying nursing autonomy, and in some cases they have been worse.

Clinical scenes on *The Mindy Project* usually occur in an outpatient setting, at a New York obstetrics and gynecology practice. Because Mindy Lahiri and her physician colleagues own the practice, they employ the nurses who work there, Morgan, Beverly, and Tamra. Of course, this is the way many health practices have traditionally operated. So it has always been a special challenge for television shows to portray the nurses who work in such settings as autonomous professionals, rather than the office assistants they are commonly understood to be. It's fair to say that those who make *Mindy* don't even know there is a challenge; a January 2014 episode found Morgan and Tamra bickering inanely over which of them a managing physician would permit to use a certain "phlebotomy desk."[84] Although the *Mindy* nurses are too bizarre and/or nasty to fit the traditional handmaiden image, there is no question that they are silly order-takers who exist solely to serve the physicians, and they rarely interact with patients about clinical matters. Granted, that is probably best for the patients, given who these nurses are.[85] In fact, it's becoming unusual to see this many registered nurses in an outpatient setting, since most practices now save money by employing more staff with less training—although those staff may still be mistaken for nurses, in part because of shows like this.

Private Practice also showed the difficulties with portrayals of nurses in the outpatient setting. The show's early episodes, in late 2007, presented nurse Dell Parker as a receptionist at a Los Angeles clinic owned by a diverse set of physicians. Dell was plainly an assistant to the physicians, with no unique scope of practice. Because he was studying to be a midwife, he was eager to learn what the main character, star obstetrics and gynecology physician Addison Montgomery, could teach him. However, in the series premiere Dell was no more than a willing but ignorant layperson. Well, he did hold a patient's hand on his own initiative and notice that she had passed out.[86]

In later years, the show suggested that Dell had promise as a midwife, particularly after he actually became one and managed a few solo deliveries. But on the whole he remained essentially a helper, continuing to act as an office administrator. Although several episodes in the show's final season included the more assertive nurse Stephanie, other nurses in that season were even more extreme versions of the show's usual handmaidens. In a December 2012 episode, two nurses caring for pregnant physician CEO/chief of medicine Charlotte King were inept—unable to start an intravenous line correctly or even get a pillow—and absolutely terrified of Charlotte. Although Stephanie claimed in passing to be the "floor manager," she also correctly described herself as Charlotte's "beck and call girl."[87]

To the extent *Hart of Dixie* has clinical scenes, they are mainly set in the small town general practice of Zoe Hart, a young New York physician who has taken over her dead father's family practice in Bluebell, Alabama.[88] In the show's first season, some episodes included down-home nurse Addie Pickett. In an October 2011 episode, Addie was introduced as a nurse with 15 years of experience and knowledge of Zoe's father's practice. She donned gloves to help Zoe and collected laboratory results. But mostly Addie acted as Zoe's adoptive older sister, giving her advice about how to fit in with the locals, such as by going to the hair salon to gossip and show that she's real! Addie was a positive character, but her role reinforced the idea that physicians control health care, with basic assistance from nurses who have practical knowledge based on their years on the job.

The patheticomic HBO series *Getting On* has sent mixed messages about nursing autonomy. The weak nurse character Dawn Forchette has often been pushed around by the physician Jenna James, to whom Dawn is far too deferential. Despite that, in one December 2013 episode, Dawn actually told off an emergency physician, somewhat quaveringly, after he had dumped a homeless patient on the geriatric unit. When the emergency physician pushed back, James stood up for Dawn and apparent licensed vocational nurse Didi Ortley. Yet in doing so, James called her colleagues "my nurses."[89]

Getting On has had nurse managers. In the November 2013 premiere, a nursing supervisor challenged James's use of the nursing staff to collect samples for her fecal study. In retaliation, James got the nursing supervisor transferred to another part of the hospital.[90] That is sadly plausible because of the weakness of some nurse managers, but the show failed to make clear that it would at least be a nursing decision. The nursing supervisor for the rest of the first season, Patsy De La Serda, tried to project professionalism and authority. And it was clear that he supervised the nursing staff and did not report to

James. But Patsy was woefully ineffective, as his name would suggest, and the show mocked his customer service sloganeering, abysmal people skills, and self-pitying vulnerability. Patsy's clashes with James about unit policy seemed to end in nil-nil draws, because both characters were so dysfunctional and lacking in real concern for others.

Scrubs, which was generally set in a hospital, presented its physician characters as directing nurses and nursing care.[91] It repeatedly told viewers that the nurses ultimately report to the chief of medicine, although it also suggested that nurse Carla Espinosa, who provided direct care, was a "head nurse." February 2009 episodes highlighted the problem of physician disrespect of nurses, but in these same episodes, Carla reported to chief of medicine Perry Cox on nurse staffing issues, including nursing schedules.[92] One physician told a nurse that the "M.D." on his I.D. badge meant he "makes the decisions." (Maybe *badges* are the secret source of physician power!) The episode suggested that the badge statement was unhelpful, but that the underlying assumption about physician authority was correct. With Carla gone for the show's final season, the few nurse characters were standard Hollywood handmaidens. In a December 2009 episode, a mute nurse in a code scene waited for the physicians to tell her to get a crash cart, fiddled with the patient's bed covers, and then scurried out of the way so the physicians could save the patient by themselves.[93]

An extraordinary November 2003 *Scrubs* episode purported to teach Carla that nursing is all about shutting up and doing what physicians tell you. In that episode, Carla advised resident physician Elliot to give a patient a certain drug, which Elliot did. The patient developed a paradoxical reaction, and Elliot was furious. She told Carla that Elliott's job was to ignore Carla and do whatever Elliott thought was right. Carla's fiancé, surgical resident Turk, told Carla how a surgical nurse with twenty years experience had recently tried to tell him what kind of suture knot to tie. Turk said he had kicked the nurse out of the OR and made her cry, because in the hospital, physicians are in charge. Turk said the job of nurses is to follow physician "orders," because ultimately the physicians are responsible for the patients (and presumably nurses are not). Carla accepted this. A later scene found Elliott and Carla at a patient's bedside. When Elliot asked for a certain treatment, Carla meekly obeyed, smiling, clearly relieved to have learned her proper role as physician helpmate. There was no irony in this megalomaniacal fantasy, which was especially insidious because Carla endorsed it.[94]

Strong Medicine was a hospital show that focused on two female physicians but also included nurse midwife character Peter Riggs, who at times displayed limited autonomy. But even his intermittent appearances were undermined by a persistent vision of physicians as the masters of all health care. Other nurses—when they appeared at all—were almost always faceless servants, silent and submissive. One January 2002 episode about a nursing strike actually did show that nurse short-staffing was deadly and that physicians could not easily do nurses' jobs. But even that episode clearly conveyed that the physicians were in charge. As one striking nurse said (wrongly), physicians are management and nurses are labor. Riggs led the striking nurses, negotiating directly with a physician who appeared to be both chief of medicine and hospital CEO, but no nurse manager ever appeared.[95]

Apart from the 2009 nurse shows, the slew of short-lived recent US hospital dramas have shown no improvement. Recent US shows lasting one season or less that show brilliant physicians directing meek nurse handmaidens include *Monday Mornings; Emily Owens, MD; Do No Harm; The Mob Doctor; A Gifted Man; Off the Map; Miami Medical*; and *Three Rivers*. On these shows, which focused on surgery and trauma, the producers managed to present most clinical interactions with no nurses at all. But when nurses did appear, they were generally deferential order-takers. In an October 2009 episode of *Three Rivers*, no nurse uttered a word that reflected knowledge of patient conditions, but we did count three submissive "yes, doctor!"s from invisible nurses and forearm nurses.[96] In a February 2013 episode of *Emily Owens, MD*, after two nurses complained helplessly that a difficult patient had disconnected her intravenous line and disappeared, the lead physician character had to instruct them to call the police and have maintenance come clean up the mess in the room.[97]

Even on the minority of these shows that included a regular nurse character, the best the nurse could do was to be a respected aide-de-camp of the dominant physicians. On *The Mob Doctor*, lead physician Grace Devlin's best friend was nurse Rosa Quintero, but Rosa's role consisted mainly in looking worried about Grace's mysterious Mob activities and covering up for her at the hospital.[98] *Miami Medical*'s Tuck Brody was the strongest nurse character on any of these shows, a real swaggerer with some clinical knowledge and authority over other nurses. But he still seemed to serve mainly as an executive assistant and head cheerleader for the trauma surgeons he himself glorified as "rock stars." Meanwhile, many of the show's more minor nurse characters were mute ciphers, handing the physicians gloves and wheeling gurneys.[99]

"I'll Go Get the Doctor!": Nursing on Non-Healthcare Shows

As you might expect, some of the worst handmaiden portrayals of nursing appear on shows that are not mainly about health care. In a September 2013 episode of *NCIS: Los Angeles*, two agents who had been tortured arrived at a hospital. In the ED, silent nurses stood by to receive impressive-sounding physician orders for drugs, tests, and even the timing of a gurney transfer in which the commanding physician was not participating. At the time of this episode, the show had producers who had previously worked on *ER* and other hospital dramas.[100]

An April 2008 episode of ABC's *Desperate Housewives* presented a nurse as a mousy physician lackey who could be bribed into revealing sensitive patient information with a free lunch.[101] In the episode, character Gaby's boyfriend Carlos was an inpatient with an eye injury, which only Carlos knew would mean permanent blindness. Another of Carlos's girlfriends, the notorious Edie, visited him in the hospital. But Edie got angry with Carlos and left. Walking down the hall, Edie spotted a nurse eating a sad sandwich. Edie asked when Carlos would get his sight back. Nurse: "I don't know . . . Mr. Solis's condition is very serious. . ." Edie: "Serious? What's wrong?" Nurse: "Well . . . you know, you should really talk to the doctor about this. I don't even think his girlfriend knows." The nurse suggested she had "said too much already," but then she succumbed to Edie's offer to treat her to lunch at a "great little French bistro." Edie easily got information out of the unsophisticated nurse and used it against Gaby and Carlos. The timid nurse could not speak with any real authority, even to say the law and her own ethics limited her ability to speak about the patient. Instead, she tried to pass the buck to the physician who had real power and expertise.

Late 2007 episodes of Larry David's HBO sitcom *Curb Your Enthusiasm* also portrayed nurses as handmaidens. In an October episode, "The N Word," a black surgeon overheard Larry relating a story in which another white man had used that racist word. The furious surgeon, wrongly assuming Larry was the bigot, took revenge on the next white man in his path by shaving the head of his patient, who happened to be Larry's friend Jeff. In the OR, a nurse weakly tried to stop the surgeon but ended up obediently handing him the clippers after the surgeon ordered her to do so. Another nurse tried to cover up what the surgeon did, suggesting to Jeff's wife that it was accidental, before the surgeon ordered the nurse to leave the room so he could apologize.[102]

A July 2005 episode of HBO's *Six Feet Under* suggested that nurses basically help the smart physicians who provide all important care. In the episode, character Nate Fisher was taken to a Los Angeles area hospital after collapsing from a brain hemorrhage. Nate had an operation to stop the bleeding, although he remained in a possibly lengthy coma. Meanwhile, family and friends gathered, including Brenda, his pregnant wife. The family dealt almost entirely with seemingly skilled physicians about Nate's condition. But there was a telling nurse interaction the morning after the operation, when Nate was on a medical-surgical floor with only Brenda present. Nate suddenly woke up. Brenda called for the nearby nurse. The nurse saw Nate and responded, "I'll go get the doctor!" No smile, no support, no assessment, no patient interaction, and no ability to respond to change. The nurse fled the room. She was a terrified flunky.[103]

News Media Helpers

The entertainment media is the leading source of explicit handmaiden imagery, but echoes of it can be found in the news media, which often at least implies that physicians direct all hospital care. Even some articles that highlight nursing skill, such as Scott Allen's October 2005 *Boston Globe* report about the training of a new intensive care unit nurse, fall into this trap to some extent.[104]

For example, recent press reports show that nurses saving lives outside of the clinical setting is news, as we noted in Chapter 3, but if there is a physician present, the nurses will likely be seen as the physician's assistants regardless of what actually happened. In July 2011, the Raleigh, North Carolina area television affiliate WRAL posted a fairly good item by Ken Smith reporting that a nurse driving down a local highway had stopped and helped to save the life of a police officer who had been gravely injured when a truck struck his motorcycle. The nurse, who was quoted, directed others to make tourniquets and made sure the officer's airway remained clear.[105]

But news items about another save the previous month were more problematic. On June 29, 2011, the *Sun Journal* of Lewiston, Maine, reported that a man had had a heart attack *while attending a lecture about heart problems* at a local hospital. Daniel Hartill's piece at least credited not only the cardiologist giving the lecture with saving the man, but also several named nurses in the audience. Based on this report, the nurses seem to have done all of the actual saving, including defibrillation, without much input from the physician. Still, the piece got extensive quotes from the physician, and it offered a photograph of the nurses surrounding him doing "their 'Charlie's Angels' impression," pretending their hands were guns, suggesting that the physician had directed their exploits. The June 29 MSNBC item about the incident was less subtle, leading with a headline that included the phrase "Maine cardiologist saves the audience member's life," although the piece did at least note that a "team of nurses" was part of the effort. A June 30 NPR item said that the patient "was surrounded by cardiac nurses who grabbed a defibrillator and saved his life," but the item also claimed that "Dr. Phillips oversaw the rescue." Perhaps it's natural that the person giving the heart lecture would get more credit than those in the audience, but no piece quoted any of the nurses, and overall the reports show how media assumptions work to reinforce the handmaiden image.[106]

Or consider a story posted in September 2006 on the ABC News website about dangerously long ED waits. An Illinois woman was reportedly found dead in an ED waiting room two hours after a nurse had told her to wait.[107] The coroner found that the woman had shown "classic symptoms of a heart attack" and the coroner's jury ruled the death a homicide. The piece highlighted the serious potential consequences of triage errors, and it also linked the apparent problem in that case to ED overcrowding. But the report seemed to wrongly assume that physicians are ultimately responsible for all ED care. It relied solely on comments from the American College of Emergency Physicians. (We guess ABC News couldn't quite find room on its website for comments from the Emergency Nurses Association; data storage is expensive.) A statement attributed to the president of the American College of Emergency Physicians advised dissatisfied patients to talk to the triage nurse, but if that "doesn't work," to "ask to speak to the emergency physician." This advice gives the mistaken impression that ED nurses report to physicians. In fact, patients in such a situation should generally ask to speak with the charge nurse, the clinical nurse specialist, or the ED nurse manager. *Nurses* are the triage leaders—and the nursing leaders.

Notes

1. L. Okey Onyejekwe Jr., "Doctor of Law and Medicine," *California Lawyer* (May 2008), http://tinyurl.com/okt3s2z.
2. TNN, "Doctors, Nurses Clash at NRS Hospital," *Times of India* (December 10, 2004), http://tinyurl.com/ldtut3v.
3. Joe Kita, "Doctors Confess Their Fatal Mistakes," and Sunnie Bell, "I Didn't Question a Doctor I Knew Was Wrong," *Reader's Digest* (October 2010), http://tinyurl.com/ppjs3z6, http://tinyurl.com/m5hkvgd; TAN, "Death by Disrespect" (October 2010), http://tinyurl.com/qcurmta.

4. Peter Pronovost, "I Could Have Caused Permanent Brain Damage," *Reader's Digest* (October 2010), http://tinyurl.com/ob6pohh.
5. Kevin Keane, "Nurse Snatched Scalpel Off Doctor about to Cut Vein," *Irish Examiner* (December 14, 2013), http://tinyurl.com/p9twqv4; TAN, "Nurse X Confronts a Cutting-Edge Technique" (December 14, 2013), http://tinyurl.com/n55kq58.
6. Jordan Robertson, "Deputies Tackle Neurosurgeon Outside Oakland Operating Room," Associated Press (March 2006), http://tinyurl.com/mfr8tta; CFNA, "McDrunky," TAN (March 9, 2006), http://tinyurl.com/oogtblv.
7. Di Caelers, "Nearly Half of Our Nurses Suffer Abuse" (November 10, 2005), http://tinyurl.com/oxb4bes; CFNA, "A Short Herstory of Violence," TAN (November 10, 2005), http://tinyurl.com/oxf3ldg.
8. John Ensslin, "Nurse Sues Memorial, Claims Surgeon Threw Human Tissue at Her," *Colorado Springs Gazette* (June 26, 2009), http://tinyurl.com/kh6mdqk; TAN, "Can We Get Cultures on That?" (June 26, 2009), http://tinyurl.com/odyp44l.
9. Kevin Sack, "Whistle-Blowing Nurse Is Acquitted in Texas," *New York Times* (February 11, 2010), http://tinyurl.com/mdvy889; TAN, "Remain in Light" (February 11, 2010), http://tinyurl.com/o9khkr7.
10. US Department of Health and Human Services, Health Resources and Services Administration (HRSA), "The Registered Nurse Population: Findings from the 2008 National Sample Survey of Registered Nurses" (2010), http://tinyurl.com/7zgyet7; Jane Kirschling, "Designing DNP Programs to Meet Required Competencies—Context for the Conversation" (2012), http://tinyurl.com/oajvwx8.
11. California Nursing Practice Act, Business & Professions Code § 2725, accessed March 23, 2014, http://tinyurl.com/orpl2dc. See generally Cal. Bus. & Prof. Code §§ 2725–2742 (Nursing—Scope of Regulation), http://tinyurl.com/6sxdroo.
12. Chuck Reuter and Virginia Fitzsimons, "Physician Orders," *American Journal of Nursing* 113, no. 8 (August 2013): 11, http://tinyurl.com/nxetllw.
13. Ellen K. Murphy, "Judicial Recognition of Nursing as a Unique Profession (OR Nursing Law)," *Association of periOperative Registered Nurses Journal* (November 2004), http://tinyurl.com/ktwgqt4.
14. Sullivan v. Edward Hospital, 806 N.E.2d 645 (Ill. 2004), http://tinyurl.com/4gckg.
15. Smith v. Pavlovich, 914 N.E.2d 1258 (Ill. App. Ct. 2009), http://tinyurl.com/ox46fsf.
16. Bernice Buresh and Suzanne Gordon, *From Silence to Voice*, 3rd ed. (Ithaca: Cornell University Press, 2013).
17. Suzanne Gordon, *Nursing Against the Odds: How Health Care Cost-Cutting, Media Stereotypes, and Medical Hubris Undermine Nursing and Patient Care* (Ithaca: Cornell University Press, 2005).

18. Dana Beth Weinberg, *Code Green: Money-Driven Hospitals and the Dismantling of Nursing* (Ithaca: Cornell University Press, 2003).
19. Theresa Brown, "Healing the Hospital Hierarchy," *New York Times* (March 16, 2013), http://tinyurl.com/dxlcs2r.
20. Theresa Brown, "Physician, Heel Thyself," *New York Times* (May 7, 2011), http://tinyurl.com/lav3rxw.
21. TAN, "The Stuff of Life" (October 29, 2012), http://tinyurl.com/pcpkq5b.
22. Heidi Thomas and John Martin Johnson, writers, Roger Goldby, director, "Episode 3, Season 2," *Call the Midwife,* BBC/PBS (February 3, 2013), http://tinyurl.com/lrz6l2t.
23. TAN, "*Nurse Jackie* Episode Analyses," accessed February 2, 2014, http://tinyurl.com/kqm3k6b.
24. TAN, "Thank You Nurses!: These Nurses That Stay in One Place . . . They're Off Their Game" (May 2, 2011), http://tinyurl.com/o5duqvr; TAN, "Every Day Is Doctor Day" (June 6, 2011), http://tinyurl.com/npbesmy.
25. TAN, "Cunning, Baffling, Powerful" (April 14, 2013), http://tinyurl.com/kgrdrne.
26. Daniele Nathanson, writer, Jesse Peretz, director, "Teachable Moments," *Nurse Jackie*, Showtime (May 26, 2013).
27. Gina Gold and Aurorae Khoo, writers, Randall Einhorn, director, "Forget It," *Nurse Jackie*, Showtime (June 2, 2013).
28. TAN, "*HawthoRNe* Episode Reviews" (2011), http://tinyurl.com/jwd7neg.
29. TAN, "Chief Nursing Officer" (June 16, 2009), http://tinyurl.com/o5ce4yw.
30. TAN, "Christina Saved Her Life" (August 2011), http://tinyurl.com/ncmz5dv.
31. Liz Heldens, writer, Adam Bernstein, director, "Can We Get That Drink Now?," *Mercy*, NBC (September 23, 2009); TAN, "Traffic Is Backed Up in the Tunnel Heading into Respect" (September 23, 2009), http://tinyurl.com/kaqvmo7.
32. Toni Graphia, writer, Adam Bernstein, director, "Hope You're Good, Smiley Face," *Mercy*, NBC (October 7, 2009), http://tinyurl.com/mcf3tcv.
33. Veronica Becker and Sarah Kucserka, "I'm Not That Kind of Girl," *Mercy*, NBC (November 18, 2009); TAN, "Putting Ideas in Her Head" (November 18, 2009), http://tinyurl.com/pnlpnkj.
34. TAN, "*Mercy* Episode Reviews" (2010), http://tinyurl.com/kj3t63s.
35. TAN, "An R and an N" (October 21, 2009), http://tinyurl.com/q8k63xt.
36. TAN, "It Droppeth as the Gentle Rain from Heaven" (May 2010), http://tinyurl.com/psomrge.
37. CFNA, "Peyton Place," TAN (October 20, 2005), http://tinyurl.com/p8239cy.
38. CFNA, "A Lump of Coal," TAN (December 8, 2005), http://tinyurl.com/kk2h69z.
39. CFNA, "Midnight in the Garden of Nurses and Murses," TAN (February 2007), http://tinyurl.com/paeq4lo.
40. Greg Daniels, Michael Schur, and Norm Hiscock, writers, Randall Einhorn, director, "Ron & Tammys," *Parks & Recreation*, NBC (September 29, 2011).

41. John Alsop, Sue Smith, and Alice Addison, writers, *RAN: Remote Area Nurse*, SBS (Australia) (January 2006), http://tinyurl.com/pecma9w; CFNA, "Dogged, Petulant, Bloody-Minded Renegade . . . Nurses," TAN (January 4, 2006), http://tinyurl.com/nq75wkb.
42. Tom McDonald and Nick Curwin, executive producers, *24 Hours in A&E*, Channel 4/BBC America, accessed March 22, 2014, http://tinyurl.com/3onwxsw; TAN, "*24 Hours in A&E* Episode Reviews," accessed March 22, 2014, http://tinyurl.com/k7wjryz.
43. Dan Cutforth, Jane Lipsitz, and Alexandra Lipsitz, executive producers, *Time of Death*, Showtime (2013–2014), http://tinyurl.com/onzor26.
44. Richard Kahn and Linda Martin, directors, *Lifeline: The Nursing Diaries*: Part 1: *The Rookies*, Discovery Health Channel (2004); CFNA, "Part 1: *The Rookies*," TAN (December 16, 2004), http://tinyurl.com/ob9df8c.
45. Greg Rienzi, "TV Documentary Explores Nursing," *The Gazette Online* 29, no. 42 (July 31, 2000), http://tinyurl.com/q8kqald; CFNA, "Nurses" TAN (2002), http://tinyurl.com/qzjaldh.
46. Glenda Hersh, John Bowman, and Stephen Weinstock, executive producers, "Cool Hand Luc," *Doctors Without Borders: Life in the Field*, National Geographic Channel (July 2, 2003); CFNA, "Geographic's 'Doctors Without Borders' Episode Focuses on . . . Nurses!," TAN (July 9, 2003), http://tinyurl.com/kl3fjc2.
47. John Hamburg and Larry Stuckey, writers, Paul Weitz, director, *Little Fockers*, Tribeca/Everyman Pictures (2010); TAN, "Little Fockers" (August 4, 2011), http://tinyurl.com/oko5yzw.
48. James Gunn, screenplay, Zack Snyder, director, *Dawn of the Dead*, Universal Pictures (2004); CFNA, "Dawn of the Dead," TAN (April 7, 2004), http://tinyurl.com/py9holr.
49. Tony Kushner, writer, Mike Nichols, director, *Angels in America*, HBO Films (2003); CFNA, "Angels in America," TAN (April 4, 2004), http://tinyurl.com/mqcbd3l.
50. Margaret Edson, playwright, Emma Thompson and Mike Nichols, screenplay, Mike Nichols, director, *Wit*, HBO Films; CFNA, "Wit," TAN (January 5, 2003), http://tinyurl.com/q2rfz8s.
51. Ian McEwan, *Atonement*, Nan Talese/Doubleday (2001); Christopher Hampton, screenplay based on the novel by Ian McEwan, Joe Wright, director, *Atonement*, Working Title Films, Relativity Media (2007); CFNA, "Atonement" (film review), TAN (January 13, 2008), http://tinyurl.com/ooxmyvm; CFNA, "Atonement" (book review), TAN (May 10, 2003), http://tinyurl.com/l54xzko.
52. Julian Guthrie, "Nursing School Dean Brings His Career of Caring," *San Francisco Chronicle* (March 11, 2012); TAN, "You Just Have to Listen" (March 11, 2012), http://tinyurl.com/ncsmen2.
53. John Blanton, "Care and Chaos on the Night Nursing Shift; in a Search for Purpose, an Editor Changes Careers; 'He's Asking for You Again,'" *Wall Street*

Journal (April 24, 2007); CFNA, "There and Back Again," TAN (April 24, 2007), http://tinyurl.com/ndu5dx8.

54. Julia Bucher, "Advice for Caregivers of Relatives with Cancer," *New York Times* (July 3, 2013), http://tinyurl.com/nxce4y6; TAN, "Diplomacy: This Message Is Important to Share" (July 3, 2013), http://tinyurl.com/o6rcwda.
55. Kerry Cullinan, "Now They Have Sheets on the Beds, but No Money," *South Africa Star* (December 6, 2004), http://tinyurl.com/ngxcgeb; CFNA, "Nurses Power Legendary South African Clinic," TAN (December 6, 2004), http://tinyurl.com/qfmy8pr.
56. Philippa Stevenson, "Nurse Ward Helps Families See the Colour of Caring," *New Zealand Herald* (December 7, 2004), http://tinyurl.com/ozo86tf; CFNA, "True Colours," TAN (December 7, 2004), http://tinyurl.com/l5ekgyf.
57. Carolyn Thompson, "School Nurses Have Come a Long Way Since 1902," Associated Press (August 20, 2013), http://tinyurl.com/ngnrcng.
58. UPI, "Program: Teen Depression, Suicide Drops" (August 13, 2011), http://tinyurl.com/kbayl8l; TAN, "Surviving the Teens" (August 2011), http://tinyurl.com/osmv6dw.
59. Adam Brimelow, "Dutch District Nurses Rediscover 'Complete Care' Role," *BBC News* (May 27, 2013), http://tinyurl.com/nj9tsq6.
60. *Copenhagen Post*, "Nurses Make House Calls on Bike" (July 7, 2013), http://tinyurl.com/ltlzfx4.
61. Scott Simmie, "Street Nurse Earns Prestigious Honour," *Toronto Star* (January 22, 2004); CFNA, "Street Nurse Earns Prestigious Honour," TAN (January 22, 2004), http://tinyurl.com/mppmcc6.
62. William Brangham, producer, "Nursing the Wounded," *Need to Know*, PBS (June 22, 2012), http://tinyurl.com/7rxmhm2; TAN, "Heroes Among Us" (November 3, 2012), http://tinyurl.com/nezoh9j.
63. NPR, "Clara Adams-Ender: Army Achiever" (March 27, 2007), http://tinyurl.com/oaoqxrd; CFNA, "Army Achievers," TAN (March 27, 2007), http://tinyurl.com/pkznojr.
64. Holly Hobbie, *Fanny* (New York: Little, Brown and Company, 2008); TAN, "Fanny" (June 4, 2010), http://tinyurl.com/klpmcpv.
65. TAN, "*Grey's Anatomy* Episode Analyses and Action," accessed March 22, 2014, http://tinyurl.com/pgayg7h.
66. William Harper, writer, Tony Phelan, director, "Get Up, Stand Up," *Grey's Anatomy*, ABC (December 12, 2013), http://tinyurl.com/q2eawfp.
67. TAN, "Who's the Man" (October 13, 2011), http://tinyurl.com/onha8uc.
68. Tony Phelan and Joan Rater, writers, Michael Pressman, director, "I Always Feel Like Somebody's Watchin' Me," *Grey's Anatomy*, ABC (October 1, 2009), http://tinyurl.com/oawjco3.

69. Tony Phelan and Joan Rater, writers, Julie Anne Robinson, director, "The Becoming," *Grey's Anatomy*, ABC (May 8, 2008); CFNA, "Looking for Mr. McSteamy," TAN (May 8, 2008), http://tinyurl.com/oj3ybyy.
70. Krista Vernoff, writer, Jeff Melman, director, "I Am a Tree," *Grey's Anatomy*, ABC (September 28, 2006); CFNA, "We're All 17 Years Old," TAN (September 28, 2006), http://tinyurl.com/pxne9to.
71. Zoanne Clack, writer, David Paymer, director, "Break On Through," *Grey's Anatomy*, ABC (January 29, 2006); CFNA, "Weird Scenes Inside the Gold Mine," TAN (January 29, 2006), http://tinyurl.com/nzl6ohf.
72. James Parriott, writer, Adam Davidson, director, "No Man's Land," *Grey's Anatomy*, ABC (April 17, 2005); CFNA, "The Scrubbed Nurse," TAN (April 17, 2005), http://tinyurl.com/mbrs72r.
73. Alden Oreck, "Modern Jewish History: The Golem," Jewish Virtual Library, accessed January 30, 2014, http://tinyurl.com/5f9gt.
74. Sara Hess, writer, Fred Gerber, director, "Spin," *House*, Fox (November 15, 2005); CFNA, "And on the Eighth Day, the Lord Physician Created Nurses, to Clean Up the Mess," TAN (November 15, 2005), http://tinyurl.com/o4qdogh.
75. TAN, "*House* Single Episode Reviews" (February 2011), http://tinyurl.com/py4b5ug.
76. David Shore and David Hoselton, writers, Deran Sarafian, director, "No More Mr. Nice Guy," *House*, Fox (April 28, 2008); CFNA, "I Don't Use Nurses," TAN (April 28, 2008), http://tinyurl.com/no4vmg4.
77. Leonard Dick, writer, Daniel Sackheim, director, "The Jerk," *House*, Fox (May 15, 2007); CFNA, "Yes, Doctor. Right Away. I Was Just Trying to Get a Urine Sample, and He Went Crazy!," TAN (September 7, 2007), http://tinyurl.com/o32szd4.
78. CFNA, "Golem," TAN (May 23, 2006), http://tinyurl.com/o9ydmvo.
79. TAN, "*ER* Episode Analyses" (2009), http://tinyurl.com/odsbmqw.
80. CFNA, "Orders," TAN (November 8, 2007), http://tinyurl.com/necev3r.
81. Ibid.
82. CFNA, "A Lump of Coal," TAN (December 8, 2005), http://tinyurl.com/kk2h69z.
83. CFNA, "Stop Me Before I Empathize Again," TAN (October 9, 2003), http://tinyurl.com/qf2gugj.
84. Mindy Kaling and Charlie Grandy, writers, Rob Schrab, director, "Danny Castellano Is My Personal Trainer," *The Mindy Project*, Fox (January 7, 2014).
85. TAN, "*The Mindy Project* Reviews," accessed March 24, 2014, http://tinyurl.com/pu8wxuv.
86. TAN, "*Private Practice* Episode Analyses" (2013), http://tinyurl.com/lecehka.
87. TAN, "The Beck and Call Girls" (January 22, 2013), http://tinyurl.com/qxlcfpp.
88. TAN, "*Hart of Dixie* Reviews," accessed March 24, 2014, http://tinyurl.com/onhnqbx.

89. Jo Brand, Vicki Pepperdine, Joanna Scanlan, Mark V. Olsen, and Will Scheffer, creators, *Getting On*, HBO, accessed March 24, 2014, http://www.hbo.com/getting-on.
90. Mark V. Olsen, writer, Miguel Arteta, director, "Born on the Fourth of July," *Getting On*, HBO (November 24, 2013).
91. TAN, "*Scrubs* Episode Analyses" (2009), http://tinyurl.com/p9n8e58.
92. Bill Lawrence and Debra Fordham, writers, Mark Stegemann, director, "My Lawyer's in Love," *Scrubs*, NBC (February 3, 2009); TAN, "What *Does* That M.D. Mean?" (February 3, 2009), http://tinyurl.com/pyjb4s4.
93. Bill Lawrence, Steven Cragg, and Brian Bradley, writers, Gail Mancuso, director, "Our Role Models," *Scrubs*, NBC (December 8, 2009); TAN, "Fiddling with the Covers while Rome Burns" (December 8, 2009), http://tinyurl.com/q66o9vm.
94. Mark Stegemann, writer, Ken Whittingham, director, "My Fifteen Seconds," *Scrubs*, NBC (November 20, 2003); CFNA, "*Scrubs* Defines Nursing: It's All About Shutting Up and Following Physician 'Orders,'" TAN (November 20, 2003), http://tinyurl.com/py7rrdo.
95. CFNA, "*Strong Medicine* Episode Reviews," TAN (2006), http://tinyurl.com/o5q2awp.
96. TAN, "*Three Rivers* Episode Analyses" (2009), http://tinyurl.com/pm7wszo.
97. Paul Sciarrotta, writer, Jann Turner, director, "Emily and . . . the Leap," *Emily Owens, MD*, The CW (February 5, 2013).
98. Josh Berman and Rob Wright, creators, *The Mob Doctor*, Fox (2012–2013), http://tinyurl.com/nq8e5c4.
99. TAN, "*Miami Medical* Episode Reviews" (April 2010), http://tinyurl.com/pveg9xt.
100. Frank Military, writer, Terrence O'Hara, director, "Ascension," *NCIS: Los Angeles*, CBS (September 24, 2013)
101. Alexandra Cunningham and Lori Kirkland Baker, writers, David Grossman, director, "Sunday," *Desperate Housewives*, ABC (April 13, 2008); CFNA, "Desperate Nursemaids," TAN (April 13, 2008), http://tinyurl.com/nm9vze7.
102. Larry David, writer, Tom Kramer, director, "The N Word," *Curb Your Enthusiasm*, HBO (October 28, 2007); CFNA, "The N Word," TAN (November 11, 2007), http://tinyurl.com/nuvh6gy.
103. Alan Ball and Nancy Oliver, writers, Daniel Minahan, director, "Ecotone," *Six Feet Under*, HBO (July 31, 2005); CFNA, "An A + in Getting the Doctor," TAN (July 31, 2005), http://tinyurl.com/njxdxs9.
104. Scott Allen, "A Crash Course in Saving Lives," *Boston Globe* (October 23–26, 2007), http://tinyurl.com/yje5d62; CFNA, "As I Lay Dying," TAN (October 23–26, 2007), http://tinyurl.com/mnm2zkh.

105. WRAL, "Virginia Nurse Helps Save Injured Cary Officer" (July 17, 2011), http://tinyurl.com/3uva9xm; TAN, "Kicking In: He Needed Me" (July 17, 2011), http://tinyurl.com/pc8ek85.
106. TAN, "Kicking In: Overseeing the Rescue" (July 17, 2011), http://tinyurl.com/k3n3wvc.
107. ABC News, "Illinois Woman's ER Wait Death Ruled Homicide" (September 17, 2006), http://tinyurl.com/nbv9t; CFNA, "Errors and Omissions," TAN (September 17, 2006), http://tinyurl.com/noz2vsu.

5 THE NAUGHTIEST NURSE

In the early 1990s an inebriated homeless patient assaulted an emergency department nurse at a public hospital in San Francisco. The patient grabbed the nurse's breast. In the late 1990s the same thing happened to that nurse while she was working at a major private hospital in Washington, DC—except that the assaulting patient was an inebriated United States ambassador to a foreign nation. The nurse was Sandy.

She is not alone. In October 2009 the *Salt Lake Tribune* reported that a Utah man had allegedly grabbed the breast of a hospital nurse he found "cute."[1] The man was at the hospital for the impending birth of his child. Police said that the nurse he assaulted was wheeling the mother of his unborn baby to the delivery room. The man was arrested, so he missed the birth.

In December 2010, an MSNBC item reported that an Allentown, Pennsylvania man had twice grabbed an emergency room nurse's buttocks, but claimed he did so to say "thank you" for her care.[2] After the nurse gave him some negative feedback, the man apparently told her: "Well, you're a nurse, right?" In other words, you're a slut and it's part of your job to provide sexual services, or at least to endure sexual abuse.

Contrary to the "naughty nurse" image, nurses do not wish to be sexualized, harassed, or assaulted. But they are—a lot. In a December 2005 study, University of Missouri communications professor Debbie Dougherty found that more than 70 percent of the nurses she surveyed in four US states had been sexually harassed by patients.[3] In March 2006, Dougherty told a writer for the *Monster* website that she was "surprised" at the aggression the nurses faced: "Patients threatened to attack nurses sexually and called them prostitutes." A 2009 study indicated that 56 percent of Japanese hospital nurses had been sexually harassed at some point in their careers.[4] A 2012 study in Pakistan found that more than

31 percent of nurses at three Karachi hospitals had experienced "physical violence, and verbal and sexual harassment" in the preceding year, but only 3 percent reported the incidents, because they "feared retaliation and lack of support."[5]

Indeed, abused nurses often do not receive adequate support from their hospital employers. In February 2009 the *New York Daily News* reported that a Queens jury had awarded a nurse $15 million after Flushing Hospital had allegedly allowed a physician to sexually abuse her and other nurses for years, even though hospital officials were aware of the physician's history of misconduct.[6] The physician finally lost his admitting privileges after two 2001 incidents, including one in which he had allegedly chased the nurse through the halls, cornered her, and "aggressively groped her below the waist." Some employers seem to view that kind of abuse as part of nurses' jobs. Just get over it!

In all this excitement, even a few nurses seem to have forgotten the real nature of their work. In March 2010, Reuters reported that a Dutch nurses union had launched a national campaign to remind everyone that sexual services were actually *not* part of nurses' jobs.[7] Apparently, a young female nurse had complained that a disabled patient had demanded that she provide sex as part of his care, then threatened to have her fired when she refused. What might have given him the idea that sexual services were part of nursing? Well, there is that global naughty nurse stereotype, but the complaining nurse also said she saw "some of her peers performing sexual acts with the patient."

Sexual abuse has a negative impact on patient care, as a December 2005 Associated Press item about Dougherty's study explained.[8] A nurse traumatized by abuse cannot provide her best care. She is less likely to provide good psychosocial care and to notice important changes in patient conditions, but more likely to make errors, miss work, burn out, and leave the bedside.

Much of global society continues to regard nurses as sex objects. A 2006 Agence France-Presse item reported that a recent poll had found that 54 percent of British men had sexual fantasies about nurses—more than about any other profession.[9] Nursing led a list of traditionally female, service-oriented jobs; it was followed by maids and flight attendants. By contrast, the poll found that women's popular fantasies focused on traditionally male jobs associated with heroism and/or socioeconomic power, including medicine. Leading that list were "firemen," about whom 47 percent of British women dreamed. For men, it seems, to be the object of fantasies is a mark of power and prestige. For women, it is a mark of perceived submissiveness and low status.

In May 2009 the *New York Times* reported that clinics in Prague were offering inducements including free plastic surgery in order to recruit scarce nurses, because many had left the Czech Republic for better paying jobs elsewhere in Europe. The report made clear that Czech nurses were evaluated in part by how sexually attractive they were. One nurse reported that at one nursing job interview, a male recruiter had asked her to walk in a straight line, as if she was seeking a modeling position.[10]

The naughty nurse remains a common cultural reference. In March 2007, on *Live with Regis and Kelly*, Kelly Ripa repeatedly promised to be a "sponge bath nurse" in her "little nursey costume" for cohost Regis Philbin, who was undergoing bypass surgery.[11] Ripa's comments were enthusiastically amplified in press stories about Philbin's condition, from the Associated Press to the *New York Post*.

Some celebrities seem a bit obsessed with the naughty nurse. After nurses persuaded shoe company Skechers to stop including images of pop star Christina Aguilera dressed as a naughty nurse in global advertising campaigns in 2004,[12] Aguilera posed for photographs in a naughty nurse costume the following year at her Las Vegas Halloween party.[13] As *People* reported and the photographs confirmed, she was "playing doctor" with her scrubs-clad music executive fiancé. Take that, little nursies!

In December 2006, sometime Italian prime minister and media mogul Silvio Berlusconi found a novel way to thank his nurses at the Cleveland Clinic, where he had just had a pacemaker implanted: "Italian nurses are better-looking. . . . These ones scare me a bit. Don't even think about leaving me alone at night with one of them."[14] Don't worry—we wouldn't! Of course, the public got valuable detail about Berlusconi's vision of nursing from January 2011 reports about the investigation into his alleged corruption and sexual misconduct. The *London Evening Standard* reported that he had hosted parties at which young women were asked to don naughty nurse attire for "lesbian stripper acts."[15]

Some consider nursing to be comparable to sex work. In August 2004 the *Times* of London reported that in "some Asian cultures, nursing is considered on a par with prostitution."[16] In June 2006 the Inter Press Service News Agency quoted the press secretary of the Pakistan Nurses Association as noting that "the majority of patients and their relatives regard us as sex symbols."[17] That story described sexual assaults by patients and physicians about which nothing was done. One nurse found that "not even paramedics" would marry her because, she explained, her hospital colleagues "think I am a prostitute." One striking expression of this problem was Dame Helen Mirren's June 2010 comment, in promoting a film about a Reno brothel on CBS's *Late Show with David Letterman*, that "a lot of girls who work in that [prostitution] industry actually come from the nursing industry, which kind of makes sense, because they're used to naked bodies. It's not intimidating to them, you know, the body and the bodily functions, if you like."[18]

The media plays a central role in perpetuating the global vision of nurses as prostitutes or half-dressed nymphomaniacs. From the time the modern naughty nurse image emerged in the 1960s, as discussed in Chapter 2, the prevalence of the image has been staggering. It appears in television shows, pop music videos, sexually-oriented products, and the news media. Major corporations have used the image to sell such products as beer, vodka, razor blades, cosmetics, shoes, men's underwear, milk, cell phone service, gum, vodka, and beer. In October 2011, the family-oriented Williamsburg, Virginia theme park Busch Gardens celebrated Halloween with a show featuring naughty nurse dancers; later, the "nurses" reportedly sold park patrons shots from their "syringes."[19]

How sexualized is the media image of nurses? Table 5.1 shows how nursing compares to other professions.

Table 5.1 Google results for selected English language phrases—July 2014[133]

	"Sexy ______"	"Hot ______"	"Naughty ______"
"Lawyers"	13,200	16,600	2,050
"Doctors"	97,800	131,000	33,300
"Nurses"	1,150,000	1,290,000	1,200,000

The naughty nurse image is not limited to straightforward indications that nurses are total bimbos. It encompasses more subtle messages that nurses, who are primarily women, are mainly focused on the romantic pursuit of men, particularly physicians. In November 2004 psychologist Dr. Phil ran a segment on his syndicated show about the damage a physician had done to his family by having an affair with a nurse. Dr. Phil offered these pearls of wisdom:

> I spent a lot of years in the health care delivery system, and I watched doctors and nurses play footsie back and forth. And I watched doctors whose wives worked, put them through medical school, all this, and they come up there with a cute little nurse and they start playing footsie with her. I've seen lots of cute little nurses go after doctors, because they're going to seduce and marry them a doctor, because that's their ticket out of having to work as a nurse.[20]

Dr. Phil's statement is a persuasive, insider's vision of nurses as physician gold diggers—the "little" things' bodies are the only way they have to escape their dead-end jobs. Similarly, in an August 2010 report by the news service *Al Bawaba* about a protest over an Egyptian naughty nurse television character, Dr. Nihad Abd Al Salam of the International Nurses Academy observed that the Egyptian media reinforces the widespread perception that nurses are "girls with bad reputations who try to seduce doctors and rich patients."[21] In *A Young Doctor's Notebook*, the Sky Arts show about rural Russia in 1917 airing in the United States in late 2013, veteran midwife Pelagaya at first seemed to feel it was part of her job—a mildly annoying one—to provide the Young Doctor with a sexual release.[22] By the show's second season, the unfortunate Pelagaya seemed to be more interested in the caddish Doctor than he was in her.

Why are nurses so naughty? As explained in Chapters 1 and 2, nurses have struggled since the founding of the modern profession to put society at ease with the idea of females providing intimate care to men. The profession's image has long teetered between extremes of femininity, from the angel to the harlot. It may be that some cannot get past the "Madonna and whore" dichotomy: as females who provide intimate care, nurses must be one or the other. The research suggests, and even a cursory look at the Internet confirms, that male sexual fantasies often focus on traditionally female professions that are seen as involving basic personal services. These workers may be perceived as submissive females who are more sexually available or ripe for abuse because they have no strong, independent professional identity—not much else going for them. Some have also suggested that regarding nurses as sluts may help vulnerable male patients handle the fact that female nurses have some power over them. Illness and incapacity are frightening, and some may express that fear by diminishing the nearest available women.

Whatever the reasons, such social contempt discourages practicing and potential nurses, undermines nurses' claims to clinical and educational resources, and encourages workplace sexual abuse. The naughty nurse image is a factor in the global nursing crisis, and overcoming it is a critical part of resolving the shortage. Nurses have urged the media to reconsider its rampant use of the image. We just hope there's some other way to sell men beer and stuff.

"Penny Shots for Naughty Nurses": Why the Naughty Nurse Matters

In April 2008 nursing student Emily Pirie reported that a bar on Pittsburgh's South Side had been running the following promotion: "Penny Shots for Naughty Nurses."[23]

The naughty nurse image might be good for some free drinks and social activities tonight, but nurses and their patients pay in the long run. One way they pay is in the loss of respect and resources nurses really need—pennies for nurses!

Naughty nurse images add to the chronic underfunding of nursing research, education, and clinical practice. Healthcare decision makers—many of whom are sadly uninformed about what nursing really is—are less likely to devote scarce resources to a profession that has become so degraded in the public mind. This negative image also holds little appeal for career seekers. The naughty nurse isn't just promiscuous. She's either submissive and dim, or comically aggressive or evil. And she's always female. If a profession is constantly associated with female sexuality, it's not going to attract and retain many men. Nursing remains at least 90 percent female.[24] When you combine the lack of respect, the low appeal to the more powerful gender, the intense training nursing actually requires, and the difficulty and stress of real nursing practice, it's no surprise that the profession remains in the midst of a global shortage. This is the difference between sexual images of female nurses and, say, female FBI agents, or for that matter, male firefighters. Those challenging professions are not being undermined by the idea that their members are sex-crazed twits. Nursing is.

Of course, there's nothing wrong with being seen as sexy—as long as that's not your dominant image in the workplace. An article published in *Psychology of Women Quarterly* in 2005, based on research by Lawrence University professor Peter Glick, suggested that more sexualized work attire actually lessens respect for female workers in responsible jobs like management, causing others to see them as less competent and intelligent.[25] In 2009, Melissa Wookey and colleagues found that dressing sexually harmed people's perception of the social competence of professional women, although apparently it did not cause similar harm to nonprofessionals.[26] Thus, to the extent nurses are correctly seen as professionals, constantly associating them with sex lessens respect for them. If sexual imagery does not lower the opinions of nurses held by those who do *not* see nurses as professionals, that may be because those opinions are so low to begin with.

Consider the inordinate amount of sexual abuse that nurses suffer at work. It's hard to prove the extent to which such abuse is caused by naughty nurse stereotyping. But if a profession is an object of frequent sexual mockery and contempt, that status will invite sexual abuse, especially from those who are mentally altered, such as by drugs or mental illness.

Some say that naughty nurse imagery is just a "joke" or "fantasy" and no one believes nurses really are that way. Of course most people probably don't think the average nurse goes to work in lingerie, looking for sex. And it may be hard to see how one naughty nurse image could matter. But each image is a tiny part of a global wave of media imagery, all suggesting nursing consists of hot females satisfying the sexual needs of patients and/or physicians, or at best, that nursing is so unimportant that nurses have time to focus on sex while caring for patients. In the aggregate, decades of that message will have an impact. Few people would accept "just joking" as an excuse for stereotyping other disempowered groups.

Even humor and fantasy images affect how people act, as explained in Chapter 2. In fact, a study by researchers at the University of Granada (Spain), published in the *Journal of Interpersonal Violence* in 2010, found that men who had listened to a series of "sexist jokes" later displayed more tolerance for violence against women than those who had not listened to the jokes.[27] In a related vein, psychologist and anthropologist Gil Greengross explains the "normative window theory of prejudice" proposed by Chris Crandall and colleagues: When the prejudice against a given group is shifting in society, and you hold negative views about a group, "hearing disparaging jokes about them releases inhibitions you might have, and you feel it's ok to discriminate against them."[28] Under Thomas Ford and Mark Ferguson's "prejudiced norm theory,"[29] which Tendayi Viki and colleagues have evaluated favorably,[30] delivering prejudice in a joke (disparagement humor) discourages criticism of the discriminatory message, encouraging the receiver to accept that message as the norm; repeated joke exposures create a greater tolerance of future discriminatory events in those who are already prejudiced. Ford asserts that "the acceptance of sexist humor leads men to believe that sexist behavior falls within the bounds of social acceptability."[31] Ford and colleagues at Western Carolina University published a 2008 study in the *Personality and Social Psychology Bulletin* suggesting that exposure to sexist humor also decreased the amount of money sexist men were willing to give to a women's organization.[32] It's not hard to relate that finding to the low funding nursing receives compared to medicine.[33]

Some also claim that objections to the constant association of nursing with sex indicate prudishness. But there is a big difference between objecting to sexual images generally and objecting to the use of nursing as a marker for shallow, servile, sexually available females.

Of course, sexual desires and fantasies do not instantly go away just because certain media images become less prevalent. But we doubt that something as specific in time as the naughty nurse image of recent decades is biologically predetermined or unchangeable, at least on a society-wide basis. It seems to us that the image is largely the result of specific cultural information, although it may incorporate some broader elements, such as the eroticism of apparent innocence. Some aspects of human attraction may evolve over time. For instance, common standards of human beauty do not appear to be the same today as in past centuries. It is in humanity's long-term interest to consider new ways to think about nurses.

One could argue that the work of nurses is so intimate that it will always be subject to some level of sexual fantasy. But the work of physicians is intimate, and they don't seem to suffer from the idea that they are submissive and sexually available.

At ground level, the devaluation of nursing translates into an underpowered profession that may not be strong enough to save your life when you need it to do so. The naughty nurse isn't going to catch deadly medication errors, intervene when a patient is about to crash, or teach a patient how to survive with a life-threatening condition. It's time for her to change into something a little more comfortable.

Call Me Magdalene: Is Nursing the World's Oldest Profession?

Naughty nurse images circle the globe. As the rest of this chapter shows, virtually all are just variations on the tired bimbo nurse imagery that has permeated pop culture since the 1960s. However, recently there have been fairly thoughtful media explorations of the naughty nurse image. Well, actually, we can think of just two examples. But hey—there are two!

One is Richard Prince's "nurse paintings," which were the subject of prominent exhibitions worldwide throughout the 2000s and early 2010s. Prince starts with the covers of mid-twentieth-century pulp novels that show the standing figure of a white-uniformed nurse. Then he covers much of the nurses' faces with white mask-like paint blobs. In many cases, red paint bleeds off different parts of the figures. Parts of the original book cover backgrounds emerge in vague, often ominous forms. Thus we get *Nympho Nurse, Tender Nurse*, and the especially gory *Man Crazy Nurse #2*—which sold at Christie's New York for $7.4 million in May 2008. Some nurses object to Prince's paintings, and the artist could be accused of using misogynist iconography to score cheap pop art shock points. But it is hard to miss the irony driving the works. Prince's nurses are effectively gagged; they are defined by the large, aggressively ridiculous book titles, and they are alone in a world of scary shadows and blood. Trapped in their oppressive clothes and our oppressive attitudes, the pulp nurses may reflect the plight of today's real nurses and of women generally. The blood spots on their bodies are stigmata of caring. The masks point to critical problems today's nurses face, namely their invisibility and difficulty in speaking up. In some of the paintings, the nurses' eyes burn out over the masks, suggesting sentient beings struggling to assert a genuine identity.[34]

A related example is the alternative band Sonic Youth's 2004 album *Sonic Nurse*, which used Richard Prince's nursing imagery to explore troubling aspects of women's lives. The CD package art has images of the nurse paintings. Maybe Sonic Youth saw nursing as a busy intersection on the boulevard of broken female dreams. The album title may also suggest that the band is not unlike a nurse, assessing a given environment and, in some sense, intervening. The song "Dude Ranch Nurse" is based on a Richard Prince painting that in turn seems to be drawn from a 1953 Cherry Ames novel, one in a series of nursing adventures aimed at schoolgirls. The band's Kim Gordon sings that the "dude ranch dream has fallen apart," but still, "I could love him."[35]

Unfortunately, the vast majority of naughty nurse imagery won't be telling the public anything useful about nursing. Consider some examples from recent advertising, television and film, sexually oriented media, pop music, and news media.

Catching "Lusty-Nurse Fever": The Nurse in Global Advertising

The naughty nurse is especially adept at selling products to young men. But it seems she can sell anything, including women's shoes. She has even volunteered to promote nonprofit endeavors, from hospitals to health awareness campaigns.

The naughty nurse is eager for men to buy alcohol, even though real nurses spend much of their time handling the damage caused by alcohol abuse. Maybe it's all about nursing job security! First, of course, there's beer. During the mid-2000s, Coors's Canadian division relied heavily on naughty nurse imagery in its Coors Light Trauma Tour, a marketing campaign based on sponsorship of extreme sports events. Naughty nurse models appeared in visual advertisements and interacted with spectators at the events.[36]

Meanwhile, the maker of Gzhelka vodka (which appears to be the Russian government) crafted our favorite naughty nurse ad *ever*. In the television spot, which apparently started airing in 2006, an attractive young female nurse entered a hospital room. The ominous theme from the 1968 thriller *Twisted Nerve* played; the evil character Elle Driver had whistled that theme in

Quentin Tarantino's *Kill Bill* (2003) when, disguised as a nurse, she prepared to assassinate the film's hospitalized Bride character by lethal injection. But the Gzhelka nurse had something else in mind. She set up an intravenous bottle of vodka to infuse into her unconscious male patient. Once the vodka started infusing, the patient became very aroused under the sheet. The nurse mounted and had energetic intercourse with the still-unconscious patient. Onscreen text said there was "no prescription needed," and the nurse asked why anyone would need medicine at all.[37] Note the cool public health themes of a nurse/prostitute pushing huge quantities of vodka as a sexual aid and overall health promoter.

The naughty nurse has also sold young males drinks with more serious claims of health benefits. In 2008 Canada's Neilson Dairy marketed its Ultimate flavored cow milk products with a campaign that was remarkably similar to the earlier Coors Light Trauma Tour. Naughty nurse models appeared in advertisements and at an extreme sports tour. Neilson advertisements matched the "nurses"—the "Ultimate Recovery Team"—with sports-related sexual innuendo.[38] In August 2008 we and the Registered Nurses Association of Ontario helped Neilson recover from its naughty nurse workout, persuading the company to remove the nurse element from the campaign.

We've noticed that the naughty nurse wants her man to be well-groomed and sweetly scented before she provides her, you know, "nursing services." In late 2006 a print advertisement campaign for Schick's Quattro Titanium razor featured an injured male skateboarder in a research facility bed. He was surrounded by white-coated researchers—and three naughty "nurses" giving him "more intensive care."[39] Schick placed the advertisement in *Sports Illustrated* and also distributed it at college bookstores, perhaps as an inspiration to nursing students. In a late 2005 television spot, Gillette's TAG Body Spray caused a provocatively-dressed "nurse" to develop "highly contagious lusty-nurse fever" and climb into bed with a male patient wearing the product.[40] In September 2007 Cadbury Schweppes Canada ran television advertisements for Dentyne Ice chewing gum that showed female nurses being lured into bed with male patients the instant the men popped the product into their mouths. The tag line: "Get Fresh."[41]

The naughty nurse also wants to show you a good time at restaurants, bars, and sporting events, often as part of an ironic health-related theme. In January 2014, the RocketNews24 site reported that a McDonald's outlet in Taiwan had started the new year with female staff dressed in "sexy" "nurse" outfits that featured short dresses "and thigh-high stockings." That prompted "many hopeful men to [take] the chance while it was their turn at the counter to ask if the girls had boyfriends."[42]

Of course, "nurses" can't be underdressed at "breastaurants." For example, in March 2011, the popular chain Hooters declared "National Hooky Day" in honor of the start of the US men's college basketball tournament. The company's website featured photos of naughty nurse "Ashleigh," who wanted to send you a "Doctor's Note" so you could take the day off work to recover from "Basketball Fever" and enjoy a free appetizer. In a related television commercial, Ashleigh quickly diagnosed broadcasting legend Dick Vitale with this fever and treated him with the free appetizer. Then Vitale, bellowed: "Hooters! It's the cure, baby!"[43]

But no national restaurant group could top the Heart Attack Grill. In 2005 the Phoenix-area restaurant began using scantily dressed naughty nurse waitstaff. The restaurant flaunted its antihealth menu, which included "quadruple-bypass" burgers and "flatliner fries." The "nurses" did "role playing": helping diners with "heart attacks," sitting on their laps, and pushing the overfed in wheelchairs. Grill owner "Dr. Jon" Basso's "role" was to remain fully dressed, in a laboratory coat and tie. The Grill was a striking example of the naughty nurse image, so in October 2006 we generated global press coverage about it. Since then, the culinary landmark has survived moves to Dallas and finally to Las Vegas, as well as the (actual) early deaths of two Grill spokesmen[44] and other diet-related casualties. But Basso and the "nurses" are still there. In 2014, the nurses were "spanking" customers who didn't finish their food, with a "spank cam" on the Grill's website recording the events.[45]

As you might expect after all that hard work, when night falls the naughty nurse wants to party. In 2004 Los Angeles's Club Good Hurt began attracting patrons with local bands and "nurse" bartenders. In 2013, the club's website advised potential customers to "let our Signature Naughty Nurses[TM] write your prescription for one of our Prescription Cocktails[TM], like the Transfusion, and find out the true meaning of a Good Hurt."[46] Really—*trademarking* the "signature naughty nurses"? What an honor. By 2009 the City Steam Brewery Café was selling its Naughty Nurse Amber Ale, the popular brew pub's "best seller," throughout the Hartford, Connecticut area.[47]

At a professional basketball game in February 2012, when the Dallas Mavericks hosted the New Jersey Nets, the Mavericks Dancers entertained the crowd and a large television audience at half-time by dressing in naughty nurse outfits and doing a sexually-oriented dance to the tune of Robert Palmer's "Bad Case of Loving You."[48]

Virgin Mobile often calls on the naughty nurse. Starting in 2008, Virgin Mobile India's "Think Hatke" (Think Differently) campaign included an advertisement in which a supposedly immobilized male hospital patient tricked a scantily-dressed female "nurse" into reaching around in his pants pockets, searching for his cell phone, to help him answer a call strategically placed by the patient's friend.[49] There was no word on whether Mohandas Gandhi, whose image appeared in the classic 1980's Apple "Think Different" campaign, would also appear in this innovative new marketing. In 2005, Virgin Mobile Canada introduced a multimedia campaign with naughty nurse models who would supposedly help customers avoid "The Catch," a venereal disease associated with rival companies. Virgin tycoon Richard Branson frolicked with some of the "nurses" at the March 2005 kickoff event in Toronto.[50]

The 2004 Skechers campaign, which was called "Naughty and Nice," featured Christina Aguilera wearing Skechers footwear in three different advertisements, including one in which she appeared both as a dominatrix naughty nurse and as the nurse's patient. Nurse Christina seemed ready to inject patient Christina with a huge metal syringe connected to a big needle. This campaign ran in youth magazines and point-of-sale retail displays around the world, although nurses persuaded the company to drop the nurse advertisements.[51]

But the naughty nurse would be hurt if you thought she was all about money. Behind that sexy bra beats a passionate heart of caring! She helps healthcare-related companies. In March 2010, the *Daily Mail* (UK) reported that the Diamond Bus Company in the West Midlands was using a large naughty nurse advertisement to promote its route to a hospital. Nurses and government health officials asked Diamond to pull the advertisement, but the company refused, stating that it had been "vetted" by a group of nurses who agreed it was "funny."[52] And in July 2005 Reuters reported that the Spanish cosmetic surgery firm Corporación Dermoestética had used "50 mini-skirted models" dressed as nurses at its stock market launch.[53] It was unclear whether the models would also be caring for the firm's patients.

In other cases, the naughty nurse's work is more altruistic. Lionsgate's *SAW* movies, released from 2004 to 2010, were reportedly the most successful horror film franchise of all time. To promote the films' releases, the company sponsored blood drives and advertised them with eye-catching posters featuring sexy/scary naughty nurse imagery. The company boasted of the lives the blood drives saved, but the nurse images it used degraded the very professionals who use the blood collected to save those lives.[54]

In November 2009 the naughty nurse actually appeared in a major public awareness campaign by the Lung Cancer Alliance, a prominent US charity. In the lead campaign video, "Dr. Lung Love" rapped about the danger lung cancer poses to women, as hot "nurses" caressed and danced suggestively with him. The nurses wore scrubs, in contrast to the Pitbull video on which the Lung Cancer Alliance video was based, which had sexy women in lingerie but no nursing element. But the Lung Cancer Alliance video still presented female nurses as the submissive sexual playthings of commanding male physicians.[55]

"Ranking Nurses in Order of Do-Ability": Modern Hollywood's Tribute

The naughty nurse has been a plot device on some of the most widely seen recent television dramas. In a February 2011 episode of *NCIS: Los Angeles* (CBS), a helpful and attractive Nurse Debbie was the subject of two playful "ready for my sponge bath!"-type remarks from a wounded detective named Deeks. Debbie did not act provocatively, and she was not even present for the sponge bath comments; they were a stock dramatic device the show's writers used mainly to further Deeks's ongoing flirtation with a female detective colleague—a peer.[56] In an October 2007 episode of *Desperate Housewives*, the sexy character Gaby donned naughty nurse attire as a cover to rub lotion on her husband and covertly heal a case of pubic lice that she had given him.[57]

The most notable recent prime-time television examples of naughty nurse imagery have been on *Grey's Anatomy*. It's not just the occasional "comic" appearance, as in an October 2011 episode with a woman dressed as a "sexy zombie nurse" who arrived at the hospital after being injured at a comics convention.[58] On *Grey's* it goes deeper. Nurse characters have often been vehicles through which the show's pretty female physicians confront latent fears about female subservience and sexual virtue. December 2005 episodes displayed the fury of intern Izzie because the object of her affection, intern Alex, had had call-room sex with less attractive nurse Olivia. Alex wanted to talk, but Izzie snapped that he was "too busy screwing nurses to talk—just get out." At another point, intern Cristina marveled that "hell hath no fury like a girl whose non-boyfriend screws a nurse." Izzie also accused Alex of having cheated on her with the "skanky syph nurse," a reference to the fact that Alex had previously given Olivia syphilis, which Olivia later passed on to intern George. Olivia had not known about the Alex and Izzie romance, and she was meekly apologetic to Izzie. In response, Izzie projected seething contempt.[59]

These episodes reveal the interns' fears of sexual degradation and even of a kind of class miscegenation. Alex has not just cheated on Izzie, he has "screwed" a *nurse*, the low-rent embodiment of everything a smart, ambitious modern woman must avoid. Let's face it: some people just don't belong. Consider that Izzie called Olivia a "skanky syph nurse" even though it was actually *Alex* who gave Olivia syphilis. And although Olivia slept with two interns, intern Meredith had apparently been getting drunk and sleeping with a different guy every night. Izzie did briefly call attention to this, but no one used the expression "skanky syph doc."[60]

The show has also relied on the nurse-grasping-for-physician-love theme, as in the May 2008 plotline in which jilted nurses boycotted Mark "McSteamy" Sloane's surgeries, as discussed in Chapter 4.[61] Even the Rose plotline that aired in late 2007 and 2008 presented the nurse as wide-eyed about romance with neurosurgeon Derek "McDreamy" Shepherd. Rose confessed to being intimidated by the "legend" of the prior romance between Derek and Meredith, and in one intensely embarrassing April 2008 episode, Rose expressed amazement that she was actually dating the great man: "I'm trying to play it cool. I *am* playing it so, so cool. I love him!"[62]

House has not bothered with nurses enough to have as many naughty nurse images as *Grey's*. But a February 2011 episode did include a visualization of a story House told in which a nameless female nurse served as a physician sex object. In House's semi-apocryphal story, told to a class of precocious fifth graders and parents, part of House's physician team was at a patient's bedside. One male physician asked an attractive nurse if she wanted to have an affair, and another physician asked if she wanted to have a threesome. The nurse looked a bit intrigued, but a female medical student objected.[63] As with the *NCIS* detective, House's real goal in telling the story may have been to tweak others, especially females. Nurses' apparent sexual availability is convenient! A February 2007 episode invited viewers to chuckle at the witty House's suggestion that if a physician friend would just stop annoying him, they could be "ranking nurses in order of do-ability."[64] In a November 2005 episode, the resourceful House coerced a reluctant surgeon into performing a risky liver transplant by threatening to tell his wife what the surgeon had secretly been doing with lots of nurses.[65] Skanky syph nurses, we bet!

Sitcoms are a natural home for the naughty nurse. For example, in a January 2014 episode of *The Mindy Project*, physician character Jeremy played "nookie hookie" from work, an activity that seemed to involve partying with two attractive young lingerie-clad women. When a fellow physician tried to persuade Jeremy to return to work, he demurred, noting that "my nurses have a few more tests to run."[66] That's really all we got, so we were left to wonder: Were they really nurses? Or was that just a joke with a health care theme? Either way, it's naughty nursing.

In the September 2011 pilot of NBC's *Whitney*, the lead character tried to seduce her boyfriend Alex with a revealing naughty nurse outfit. It worked well until Alex fell while trying to get out of his pants, hit his head on a table, and lost consciousness.[67] In an October 2010 episode of ABC's *Modern Family*, the naughty nurse was one of a series of Halloween costumes worn by the teenage character Haley Dunphy that her mother found too sexually explicit.[68]

An April 2004 episode of *Will & Grace* was a naughty nurse landmark. The episode focused on the frivolous Jack graduation from "nursing school." At the tiny ceremony, one of the nurse speakers was a very attractive woman whose sheer white uniform was unbuttoned below the level of her bright blue bra. Jack began to read the speech he got to deliver because he was voted "most popular," but he decided in the middle that he would follow his original dream of being an actor. Later Will delivered the rest of the speech privately to the blue bra nurse, who was moved by its "follow your dream" theme to muse, "Maybe I will get back into porn."[69]

The naughty nurse has even appeared briefly in one of the 2009 nurse shows. The June 2009 series premiere of *HawthoRNe* introduced an attractive nurse character named Candy Sullivan who saw it as part of her job to provide manual sex to injured Iraq war veterans, as a "thank you" for their service.[70] Even the show seemed embarrassed, backing away quietly from the plotline several episodes later, and Candy was later shown to be a competent nurse. By contrast, although *Nurse Jackie* and *Mercy* have featured lead characters who were adulterous, no reasonable viewer could interpret those smart, strong women as "naughty," certainly not by current television standards.[71]

MTV's reality show *Scrubbing In*, which focused on travel nurses in California, included plenty of sexual situations and discussions. In an October 2013 episode, several female nurses giggled about finding some "hot doctors." Other scenes touched on pressing public health issues of the day (e.g., "I have big fake boobs!"; "Did you guys bring your vibrators?").[72] In a December 2013 episode there was skinny dipping, including naked "chicken fighting," with some flirtatious behavior involving one nurse and another who was engaged to marry someone else![73] Of course, although nurses should be permitted the same social activities as anyone else, associating the profession with frank sexual imagery can reinforce the naughty nurse image.

Beyond prime time, the landscape is hardly better. Even David Letterman, who gave nurses credit following his heart bypass surgery in 2000,[74] has been unable to resist the naughty nurse's charms. In December 2005, his CBS *Late Show* included a segment about an injury to his hand. Robert Hotchkiss, a real hand surgeon, strode out followed by two models dressed as "nurses" in short white dresses and caps. Hotchkiss examined the wound and bantered with Dave. The "nurses" giggled. Preparing for Hotchkiss to remove the stitches, Dave asked if there would be any disrobing. Paul Shaffer interjected, "Just the nurses!" The physician was the witty expert. The "nurses" were sex props.[75]

It's no surprise that the naughty nurse appears on soap operas, which feature a toxic stew of nurse stereotypes, including vacuous handmaidens, gossiping twits, and, uh, monkeys. From 2004 to 2005, the CBS daytime drama *As the World Turns* featured nurse character Julia Larrabee, memorialized in a December 2004 *TV Guide* piece entitled "'Nurse Skank Strikes Again."[76] The character was a "needy, man-hungry nurse" whom fans hated for breaking up some of the soap's most popular couples.

But some might be surprised that the naughty nurse has appeared on respected daytime talk shows. In November 2010, the globally popular program *The Dr. Oz Show* offered viewers a short segment about Angel Williams, who lost 200 pounds by dancing. Williams, dressed in a short white nurse's dress, told host Mehmet Oz she was going to "get sexy" and unbuttoned the top of the dress as she prepared to lead him in some dancing. She also told Oz that she and a group of similarly attired dancers would be "your nurses—we're gonna keep America moving for you." Oz himself referred to the dancers as Williams's "fellow nurses."[77] No doubt the show thought it would be fun to present these women as Oz's sexy nurse backup dancers—doesn't every celebrity physician have those? After a Truth About Nursing campaign, Oz did publicly apologize to nurses.

The naughty nurse has even seduced animated television programs for children. On *Steven Spielberg Presents Animaniacs* (1993–1998), the very voluptuous character "Hello Nurse" was a "sex kitten" in a tight white dress who apparently aroused even the very young. Main characters Yakko and Wakko used the hilarious "Hellooooo Nurse!" cat call when attractive females appeared.[78]

The sexually available nurse remains welcome in major Hollywood film productions. Consider Ron Howard's successful *Rush* (2013), which dramatized the real-life rivalry between two leading 1970s Formula One racers, the free-spirited British playboy James Hunt and the brilliant, driven Austrian Niki Lauda. In one scene, Hunt arrives at an emergency department for a minor patch-up and immediately seduces an attractive young nurse—the two hook up on the spot in a treatment room.[79] Just a bit of history? Apparently not; reviews suggest the nurse scene is not part of the historical record.[80]

The naughty nurse isn't afraid of horror films, in which the naughty image has often been mixed with malevolence, as in the *Saw III* promotions. You might think nurses are harmless sluts—the conventional view—but here, they're forces of evil, seeming to embody male fears about female sexuality generally and female nurses in particular.[81] In the 2014 erotic thriller *Nurse 3D*, the main character was an attractive female nurse—and a sadistic, sexually aggressive killer with severe psychological issues who targeted cheating men.[82] Nurses figured in the successful *Silent Hill* horror film franchise, which was based on popular Konami video games about a haunted town. In the video games, the "nurses" were monsters, deformed manifestations of human fears who only occasionally presented sexually.[83] But in the films *Silent Hill* (2006) and *Silent Hill: Revelation 3D* (2012), the nurses were provocatively-dressed as they blindly struck out at others and even killed each other—capturing the effect of naughty nurses pretty well.[84] *Candy Stripers* (2006) was about a hospital full of sexy, horny "candy striper nurses" who had been infected with an alien virus, which they spread through . . . close contact.[85] *Sick Nurses*, a low-budget 2007 Thai film, featured seven hot nurses as what one review called a "harem" to a young hospital physician who provided cadavers to body-parts dealers.[86] The nurses liked to take most of their clothes off. But when one nurse got a little too jealous of the physician attention another was receiving, a ghostly horror plot developed. Scary!

Night Shift Nurses: Nursing in Sexually-Oriented Products

The naughty nurse often practices her love in products whose purpose is mainly sexual. This includes pornography in all its forms, as well as lingerie and Halloween costumes.

The naughty nurse thrives in hard-core pornography worldwide. Hundreds of nurse-themed feature films are available. They include *I Love Nurses* (2013),[87] *Transsexual Nurses 10* (2012),[88] *Naughty Nympho Nurses* (2011),[89] *Naughty Nurse Nancy* (2009),[90] *Lesbian Big Boob Squirting Nurses* (2008),[91] *Asian T-Girl Latex Nurses 4* (2007),[92] *Trailer Trash Nurses 7* (2003),[93] *Nasty Backdoor Nurses* (2001),[94] and *Night Shift Nurses* (1989)[95]—this last one is also the title of a popular fetishistic Japanese *hentai* (pornographic animation) series begun in 2000.[96] Some Internet sites are devoted to hardcore nurse imagery. In early 2014, examples included www.hotnakednurses.com, www.sexynurse.tumblr.com, www.lovelynurses.com, and www.linfirmiere.

com (the nurse). The images range from female models shedding clothes to multiple actors (including male "doctors") engaging in intercourse and other sex acts. The women wear, or almost wear, skimpy "nurse" outfits or lingerie, usually white—no patterned scrubs here! Hundreds of general porn sites and networks include large naughty nurse sections. It seems that no female porn star's resume is complete without some nurse imagery. Maybe it's like doing Shakespeare is for mainstream Hollywood stars.

The naughty nurse is also popular in less graphic sexually-oriented products, including "lad's magazines," newspapers, and digital media that may not include full nudity. Yes, of course there are naughty nurse applications, featuring photos of models in the standard naughty nurse attire, like the imaginatively named "Naughty Nurses" app that Ocean Red released in 2011.[97] Apple introduced apps called "A Naughty Nurse"[98] (2009) and "Sexy Nurses"[99] (2009) for the computer company's iPhone and iTouch units.

Print publications rely on the naughty nurse. In August 2005, the cover of the Australian magazine *Ralph* featured Gianna, a former contestant on the local *Big Brother* television program, in a bra and panties "nurse" outfit.[100] Gianna made a different naughty nurse outfit a major feature of her time on the reality show. At the end of 2006, 2007, and 2010, the *Sun* (UK)—the most widely-circulated English-language daily newspaper in the world—ran promotional tie-in pieces for Babes and Boys' annual naughty nurse calendars.[101] The *Sun* pictorials featured the usual lingerie-nurse outfits, but a key theme was that the models really *were* nurses. One "student nurse" told the *Sun* she posed for "a bit of a laugh" and "a bit of extra money." Plus, "People always joke about nurses looking saucy so it's fun to be the real thing."[102]

The naughty nurse is also poised to spring out of women's closets. A North Carolina company called 3 Wishes Lingerie has offered a variety of nurse-related items for many years. In late 2013 its online selection of outfits included the Bedroom Nurse, Bad Nurse, Night Nurse, Nurse Goodhands, and Doctors Orders.[103] In January 2005, the Australian Nursing Federation persuaded retailer Bras N Things to end advertising for one naughty nurse outfit, although it remained for sale in the lingerie chain's more than 150 stores. As of early 2014, the retailer's website still offered a Nurse Feelgood Costume.[104]

In fact, a naughty nurse costume may have altered the course of Western civilization! The *Daily Mail* reported in July 2013 that the British royal couple Kate Middleton and Prince William had repaired their broken relationship in 2007 when Kate wore a "naughty nurse" outfit to a "Freakin' Naughty" costume party at William's military barracks.[105]

Every year at Halloween, major US retailers sell many naughty nurse costumes. Don't miss Party City's "Adult Hospital Honey Nurse Costume"[106] or Spirit Halloween's "Nurse Heartbreaker Costume!"[107] In early 2014, the wholesale supplier Alibaba consistently had more than 3,000 different types of naughty nurse costumes for sale.[108] Yes, it's just for "a bit of a laugh." But it still undermines nursing. The Southern Poverty Law Center's highly regarded Teaching Tolerance campaign has urged the public to reconsider the use of stereotypes even in Halloween costumes.[109]

Promiscuous Girls: The Nurse in Pop Music

The naughty nurse is a bit of a pop music groupie, and she lets musicians use her to sell or accompany their music, even if the music itself makes no mention of nurses. The mixing of nursing and sexuality runs across musical styles and goes at least as far back as reggae artist Gregory Isaacs's "Night Nurse" from 1982. Sample lyrics:

> Night nurse
> Only you alone can quench this here thirst
> My night nurse, oh gosh
> Oh, the pain is getting worse
> I don't wanna see no doc
> I need attendance from my nurse around the clock
> For there's no prescription for me
> She is the one, the only remedy.[110]

The song has been covered by Simply Red (1998)[111] and Sinead O'Connor (2009),[112] among others.

In January 2010, pop star Mariah Carey released a video for "Up Out My Face" to promote her remix album *Angels Advocate*. The video featured Carey and rapper Nicki Minaj in skimpy "nurse" outfits, with white stockings and high heels. The song is actually a bitter kiss-off to a former lover, so it would seem to reverse the standard naughty nurse theme of sexual availability. But the point of the video seems to be to show the ex-lover just what he will be missing. At a couple points in the video, Minaj applied her stethoscope to Carey's chest, as if checking her heart rate.[113] The Truth About Nursing started a campaign to protest the video that received international press coverage but got no response from Carey. As of July 2014, the video's VEVO view count was more than 39 million.[114]

In March 2009 the veteran metal band Mötley Crüe announced its upcoming summer tour at a New York press conference that featured women in naughty nurse outfits and a classic Cadillac ambulance. The band evidently wanted to highlight the fact that it would be playing its popular 1989 album *Dr. Feelgood* all the way through at each show.[115]

Julie Taymor's 2007 film *Across the Universe*, a musical about the upheavals of the 1960s featuring Beatles songs, included a number in which Salma Hayek played a small group of identical "nurses," all wearing a little black nurse's dress. The sexy Hayeks appeared in a hospitalized male character's hallucination and helped him sing "Happiness Is a Warm Gun," as they danced around somewhat provocatively. Finally, one Hayek injected the bedridden man with a syringe containing a little blue naked woman. The nurses' main line: "Bang, bang, shoot, shoot!"[116]

In 2005 the UK electronic-alternative-pop duo Goldfrapp set a video for their single "Number 1" at a plastic surgery clinic where everyone but singer Alison Goldfrapp had a human body and a dog's head. In director Dawn Shadforth's video, Goldfrapp acted like a dog, danced with the clinic staff, and spun the song's tale of animalistic sexual obsession. The "nurses" were all females in short dresses who handed things to the all-male "physicians." The camera dwelled on the nurses' bottoms—on which the physicians, at one point, playfully placed their stethoscopes.[117]

Country rock singer Keith Anderson's song "XXL" (2005) is an ode to the virtues of the big and tall, including their ability to get hot babes. The song describes the singer's birth: "Took two nurses to hold me and one nurse to slap me." The music video, directed by Trey Fanjoy, featured the famously well-endowed Mötley Crüe drummer Tommy Lee as the leering "doctor." Tommy's laboratory coat said "Dr. Feelgood" (there he is again!). In the delivery room, Tommy was on intimate terms with three naughty nurses, who posed, pouted, and spilled out of their tiny dresses—as they all cared for the "XXL" infant and his mom.[118] Paging Dr. Freud to obstetrics!

Of course, an actual porn star can add naughty nurse realism. The punk-pop band blink-182's hit 1999 CD *Enema of the State* featured photographs of porn star Janine.[119] On the front cover, the front of her white nurse's uniform was open to reveal a red bra, as she pulled on a blue examining glove. On the back cover, Janine sat on a stool dressed in a short naughty nurses' uniform, holding a huge syringe and needle. The band members, facing her, were dressed only in their underwear, looking concerned. In the photographs, Janine seemed both seductive and threatening—not unlike some recent horror film nurses.

"The Nurse," a song from the White Stripes' 2005 album *Get Behind Me Satan*, offered a more subtle take on the nurse as romantic object. The Detroit garage rock duo's song isn't naughty, but it does use an unholy mix of nursing imagery to complain about betrayal. Songwriter Jack White sings, "The nurse should not be the one who puts salt in your wounds." He also mentions promises this "nurse" has broken, and laments that the "maid that you've hired could never conspire to kill," not wanting to believe it.[120]

White's metaphors compare the faithful care one would expect from a nurse to that of a close friend, presumably a female lover. Wouldn't it be tragic if a "nurse," rather than taking care of you like that "night nurse" we've heard about, instead hurt you? Yeah, man. Nurses are obligated to protect their patients, but that doesn't mean their expert care is like romance. A man may need a "maid," as Neil Young once sang, but he isn't getting a "nurse" every time he gets a lover.

Hot or Not? Sexy Nurses in the News Media

You might think the naughty nurse would hesitate to appear in the news media. But she still pops out of articles about kooky hospital policies, discussions of celebrities and current issues, and even comic strips.

The mainstream press is always ready to leap on a nurses-and-sex story. It gets the chance when health facilities seem to be either promoting or discouraging naughty nursing. In February 2012, press entities around the world gleefully reported that Stockholm's South General Hospital was seeking to hire "TV-series hot nurses." That allowed the media to embrace the naughty nurse image while seeming to be just telling the story of a notable hospital recruiting tactic. Lee Moran's *Daily Mail* (UK) piece not only reported on the summer job advertisement, but it also included an unrelated naughty nurse image (helpfully labeled "picture posed by model"), just to show curious readers what a "TV-series hot nurse" might look like. Nurse managers at the Swedish hospital stressed that they were just trying to "catch people's attention"—mission accomplished!—and that professional nursing qualifications were all that really mattered in their hiring.[121]

In March 2008 news sources worldwide reported that a clinic in Spain had told its nurses they would be docked pay if they failed to dress in miniskirts. These reports were partly wrong, as the clinic was only requiring the nurses to wear traditional outfits with a modest-length skirt and cap. That was regressive enough. But press sources (such as ABC News) embraced the miniskirt angle.[122]

Similarly, the Ananova Internet news site has aggressively covered efforts by hospitals in Southeast Europe to get unruly nurses back into skirts. In September 2006 the site's "Nurses in Romania to Wear Miniskirts" reported that "doctors" in a Romanian town had asked "officials" to order female nurses and physicians to wear miniskirts, ostensibly because it would be more "elegant."[123] Somehow, the female physicians did not make the headline. In October 2005 the *Hindustan Times* (India) site posted an Ananova-based item reporting that a Croatian hospital had ordered nurses to "go back to wearing skirts instead of trousers after complaints from patients." The hospital director was quoted as noting that the skirts' length, "be they mini skirts or otherwise," was up to the nurses. The *Hindustan Times* ran this lead: "It has long been suspected that pretty nurses doing their 'nightingale' rounds in their freshly-starched skirts, more often than not, bring a cheer to even the most woefully-ill patients, and now it seems that believers in this theory were right all along." The headline: "Patients Want Pretty, Skirt-Clad Nurses!"[124]

However, in September 2006 the *Daily Mail* (UK) was compelled to report a sad setback for the naughty nurse. "Nurses Face Ban on Thongs and Cleavage" explained that an Essex hospital was considering requiring nurses to make sure they didn't expose cleavage or underwear. In case anyone missed that message, the *Daily Mail* included an image of the Christina Aguilera naughty nurse advertisement for Skechers, with this caption: "Sorry guys: don't expect to see the likes of Christina Aguilera in this nurses uniform at Southend Hospital."[125]

People magazine's December 2010 year-end issue included Poison singer and reality television star Bret Michaels as one of its "most intriguing" people in a two-page layout dominated by a photo of Michaels surrounded by four naughty nurse models.[126] The nurse element was a reference to his well-publicized recovery from a brain hemorrhage and other health problems, but naughty nursing was nothing new for Michaels. In a blog post following an emergency appendectomy in April 2010, he had reported that he had "hot nurses" taking care of him, referring to the "nurse fantasy" that "every man has." Maybe that kind of imagery helps reduce the sense of illness-related vulnerability that could threaten a celebrity whose image is built on strength. But *People* magazine "reache[d] more adult readers (more than 45 million as of fall 2009) with each issue than any consumer magazine ever," according to its publisher Time Inc.[127] After the Truth About Nursing contacted the company, the editor of *People* apologized, published our letter to the editor about the photograph, and promised to avoid such imagery in the future.[128]

News media humorists are not above using the naughty nurse to extract cheap laughs. In an April 2008 edition of Fox News Channel's early morning show *Redeye*, host Greg Gutfeld and his guests conducted a loving, if ironic, celebration of the Spanish clinic's misreported "miniskirt" policy. Gutfeld displayed photographs of naughty nurse models and then asked his guests, including a physician, who could be against the clinic's miniskirt policy. Guess what? No one was! Gutfeld asked if "attractive nurses in short skirts might lift the spirits of male patients and increase their chances of getting better." Guest Diana Falzone, co-host of *Devore & Diana* on Maxim Sirius radio, replied, "You know what, I believe that. Every woman no matter what size or shape has something to flaunt. Especially the Latina women. They have big butts. So I say, wear the miniskirts and just save some lives."[129]

In June 2007 syndicated radio host Stephanie Miller and sidekick Jim Ward managed to work naughty nurses into a discussion of proposed federal immigration legislation. When a caller suggested that a provision easing restrictions on the entry of foreign nurses would undermine unions, Miller seemed sympathetic but also noted jokingly that "Jim will not be happy if a lot of naughty foreign nurses get in."

WARD: Naughty nurses by the boatload.

MILLER: *(with sound effect of a whip cracking)* Jim cannot . . . no. We must stop the naughty Scandinavian nurses *(whip)*, porn nurse from infiltrating America *(whip)*.

WARD: And French maids. Mmm-hmm.[130]

Miller and Ward were playing with the stereotypes, but not questioning them. Like the whip sound, they are just standard comic effects to be exploited—although, even after five decades and thousands of repetitions, that naughty nurse joke is still a *killer*.

Not even the comics page can escape sexy nurses' plans for world media domination. In March 2008 Matt Janz's syndicated *Single and Looking* strip featured a character asking his friend Zoog whether he'd like to live to be a hundred years old. Zoog: "Sure, Sammy . . . There's something hot about a young nurse giving me a sponge bath."[131] In December 2006 John McPherson's syndicated *Close to Home* comic showed an emergency medical technician, with an ambulance, giving a stretcher-bound patient a choice: "Mercy Hospital" was "20 minutes closer," but the nurses at "Saratoga Hospital" were "really hot."[132] A piece by Charles Fiegl in the *Post-Star* of

Glen Falls, New York, about the strip reported that McPherson had based it on his recent stays at nearby Saratoga Hospital, in the hope that real nurses there would email him so he could "take them out to dinner." Asked for comment, one nurse from that hospital reportedly said she and her colleagues really were "very hot," which is "how we get our patients to come to Saratoga," although she added that the nurses there "also provide great care."[133]

Whenever a real nurse describes her profession mainly in terms of physical attraction—as hot or not—the naughty nurse smiles. It's time for a penny shot!

Notes

1. Melinda Rogers, "Man Misses Birth of His Child after Fondling Nurse, Police Say," *Salt Lake Tribune* (October 9, 2009), http://tinyurl.com/lo5azqk; TAN, "Today's Childbirth Class Topic: Resisting the Urge to Grab Your L&D Nurse's Breasts!" (October 12, 2009), http://tinyurl.com/lvjbzrt.
2. Teresa Masterson, "Nothing Says 'Thank You' Like a Tush Grab or Two: Man Says He Was Trying to Show Gratitude but Faces Assault Charge for Groping Nurse Twice," MSNBC (December 2, 2010); TAN, "You're a Nurse, Right?" (December 2, 2010), http://tinyurl.com/mff95n3.
3. Tammy McGuire, Debbie Dougherty, and Joshua Atkinson, "Paradoxing the Dialectic: The Impact of Patients' Sexual Harassment in the Discursive Construction of Nurses' Caregiving Roles," *Management Communication Quarterly* 19, no. 3 (2006): 416–450, http://tinyurl.com/y9c92lc; Mildred L. Culp, "Patients Harassing Nurses? Oh, Yes! How Nurses, Administrators and Society Can Respond," *Nursing in Virginia Magazine* (Spring 2006), http://tinyurl.com/lkotkyp; John Rossheim, "How Nurses Can Fight Sexual Harassment," *Monster* (March 2006), http://tinyurl.com/yh4ozv3.
4. Y. Hibino, Y. Hitomi, Y. Kambayashi, and H. Nakamura, "Exploring Factors Associated with the Incidence of Sexual Harassment of Hospital Nurses by Patients," *Journal of Nursing Scholarship* 41, no. 2 (2009): 124–131, http://tinyurl.com/yzok6cb.
5. *New York Daily News*, "Pakistani Nurses Vulnerable to Sexual Harassment" (August 5, 2012), http://tinyurl.com/klwqa3c; TAN, "Thanking the Nurse" (August 5, 2012), http://tinyurl.com/pmfs55o.
6. Nicole Bode, "Flushing Hospital Nurse Gets $15 Million Award in Sexual Harassment Suit," *New York Daily News* (February 23, 2009), http://tinyurl.com/ljjagx7.
7. Ethan Sacks, "Dutch Nurses Need Public Service Campaign, Stat! Don't Have to Perform Sexual Acts for Patients," *New York Daily News* (March 12, 2010),

http://tinyurl.com/mgfq6sb; TAN, "Drawing the Line" (March 12, 2010), http://tinyurl.com/lksyatf.

8. Associated Press, "Inappropriate Patient Behavior Tough on Nurses: Sexual Harassment a Widespread Problem, Health Officials Say," MSNBC (December 15, 2005), http://tinyurl.com/kora4ym; CFNA, "AP: 'Inappropriate Patient Behavior Tough on Nurses,'" TAN (December 15, 2005), http://tinyurl.com/mgnjmd9.
9. Agence France-Presse, "Nurses and Firemen Top Fantasy Poll," *The Age* (August 24, 2006), http://tinyurl.com/k8vcx7e; CFNA, "Nurses Are No. 1. . . . In Male Sexual Fantasies," TAN (August 24, 2006), http://tinyurl.com/n4pyw25.
10. Dan Bilefsky, "If Plastic Surgery Won't Convince You, What Will?" *New York Times* (May 24, 2009), http://tinyurl.com/kcel3mx; TAN, "We Are Offering Free Breasts" (July 14, 2009), http://tinyurl.com/m6mrtyh.
11. Kelly Ripa, *Live with Regis and Kelly* (March 12 and 15, 2007); CFNA, "Kelly Ripa Is Your Sponge Bath Nursey in Her Little Nursey Costume! Did We Mention She Was a Nursey? With a Sponge? Ooh! She Missed a Spot over Here!," TAN (March 15, 2007), http://tinyurl.com/n8d7xct.
12. CFNA, "Skechers Pulls Christina Aguilera 'Nurse' Ad after Receiving More than 3,000 Letters from Nursing Supporters," TAN (August 17, 2004), http://tinyurl.com/lfz2ebb.
13. Getty Images, "Christina Aguilera Celebrated as a Sexy Nurse with Jordan Bratman in Las Vegas in 2005" (2005), http://tinyurl.com/msf8c7g.
14. CFNA, "Italian Nurses Are Better-Looking . . . These [U.S.] Ones Scare Me a Bit. Don't Even Think About Leaving Me Alone at Night with One of Them," TAN (December 22, 2006), http://tinyurl.com/lp66x2w.
15. Nick Pisa, "Nurses Attack Silvio Berlusconi over Striptease," *Evening Standard* (January 20, 2011), http://tinyurl.com/lbxx59e; TAN, "Neverland" (January 23, 2011), http://tinyurl.com/kb5ea6q.
16. *The Times*, "Racists Hit Drive for Nurses" (August 24, 2004); CFNA, "At Least They've Avoided that Angel Stereotype: Asian Nurses Confront Racist Abuse and Views That Their Profession Is 'On a Par with Prostitution,'" TAN (August 24, 2004), http://tinyurl.com/l335jpg.
17. Ashfaq Yusufzai, "Pakistan: Nurses Get Little Training or Respect," Inter Press Service (June 3, 2006), http://tinyurl.com/mfnodp2; CFNA, "'Colleagues at the Hospital Think I Am a Prostitute,'" TAN (June 4, 2006), http://tinyurl.com/l2wsshs.
18. Dame Helen Mirren, *Late Show with David Letterman*, "Season 17, Episode 152" (June 14, 2010); TAN, "Nursing at the Love Ranch" (June 14, 2010), http://tinyurl.com/lzolweq.
19. TAN, "Busch Gardens Teaches Kids about Nurses" (October 2011), http://tinyurl.com/lw2arck.

20. Phil McGraw, "Anatomy of an Affair," *Dr. Phil* (November 18, 2004), CFNA, "Kicking Dr. Phil's Ass to the Curb," TAN (November 18, 2004), http://tinyurl.com/mxj9d2r.
21. *Albawaba*, "Nurses Union Demands Ghada Abd Al Riziq's Drama Be Stopped" (August 16, 2010), http://tinyurl.com/lzd3rrf; TAN, "Bad Reputation" (August 16, 2010), http://tinyurl.com/khes382.
22. Mark Chappell, Shaun Pye, and Alan Connor, writers, based on the short stories of Mikhail Bulgakov, Alex Hardcastle, director, "Season 1, Episode 3" and "Season 1, Episode 4," *A Young Doctor's Notebook*, Ovation/Sky Arts (December 20 and 27, 2012), http://tinyurl.com/n2cbe6o and http://tinyurl.com/k4ebqe3.
23. Emily Pirie, personal email (April 20, 2008).
24. US Census Bureau, "Men in Nursing Occupations: American Community Survey Highlight Report" (February 2013), http://tinyurl.com/mjxgvue.
25. Peter Glick, Sadie Weber, Cathryn Johnson, and Heather Branstiter, "Evaluations of Sexy Women in Low and High Status Jobs," *Psychology of Women Quarterly* 29, no. 4 (December 2005): 389–395, http://tinyurl.com/kzhz5gu; Eric Noe, "Can Sexy Women Climb the Corporate Ladder? A New Study Suggests that Bold, Revealing Clothing May Keep You from Getting a Promotion," ABC News (December 2, 2005), http://tinyurl.com/y937x4a.
26. Melissa L. Wookey, Nell A. Graves, and J. Corey Butler, "Effects of a Sexy Appearance on Perceived Competence of Women," *The Journal of Social Psychology* 148, no. 2 (2009): 116–118.
27. Mónica Romero-Sánchez, Mercedes Durán, Hugo Carretero-Dios, Jesús L. Megías, and Miguel Moya, "Exposure to Sexist Humor and Rape Proclivity: The Moderator Effect of Aversiveness Ratings," *Journal of Interpersonal Violence* 25, no. 12 (December 2010): 2339–2350, http://tinyurl.com/n8jc37a.
28. Gil Greengross, "Humor Sapiens: The Laughing Ape and Other Insights into the Nature of Funny," *Psychology Today* (July 18, 2011), http://tinyurl.com/kr5br2k.
29. Thomas E. Ford and Mark A. Ferguson, "Social Consequences of Disparagement Humor: A Prejudiced Norm Theory," *Personality and Social Psychology Review* 8, no. 1 (2004): 79–94, http://tinyurl.com/9gwl48f.
30. G. Tendayi Viki, Manuela Thomae, Amy Cullen, and Hannah Fernandez, "The Effect of Sexist Humor and Type of Rape on Men's Self-Reported Rape Proclivity and Victim Blame," *Current Research in Social Psychology* 13, no. 10 (2007): 122–132, http://tinyurl.com/bqkdjas.
31. *Science Daily*, "Sexist Humor No Laughing Matter, Psychologist Says" (November 7, 2007), http://tinyurl.com/yg7p8r8.
32. Thomas E. Ford, Christie F. Boxer, Jacob Armstrong, and Jessica R. Edel, "More than 'Just a Joke': The Prejudice-Releasing Function of Sexist Humor," *Personality and Social Psychology Bulletin* 34, no. 2 (February 2008): 159–170, http://tinyurl.com/6j9fmb5.

33. TAN, "Just How Undervalued and Underfunded Is Nursing?," accessed January 31, 2014, http://tinyurl.com/k7m4wep.
34. Richard Prince, "Nurse Paintings," exhibit at the Barbara Gladstone Gallery (New York: September 20–October 25, 2003); CFNA, "Nurse Paintings," TAN (September 28, 2003), http://tinyurl.com/k8fkgev.
35. Sonic Youth, *Sonic Nurse*, Geffen/Interscope (2004), http://tinyurl.com/8tua6bb; CFNA, "Sonic Youth, 'Sonic Nurse,'" TAN (July 12, 2004), http://tinyurl.com/kzgl476.
36. CFNA, "Coor Slight," TAN (December 2006), http://tinyurl.com/l8wmgwp.
37. CFNA, "What the World Needs Now Is Inspiring Soulful Love Dolls," TAN (October 12, 2007), http://tinyurl.com/lq2vnj2.
38. CFNA, "Your Ultimate Recovery Team," TAN (August 2008), http://tinyurl.com/nxgj7p2.
39. CFNA, "X Games," TAN (October 15, 2006), http://tinyurl.com/mg4qhzl.
40. CFNA, "Tagged: Gillette Pulls Lusty-Nurse Fever Ad," TAN (October 3, 2005), http://tinyurl.com/k85zjmw.
41. CFNA, "Don't You Think I'm So Sexy—I'm Just So Fresh, So Clean," TAN (September 27, 2007), http://tinyurl.com/mue2geq.
42. Joan Coello, "Sexy Doctors and Nurses Serve up McDonald's in Taiwan!" RocketNews24 (January 6, 2014), http://tinyurl.com/l4z5f58.
43. TAN, "It's the Cure, Baby! Naughty Nursing with Hooters" (March 31, 2011), http://tinyurl.com/3rlpacq.
44. Carey Polis, "John Alleman Dead: Heart Attack Grill Unofficial Spokesman Dies from Heart Attack," *Huffington Post* (February 12, 2013), http://tinyurl.com/axp7whx; Courtney Hutchison, "Hefty Heart Attack Grill Spokesman Dies at 29," ABC News (March 4, 2011), http://tinyurl.com/49x5cxm.
45. Heart Attack Grill, accessed March 30, 2014, www.heartattackgrill.com; CFNA, "Worth Dying For," TAN (October 2008), http://tinyurl.com/c5ouw9m.
46. Good Hurt Nightclub, "About," accessed March 30, 2014,http://tinyurl.com/nl46hc9; CFNA, "I Feel So Good I'm Gonna Break Somebody's Heart Tonight," TAN (August 15, 2007), http://tinyurl.com/l7l5d9g.
47. City Steam Brewery Café, "City Steam: The Naughty Nurse," accessed March 27, 2014, http://tinyurl.com/lwjppb7.
48. TAN, "A Bad Case of Loving Nurses" (February 28, 2012), http://tinyurl.com/7lzjjxz.
49. Virgin Mobile, "Think Hatke," YouTube video, accessed March 30, 2014, http://tinyurl.com/pxrkg4w; TAN, "Not So Hatke" (October 2009), http://tinyurl.com/n5whptp.
50. Tyler Hamilton, "Nurses Plan Boycott of Virgin Mobile over Ads That 'Demean' Profession: Shown Wearing Short Skirts and Stilettos. Demand Branson Publicly Apologize," *Toronto Star* (March 5, 2005); CFNA, "Virgin Mobile's Merry Pranksters," TAN (March 5, 2005), http://tinyurl.com/lsluapl.

51. Skechers, "Christina Aguilera Ad Campaign," adland.tv, accessed March 30, 2014, http://tinyurl.com/n6dvdh; CFNA, "Inject Me," TAN (August 2004), http://tinyurl.com/konqwjc.
52. *Daily Mail,* "Ooooh Matron! Upset Nurses Demand Bus Company Removes 'Demeaning' Advert Promoting Bus Route to Hospital" (March 16, 2010), http://tinyurl.com/mmqr3l3; TAN, "That Joke Isn't Funny Anymore" (March 16, 2010), http://tinyurl.com/lthsu2t.
53. Reuters, "Cosmetic Surgery Firm's Stunt Riles Spanish Nurses" (July 20, 2005), http://tinyurl.com/lqgvpmf; CFNA, "That Not-Obscure-Enough Object of Desire," TAN (July 20, 2005), http://tinyurl.com/lwkwldh.
54. Laura Sweet, "The Saw VI Blood Drive Posters & All the Ones from Years Past," If It's Hip, It's Here (August 8, 2009), http://tinyurl.com/kj2nwtl; CFNA, "Blood Simple," TAN (October 27, 2006), http://tinyurl.com/nyorh4s.
55. TAN, "To Serve Dr. Lung Love" (November 2, 2009), http://tinyurl.com/lrej4bs.
56. Joseph C. Wilson, writer, Kate Woods, director, "Personal," *NCIS: Los Angeles,* CBS (February 22, 2011); TAN, "Helpful and Caring and the Whole Sponge Bath Thing" (February 22, 2011), http://tinyurl.com/mct3k24.
57. Alexandra Cunningham and Lori Kirkland Baker, writers, David Grossman, director, "Sunday," *Desperate Housewives,* ABC (April 13, 2008); CFNA, "Desperate Nursemaids," TAN (April 13, 2008), http://tinyurl.com/nm9vze7.
58. Stacy McKee, writer, Tom Verica, director, "What Is It about Men," *Grey's Anatomy,* ABC (October 13, 2011); TAN, "Who's the Man?" (October 13, 2011), http://tinyurl.com/onha8uc.
59. Krista Vernoff, writer, Peter Horton, director, "Grandma Got Run over by a Reindeer," *Grey's Anatomy,* ABC (December 11, 2005); CFNA, "Plot Devices in Scrubs," TAN (December 11, 2005), http://tinyurl.com/nhlj8nd.
60. Krista Vernoff, writer, Peter Horton, director, "Grandma. . .."
61. Tony Phelan and Joan Rater, writers, Julie Anne Robinson, director, "The Becoming," *Grey's Anatomy,* ABC (May 8, 2008); CFNA, "Looking for Mr. McSteamy," TAN (May 8, 2008), http://tinyurl.com/oj3ybyy.
62. Zoanne Clack, "Where the Wild Things Are," *Grey's Anatomy* (April 24, 2008), http://tinyurl.com/nuf38tw.
63. Thomas L. Moran, writer, Greg Yaitanes, director, "Two Stories," *House,* Fox (November 21, 2011); TAN, "Helpful and Caring and the Whole Sponge Bath Thing" (February 22, 2011), http://tinyurl.com/nlasf6l.
64. Matthew V. Lewis, writer, Deran Sarafian, director, "Insensitive," *House,* Fox (February 13, 2007); CFNA, "They Dare to Be Do-Able," TAN (February 13, 2007), http://tinyurl.com/l96xcq2.
65. Peter Blake, writer, David Semel, director, "The Mistake," *House,* Fox (November 29, 2005); CFNA, "What Do Nurses Do All Day?," TAN (November 29, 2005), http://tinyurl.com/lo9ff26.

66. Mindy Kaling and Charlie Grandy, writers, Rob Schrab, director, "Danny Castellano Is My Personal Trainer," *The Mindy Project*, Fox (January 7, 2014).
67. Whitney Cummings, writer, Andy Ackerman, director, "Pilot," *Whitney*, NBC (September 22, 2011); TAN, "Whitless" (July 2011), http://tinyurl.com/cmt47df.
68. Jeffery Richman, writer, Michael Spiller, director, "Halloween," *Modern Family*, ABC (October 27, 2010), http://tinyurl.com/q3ghqwk.
69. Sally Bradford, writer, James Burrows, director, "Speechless," *Will & Grace*, NBC (April 22, 2004); CFNA, "*Will & Grace*: The Nurse As Twit, Loser, and Porn Actress," TAN (April 22, 2004), http://tinyurl.com/o8nse2p.
70. John Masius, writer, Mikael Salomon, director, "Pilot," *HawthoRNe*, TNT (June 16, 2009); TAN, "Chief Nursing Officer" (June 16, 2009), http://tinyurl.com/o5ce4yw.
71. TAN, "*Nurse Jackie* Episode Reviews," accessed March 24, 2014, http://tinyurl.com/kqm3k6b; TAN, "*Mercy* Episode Reviews" (2010), http://tinyurl.com/kj3t63s.
72. Dave Caplan, Mark Cronin, and Shannon Fitzgerald, executive producers, "Scrubbing in the OC," *Scrubbing In*, MTV (October 24, 2013), http://tinyurl.com/kvqdsbr.
73. Dave Caplan, Mark Cronin, and Shannon Fitzgerald, executive producers, "Crazy from the Heat," *Scrubbing In*, MTV (December 13, 2013), http://tinyurl.com/l86n3uy.
74. Caryn James, "Here's David: Letterman Returns, True to Form," *New York Times* (February 22, 2000), http://tinyurl.com/mb55494.
75. *The Late Show with David Letterman*, CBS (December 19, 2005); CFNA, "The Gash Cam," TAN (December 19, 2005), http://tinyurl.com/ly74f66.
76. CFNA, "TV Guide's '*Nurse Skank* Strikes Again' Inspires Center to Announce Soap Nurse Sweepstakes!," TAN (December 12, 2004), http://tinyurl.com/p9n3hsj.
77. *The Dr. Oz Show*, syndicated television show (November 4, 2010); TAN, "Thinking Right, Thinking Bright" (November 4, 2010), http://tinyurl.com/py6oao2.
78. John P. McCann, Randy Rogel, and Tom Ruegger, writers, Barry Caldwell, Jon McClenahan, and Audu Paden, directors, "Wakko's 2-Note Song/Panama Canal/Hello Nurse . . . " *Animaniacs* (February 24, 1996), http://tinyurl.com/pqehhyo; IMDb, "Hello Nurse" (1999), http://tinyurl.com/oz9a6fa.
79. Peter Morgan, writer, Ron Howard, director, *Rush*, Universal Pictures (2013).
80. Alex von Tunzelmann, "Rush: A Thrilling but Untrusty Ride," *The Guardian* (September 18, 2013), http://tinyurl.com/pykjbpj.
81. Laura Sweet, "The Saw VI Blood Drive Posters & All the Ones from Years Past," If It's Hip, It's Here (August 8, 2009), http://tinyurl.com/kj2nwtl; CFNA, "Blood Simple," TAN (October 27, 2006), http://tinyurl.com/nyorh4s.
82. Douglas Aarniokoski and David Loughery, writers, Douglas Aarniokoski, director, *Nurse 3D*, Lionsgate (2014), http://tinyurl.com/m4tvzu6; TAN, "Nurse 0D: *Nurse 3D* Finally Released" (January 27, 2014), http://tinyurl.com/mg4kqqa.

83. Keiichiro Toyama, writer and director, *Silent Hill* Video Game, Konami (1999) http://tinyurl.com/mua5jfn.
84. Michael J. Bassett and Laurent Hadida, writers, Michael J. Bassett, director, *Silent Hill: Revelation 3D*, Open Road Films (2012); Roger Avary, writer, Christophe Gans, director, *Silent Hill*, TriStar Pictures (2006); *Silent Hill*, "Silent Hill Revelation 3D Clip—Nurse Scene," YouTube video, http://tinyurl.com/nqgngkw.
85. Jill Garson and Kate Robbins, writers, Kate Robbins, director, *Candy Stripers*, Screen Gems (2006), http://tinyurl.com/oyw3qkz.
86. Piraphan Laoyont and Thodsapol Siriwiwat, directors, *Sick Nurses (Suay Laak Sai)*, Magnolia Home Entertainment (2007), http://tinyurl.com/lxvsf2r.
87. PornStar Empires, *I Love Nurses* (2013), http://tinyurl.com/ladzzgs.
88. White Ghetto, *Transsexual Nurses 10*, Avalon Enterprises (2012), http://tinyurl.com/matzwdw.
89. NaughtyNymphoNurses.com, accessed March 27, 2014.
90. Diana DeVoe, director, *Naughty Nurse Nancy* (2009), http://tinyurl.com/lhncvso.
91. Excalibur Films, *Lesbian Big Boob Squirting Nurses*, Totally Tasteless (2008), http://tinyurl.com/qctzqsy.
92. Pandemonium Movies, *Asian T-Girl Latex Nurses 4* (2006), http://tinyurl.com/lmr6j3a.
93. Jerome Tanner, director, *Trailer Trash Nurses 7* (2003), http://tinyurl.com/kyrxua4.
94. Max Steiner, director, *Nasty Backdoor Nurses*, LBO Entertainment (2001), http://tinyurl.com/mbn4zcz.
95. Jim Holliday, John Leslie, writers, John Leslie, director, *Night Shift Nurses*, VCA Pictures (1989), http://tinyurl.com/po7j9pf.
96. Absolute Anime, "Anime Profile: Night Shift Nurses," http://tinyurl.com/o7bx8y9.
97. Ocean Red, "Naughty Nurses APK," Android.DownloadAtoZ.com (December 29, 2011), http://tinyurl.com/kqbctag.
98. iPhoneapps.com, "A Naughty Nurse" (September 29, 2009), http://tinyurl.com/n435wqf.
99. iPhoneapps.com, "Sexy Nurses" (July 28, 2009), http://tinyurl.com/k5qj2os.
100. "*Big Brother*'s Gianna," *Ralph* (August 2005); CFNA, "Can Naughty Nurse Imagery Launch a Career?," TAN (August 2005), http://tinyurl.com/k69gokt.
101. "A Naughty but Nurse Calendar," *The Sun* (January 12, 2011), http://tinyurl.com/krg4mbo; Asian News International, "Naughty Nurses in U.K. to Get Pulses Racing with Saucy Calendar Shoot," Oneindia (December 14, 2010), http://tinyurl.com/mbrhfam; Lucy Hagan, "Meet the X-Rayted Nurses," *Sun* (November 28, 2006), http://tinyurl.com/owcssyv; Lucy Hagan, "Naughty Hospital Staff," *The Sun* (November 29, 2006), http://tinyurl.com/jvngkd2.
102. CFNA, "People Always Joke about Nurses Looking Saucy so It's Fun to Be the Real Thing," TAN (November 29, 2006), http://tinyurl.com/kek574m.

103. 3Wishes.com, "Nurse Costumes," accessed March 27, 2014, http://tinyurl.com/hc7y7.
104. Bras 'N' Things, "Nurse Feelgood," accessed March 27, 2014,http://tinyurl.com/qadmaml.
105. Marcia Moody, "Secrets of the Royal Romantic Reunion that Changed the Course of History: What Really Made Kate and Wills Rekindle Their Love—and Transform the Monarchy Forever," *Daily Mail* (July 6, 2013), http://tinyurl.com/q68aexc.
106. Party City, "Adult Hospital Honey Nurse Costume," accessed March 27, 2014, http://tinyurl.com/mmz9eta.
107. Spirit Halloween Costumes, "Nurse Heartbreaker Adult Women's Costume," accessed March 27, 2014, http://tinyurl.com/lv37csm.
108. Alibaba, "Adult Nurse Costume," accessed March 27, 2014, http://tinyurl.com/pnrbp67.
109. Southern Poverty Law Center, "What Do Halloween Costumes Say?," accessed March 27, 2014, http://tinyurl.com/ktmgnew.
110. Gregory Isaacs and Sylvester Weise, composers, Gregory Isaacs, performer, "Night Nurse," from the album *Night Nurse* (1982), http://tinyurl.com/ltqqh6v, http://tinyurl.com/m3u4mxb.
111. Gregory Isaacs and Sylvester Weise, composers, Simply Red, performer, "Night Nurse," from the album *Blue* (1998), http://tinyurl.com/auhrued.
112. Gregory Isaacs and Sylvester Weise, composers, Sinead O'Connor, performer, "Night Nurse," from the album *I Do Not Want What I Haven't Got* (special edition) (1990, 2009), http://tinyurl.com/k58db2y; http://tinyurl.com/kdxo9ga.
113. Mariah Carey featuring Nicki Minaj, performers, Nick Cannon, video director, "Up Out My Face," accessed March 27, 2014, http://tinyurl.com/y8ovjmo; TAN, "Mariah Carey: 'Up Out My Face'" (February 22, 2010), http://tinyurl.com/ygu9wcf.
114. Mariah Carey featuring Nicki Minaj, performers, Nick Cannon, video director, "Up Out My Face," accessed March 27, 2014, http://tinyurl.com/y8ovjmo.
115. Jay Smith, "Crüe Fest Lineup Revealed," Pollstar (March 16, 2009), http://tinyurl.com/meq4tm7; TAN, "A Short History of Dr. Feelgood" (March 16, 2009), http://tinyurl.com/lohm82u.
116. Dick Clement, Ian La Frenais, and Julie Taymor, screenplay, Julie Taymor, director, *Across the Universe*, Columbia Pictures (2007), http://tinyurl.com/dz5hhn.
117. Alison Goldfrapp and Will Gregory, composers, Goldfrapp, performer, Dawn Shadforth, video director, "Number 1," from the album *Supernature*, Mute Records (2005); CFNA, "Goldfrapp: 'Number 1,'" TAN (March 27, 2006) http://tinyurl.com/pzseh2k.
118. Keith Anderson and Bob DiPiero, composers, Keith Anderson, performer, Trey Fanjoy, video director, "XXL," from the album *Three Chord Country and American Rock & Roll*, Arista Nashville (2004); CFNA, "Keith Anderson: 'XXL,'" TAN (December 12, 2005), http://tinyurl.com/lmwzyak.

119. blink-182, *Enema of the State*, MCA Records (1999); CFNA, "blink-182, 'Enema of the State,'" TAN (July 11, 2003), http://tinyurl.com/kay9bgp.
120. Jack White, composer, The White Stripes, performer, "The Nurse," from the album *Get Behind Me Satan*, V2 Records (2005); CFNA, "Boy You Have No Faith in Nursing," TAN (April 21, 2006), http://tinyurl.com/kmgw6sx.
121. Lee Moran, "'TV Series-Hot Nurses Need Only Apply': Swedish Hospital Spices up Summer Recruitment Search for Sexy Staff," *Daily Mail* (February 22, 2012), http://tinyurl.com/mvqd5qh; TAN, "Too Darn Hot" (February 2012), http://tinyurl.com/mp9hzzf.
122. *Público.es*, "Las Enfermeras de una Clínica de Cádiz Denunciarán a la Empresa si las Obliga a Usar Falda" (March 25, 2008), http://tinyurl.com/m48t9e6; CFNA, "Wear Skirts, Caps and Aprons . . . Or Lose 30 Euros," TAN (March 28, 2008), http://tinyurl.com/klbj7qk.
123. *Ananova*, "Nurses in Romania to Wear Miniskirts" (September 29, 2006); CFNA, "Ananova Is All over That Miniskirted Nurse Beat," TAN (September 29, 2006), http://tinyurl.com/ldobzar.
124. *Hindustan Times*, "Patients Want Pretty, Skirt-Clad Nurses!" (October 4, 2005); CFNA, "Patients Want Pretty, Skirt-Clad Nurses!," TAN (October 4, 2005), http://tinyurl.com/lmymwrv.
125. *Daily Mail Online,* "Nurses Face Ban on Thongs and Cleavage" (September 2006), http://tinyurl.com/lym5bfh; CFNA, "*Daily Mail*: 'Nurses Face Ban on Thongs and Cleavage,'" TAN (September 19, 2006), http://tinyurl.com/l2lan78.
126. Justin Stephens, photographer, "Most Intriguing: Ultimate Survivor Bret Michaels," *People* (December 27, 2010): 100–101, http://tinyurl.com/mj4qz9q; TAN, "Open Up and Say . . . Naah!" (March 7, 2011), http://tinyurl.com/l98sh9x.
127. *People*, "Stats," accessed May 10, 2009, http://tinyurl.com/lv4z4cz.
128. TAN, "Open Up and Say . . . Naah!" (March 7, 2011), http://tinyurl.com/l98sh9x.
129. Tom O'Connor, writer, "Episode Dated March 31, 2008," *Red Eye*, Fox (March 31, 2008); CFNA, "Wear the Miniskirts and Just Save Some Lives!," TAN (April 1, 2008), http://tinyurl.com/l7moqow.
130. *The Stephanie Miller Show*, syndicated radio show (June 1, 2007), http://tinyurl.com/8yelu; CFNA, "We Must Stop the Naughty Scandinavian Porn Nurses from Infiltrating America!," TAN (June 13, 2007), http://tinyurl.com/jw9mhk5.
131. Matt Janz, *Out of the Gene Pool*, Go Comics (March 22, 2008), http://tinyurl.com/m27u8qt.
132. John McPherson, *Close to Home,* Go Comics (December 18, 2006), http://tinyurl.com/l9noyth.
133. Charles Fiegl, "Cartoonist Hits 'Close to Home,'" *Post-Star* (December 18, 2006), http://tinyurl.com/kxpl92f; CFNA, "Getting Close," TAN (December 19, 2006), http://tinyurl.com/kgxa266.
134. TAN, "Google Results for Selected English Language Phrases—July 15, 2014," http://tinyurl.com/k4uktc9.

6 WHO WANTS YESTERDAY'S GIRL?

In June 2008, in Washington, DC, a female attorney we know described a problem with a friend's preschool age daughter. This poor girl insisted that she wanted to be a *nurse*! Her mother, a PhD married to an MD, PhD, was aghast. Mom tried valiantly to persuade her daughter that, if the daughter wanted to work in health care, she should do the "feminist" thing and be a physician, like Daddy. Our attorney friend shared the mother's bewilderment.

In April 2008, a Chicago artist was having dinner with two nursing leaders. The artist spoke sadly about the downward trajectory of her daughter's career aspirations. When her daughter was in elementary school, she had wanted to be a *physician*. But in middle school, her daughter decided she wanted to be a *nurse*. The artist's theme was that society still pushes women into traditional pursuits that limit them. She concluded by noting that her daughter had had four kids and become a stay-at-home mom.

Too much of society continues to believe that nursing is not good enough for smart, ambitious modern women—that it's only for yesterday's girls (we use the diminutive "girls" deliberately). The mass media continues to reinforce that view. It's not just random comments, like Whoopi Goldberg's 2009 remark that modern girls know they can aspire to be physicians and not just "helpers."[1] All of the most popular Hollywood hospital shows of recent years have sent similar messages, particularly *Grey's Anatomy*, on which young female physician characters seem to regard the word "nurse" as the greatest insult they could receive. Recent Hollywood films have emphasized that today's girls can do better than their unfortunate mothers who got stuck in nursing. The news media has conveyed similar ideas, telling women how they can escape traditionally female jobs like nursing and pursue *real* careers.

The value that society places on nursing reflects the value it places on "women's work." Ann Richards, the late governor of

Texas, was quoted in an exhibit at The Women's Museum in Dallas to the effect that recorded history has traditionally been about "men and their activities,"[2] as if those activities alone have influenced the course of human events. The Women's Museum closed in 2011 and Leslie Wagner noted in a March 2013 column in the *Dallas History Examiner* that the reason was largely a lack of financial support "from men with deep pockets, men who do not consider women's contributions to society as important as those of other men."[3] Efforts are now underway to build a National Women's History Museum in Washington, DC.[4] But the overall failure of the media to fully examine women's contributions in fields like nursing is a critical reason that women's historic and ongoing role in society remains undervalued.

The enduring view of nursing as inconsequential "women's work" underlies the profession's struggle to get adequate resources. To begin with, global nursing salaries reflect this undervaluation. The International Council of Nurses has explained:

> Once established, relationships between wages paid to different jobs change very little over time, so historical inequities tend to remain unless deliberately changed. . . . Many job evaluation systems are gender-biased and fail to capture or value the work of nurses and other women workers, thus perpetuating existing wage inequities . . . Analyses confirm that many nurses continue to be underpaid because skills and competencies used in the practice of nursing were not regarded as job-related skills but as *qualities intrinsic to being a woman*.[5]

Nurses in the United States may not feel as underpaid as nurses in most other nations. But research suggests that in much of the world, nurses' low wages relative to other professions are critical factors in attrition and international migration.[6] When we lived in Cambodia in the mid-1990s, nurses earned poverty wages. According to Apheda, an Australian trade union agency, 2002 data show that Cambodian nurses then earned the equivalent of US$591 per year, which meant that they had to work about 40 minutes for a pound of rice (one-half kilo) and 17 hours for a half-pound (250 gram) jar of instant coffee.[7] Low nursing salaries also affect more developed nations. Former International Council of Nurses leader Christine Hancock has noted that nurses in Luxembourg are paid better than those in nearby developed nations, leading to inflows of nurses from those nations. Yet the nurses are still "not paid as well as postmen in Luxembourg," so they are "frustrated and devalued."[8] Depressed nursing salaries are just one effect of the undervaluation of nursing. When decision-makers undervalue the profession, they allocate fewer resources for clinical practice, education, research, and residencies.[9]

Of course, these resource issues are common in traditionally female professions. Research shows that the higher the percentage of women in an occupation, the lower the salary.[10] Studies by Juliane Achatz, and another by Trond Peterson and Ishak Saporta, refer to the devaluation of an entire field as "evaluative discrimination."[11] Although many individual women have now pursued and succeeded in fields once considered "men's work," such as medicine, their individual gains have done nothing to resolve the undervaluation of "women's work." On the contrary, this feminist flight—and particularly the media that celebrates it—may even intensify the disrespect for the abandoned fields by suggesting that "women's work" is a type of bondage that strong women now can and should escape. Yet the traditional work of women has generally been about creating, developing, and preserving human life, with a focus on the next generation. It's hard for us to think of endeavors that deserve more respect and resources, but it's very easy to think of endeavors that get more. Reducing that disparity is a key part of the unfinished business of feminism: to help society understand and value the work that women have long done.

In light of the traditionally female makeup of nursing, it's no shock that men who pursue the profession still encounter resistance. In an extensive 2005 survey of men in US nursing, "eighty-two percent noted that nursing is plagued by common misconceptions that emphasize the view that nursing is a female profession dominated by women, that men are not suited to it because they are not caring, and that men in nursing are gay."[12] In 2000 the advertising agency JWT Communications conducted a focus group study of 1,800 school kids in ten US cities that found that when the conversation on careers changed to nursing, the males in the group stopped paying attention, saying that the conversation no longer applied to them.[13] In February 2008 nurse Robert Zavuga published "Check Bias Against Male Nurses" in the *New Vision* (Uganda). Zavuga noted that people call him a "male nurse" as if that were an oddity.[14] One nurse we know says that when someone says he is a "male nurse," he tells them that he applied to become a "female nurse," but the classes were all full. The problem with using the term "male nurse" when the subject is not the maleness itself is that it wrongly suggests that the man's work differs from the work of female nurses.

Popular media on men in nursing is certainly not free of stereotypes. In Hollywood products, men in nursing may be mocked for failing to embody gender norms, perhaps through terms like "murse," which is a cute contraction of "male nurse." Or they may simply be more likely to be presented as gay than they are in reality. In a September 2013 study in the *Journal of Advanced Nursing*, researchers at the University of Western Sydney analyzed one season each of five hospital dramas: *Grey's Anatomy, Private Practice*, and all three of the 2009 nurse shows.[15] They found that although the shows did try to "expose" some common stereotypes about men in nursing, they also reinforced them, with male nurse characters "often subject to questions about their choice of career, masculinity and sexuality and their role usually reduced to that of prop, minority spokesperson or source of comedy." Two of the three male nurse characters who initially appeared in the 2009 nurse shows were gay. Male nurse characters have also served as vehicles for "feminist" role reversal—hunky modern men whose subordination to female physicians is clear. On *Private Practice*, nurse Dell worked as a clinic *receptionist*.[16] Even positive news items, like a March 2009 CBS News report about a heroic nurse who took 27 bullets to shield others during a North Carolina shooting rampage, often use the term "male nurse" when there is no legitimate reason to do so.[17]

Yet this same media is more open to men in nursing than might be expected. Hollywood has included some surprisingly strong portrayals, such as the Belize character in *Angels in America*,[18] Mo-Mo on the first season of *Nurse Jackie*,[19] and Will Royal on *Combat Hospital*[20] (yes, all three characters were also racial minorities). Helpful press stories have detailed the work of men in nursing and efforts to attract men as a way to address the global shortage. Some of these recruitment efforts assure us that "real men" can be nurses and so may themselves reinforce harmful gender stereotypes.

The view that nursing is for women with limited options undermines nursing recruitment, retention, and practice. A 2004 survey found that many US high school guidance counselors told bright students that they were "too smart" for nursing and should instead pursue fields like medicine or business.[21] In December 2005 the *New Zealand Herald* ran a piece by Vikki Bland with the hopeful title "Nursing in Terminal Decline." The piece reported that "few secondary school pupils are interested in nursing." Some career advisers reportedly viewed nursing as "less than ideal from a feminist or masculine perspective" and steered promising students away. An adviser tried to talk New Zealand Nurses Organization chief Geoff Annals' own daughter out of pursuing nursing in favor of medicine.[22] Even those who do become nurses have internalized these social attitudes, which continue to disrupt their sense of professional well-being and self-respect. Who wants to *be* yesterday's girl?

In the United States, both men and women have become more interested in entering nursing in the last decade, as discussed in Chapter 1. However, nursing schools have often lacked the faculty, infrastructure, and other resources they need to train the students they attract.[23] A society enduring a weak economy seemed to have gotten the message that nursing had plentiful jobs but not the message that training skilled nurses requires significant resources. In 2006 one US nursing leader noted that a friend had described a wedding at which another guest mentioned that her son wanted to pursue nursing. But, said the woman, her son had been put on a three-year *waiting list for nursing school.* This mother of a future man in nursing complained: "This is ridiculous. They could train a nurse in six weeks." Right. A surge in interest from job seekers will not help nursing in the long run if the public still fails to understand that nursing is a serious modern profession for men and women.

Of course, neither women nor men should be excluded from careers on the basis of gender. Women should be able to pursue medicine or any other work. But too much of the media regards traditionally female jobs like nursing as menial and insignificant, defining success in terms of the power and status available in some traditionally male jobs.

The Work Feminism Forgot

Today even media created by women, such as *Grey's Anatomy*, often expresses overt contempt for nursing, seeming to reflect what journalist Suzanne Gordon has called "dress for success" feminism. In the 2004 article "How Hollywood Portrays Nurses" in the nursing journal *Revolution*, Gordon and nurse Ruth Johnson explained that media feminists, in their rush to embrace traditionally male fields like medicine, have failed to learn the importance and complexity of "caregiving" fields like nursing.[24] As the authors noted, nursing professor Ellen Baer had decried the "feminist disdain for nursing" many years earlier, in a 1991 *New York Times* op-ed piece.[25] Even some children's books reflect that disdain. Holly Hobbie's *Fanny* (2008), discussed in Chapter 4, surrounds a strong female "physician" doll with glamorous assisting "nurse" dolls.[26] Many media feminists treat nurses with the same explicit condescension that women in general once experienced. In some ways, nurses are the new women.

There have been press items describing the work of strong, able women in nursing, including some of the better pieces discussed in Chapters 3 and 4. But apart from the 2009 nurse shows, recent fictional portrayals of nursing as being worthy of a strong woman tend to focus on the distant past. The recent BBC series *Call the Midwife* is a great portrayal of nursing in many ways, but of course the show is set in the 1950s.[27] Joe Wright's 2007 film adaptation of Ian McEwan's 2003 novel *Atonement* likewise suggested that nursing was a way for women to break out of some of their traditional roles in the World War II era.[28] The Sky Arts television series *A Young Doctor's Notebook*, set in revolutionary-era Russia, has included portrayals of veteran nurses who are strong and knowledgeable in clinical matters, guiding the troubled main character as best they can in their difficult care setting.[29] Anne Perry's mystery novels about Victorian-era detective William Monk, published from 1990 through at least 2013, feature tough, intelligent nurse Hester Latterly. Latterly, who worked with Florence Nightingale in the Crimea and in later novels runs a clinic for poor women, is far more assertive than some characters think she should be.[30]

In other words, nursing might have been the feminist thing in the 1860s, or even the 1940s and 1950s. But you've come a long way, baby! You don't have to be a nurse anymore.

Hollywood Feminism

Major health-related television shows reflexively suggest that women achieve in health care only by pursuing medicine. It has been an obvious subtext in *Grey's Anatomy, The Mindy Project, House, Private Practice*, and other shows that have focused closely on the professional development of their female physician characters.

Grey's Anatomy presents a full landscape of female achievement in health care—from new physicians to senior physicians. Nurses represent what women have to settle for if they are not bright and ambitious like the show's physician heroes: a life of nodding along to physician commands. Recall the many expressions of contempt for nursing from the show's female interns, including the seething reactions of Meredith Grey and Cristina Yang after intern Alex called Meredith a nurse in the March 2005 premiere, as discussed in Chapter 3. The female physicians' priority is not to understand nurses but to distinguish themselves from what they see as an uneducated servant class. Consider the episodes equating nurses' work with grotesque bodily functions, as well as nurse Rose's reference to neurosurgeon Derek Shepherd's discussion of "boring science stuff." We guess that nutty *science stuff* is just for smart physician girls like Meredith![31]

Grey's makes its mean-girl contempt clear in nonclinical portrayals as well. Unlike the female physicians, the nurses are generally not substantial, interesting people. Instead they are ciphers with whom Alex and Sloane have sex when something is not going right in their relations with other physicians. That's why, as Cristina once remarked about Izzie, "hell hath no fury like a girl whose non-boyfriend screws a nurse." Although nurse Rose was a positive character in some ways, she was no real competition for Meredith.

The Mindy Project follows the personal life of a flawed yet quick-witted obstetrician/gynecologist (OB/GYN) named Mindy Lahiri, but it is also concerned with her professional development as a woman of color. Several plotlines have explored Mindy's relations with the two white male physicians who co-own her practice but seem to take her less seriously at least partly because of her gender. A May 2013 episode found Mindy trying to mentor a female Columbia medical student, to help another young female succeed in a traditionally male profession. For all its wackiness, the show has never questioned that obstetric physicians are skilled professionals worthy of respect; creator Mindy Kaling's late mother was an OB/GYN physician. But the show's female nurse characters are one-dimensional jokes: the office administrator Beverly is an inept loon from, well, yesteryear, and the young Tamra, although capable of flippant remarks, is mostly a bizarre, shallow serf. Neither has displayed healthcare skill, and the portrayals encourage viewers to regard female nurses with the same light-hearted contempt the show does.[32]

ER clearly wanted to encourage women to pursue medicine and to assume leadership roles. A February 2004 *TV Guide* cover story about the show asked us to "consider the increased enrollment of women in medical schools since *ER*'s 1994 debut." The show's physician advisor Fred Einesman noted that "once *ER* went on the air, emergency medicine became the most popular residency and the number of women who applied went up dramatically."[33] In accord with the show creators' pride in promoting female physicians, *ER* highlighted the challenges they face, while sending negative messages about nursing as a female career choice. In one April 2005 episode, intern Abby Lockhart confronted an elderly male patient who seemed to respect only older male physicians. The abusive patient, assuming Lockhart was a nurse, snapped that he did not "want some nurse calling the shots around here." So, did the episode's two female writers—one a physician—have Lockhart mount a spirited defense of nursing, the profession in which she herself spent many years saving lives? Not exactly. Lockhart responded, with measured but clear indignation, "I am not a nurse. I'm a doctor."[34] What might she have said?

"Today I am practicing as a physician. But as a nurse my opinions about your care options would be just as valuable."

"You're absolutely right—no nurse or physician should decide what happens to you. That is your right. As it happens, I am a nurse *and* a physician."

"Ah . . . I gather you don't like our nurse-centered model of care." (picking up a phone) "Hello, is this Psych?"

"Don't worry about nurses calling the shots, sir. The nurses only help the patients we want to live."

A surprising bright spot for women in nursing was the Ann Perkins character on *Parks & Recreation*. At least until the character left the show in early 2014, Ann was the best friend of lead character Leslie Knope, a local government official who also served as a city councilwoman. The show might easily have drawn a sharp contrast between Leslie's political rise and Ann being stuck in nursing, but it did not. Leslie did urge Ann to apply for an open position as the city health department's public relations director, and Ann took the job part-time, but she remained in direct care nursing at a local hospital. The sitcom is a mockumentary about zany government workers, and Ann had her weird features. But as one of the show's relatively normal characters, she also displayed intelligence, health knowledge, autonomy, and strong advocacy in both the public health and clinical settings.[35]

The three 2009 nurse shows all featured strong, smart female lead characters, as discussed in Chapters 2 and 3. *HawthoRNe* showed that a nurse can be a leader with clinical and administrative authority.[36] On *Mercy*, as an NBC advertisement helpfully noted, Veronica Callahan didn't just give shots, she often called them.[37] Jackie Peyton, despite her faults, is a clinical rock star.[38] But the shows have done little to convey that nursing is a profession for the most academically advanced women; all have suggested that nurses are essentially oppressed blue collar workers. *Mercy* did seemingly refer to nursing education once, in a passing reference to Chloe Payne's masters degree.[39] It took *Nurse Jackie* almost six full seasons to tell viewers that some nurses have graduate degrees, in a June 2014 episode in which Zoey Barkow decided to apply to a masters program to become a nurse practitioner.[40]

The reaction of female critics to the 2009 nurse shows was telling. By the time *Mercy* premiered in September 2009, some critics had already seen quite enough of its pronurse stance. Ginia Bellafante's contemptuous September 2009 *New York Times* review pronounced the nurse characters in the "angry little soap" to be bridge-and-tunnel women who had fallen pretty far from

ER's nurses, who got to marry George Clooney's physician character and even join their "superiors" by attending medical school![41] In October 2009 *Salon*'s Heather Havrilesky savaged *Mercy*'s "mercilessly self-righteous" vision of nurses "wagging their fingers" at "cartoonishly self-concerned" physicians.[42] But all three of the nurse shows actually went out of their way to highlight positive physician conduct—the lead physician in each was smart, able, and a close ally of the lead nurse—and to show that the nurses were flawed. Perhaps these critics doubted that there really are smart, educated nurses who fight for patients and challenge poor physician care.

Hollywood movies often reveal similar views. Gordon and Johnson's 2004 *Revolution* article cited Richard LaGravenese's *Living Out Loud* (1998), in which a woman named Judith dropped out of medical school to marry a medical student.[43] Years later Judith's physician husband left her for a younger physician. The film found the unfulfilled Judith practicing home health nursing. But she finally achieved rebirth in part by returning to medical school.[44] Critics and women's studies scholars saw that as a "feminist" victory.[45]

More recent films have told young females that nursing is a dead-end job that the sad women of the past may have had to settle for instead of medicine. But today, girls can actually achieve something worthwhile in work and in life! Yay.

Doug Atchison's *Akeelah and the Bee* (2006) told the story of an eleven-year-old girl from a struggling Los Angeles school who aimed for the National Spelling Bee.[46] Akeelah's widowed mother, Tanya, was barely keeping it together raising the family by herself. Tanya tried to keep her daughter focused on schoolwork by citing her own lost opportunities. But Tanya shocked Akeelah by telling her that her mother actually went to college before dropping out and becoming a nurse—evidently, college is not something nurses need. The movie's young achiever message: work hard, fear not, and things like nursing will not happen to you. *Akeelah* also reinforced the idea that persons of color—like women—achieve by joining traditionally esteemed professions, but not by questioning widely shared assumptions about what kind of work has worth.

Davis Guggenheim's *Gracie* (2007) took a similar approach. In that earnest 1970s-era sports drama, a New Jersey student was determined to honor the memory of her dead brother by taking his place on their high school soccer team.[47] But she faced obstacles including a chauvinist father who wouldn't coach her, mocking peers, and a resistant school. Gracie's mother was an unhappy school nurse who urged her moping daughter to fight to make the soccer team, using her own life as a cautionary tale. Turns out, Mom wanted to be a surgeon! Gracie was incredulous. Her mother explained:

> I wanted to be in the emergency room. So, uh, now I'm a nurse. That's as close as I could get. So if you want to limit yourself, that's fine. But don't let other people do it for you.

Duly motivated by the fear that she might otherwise be condemned to a life of nursing, Gracie fought to realize her dream. Not surprisingly, promotional efforts and reporting on *Gracie* described the mother as having had to "settle" for being a nurse."[48]

Of course, it's not irrational to assume that if an oppressed group is confined to a few specific jobs, none of those jobs is worthwhile. Not irrational; just wrong. Those who "limited" women to jobs like nursing in the past did not necessarily understand the jobs' true nature any better than "feminists" do today. Little did they suspect that nursing is not trivial scut work, but a vital scientific profession whose members save lives and improve outcomes.

Escaping the Pink Ghetto: The News Media Tells You How!

There certainly have been press pieces about strong modern women in nursing. But we're not aware of any directly suggesting that a nursing career would advance the interests of society as a whole, the female gender, or any particular female as much as would a medical career. On the contrary, some in the news media have suggested that females who want a real modern career avoid nursing—a view that seems particularly common among those who claim to be advancing the interests of women.

In December 2005, Carol Kleiman's career column in the *Chicago Tribune* examined how women can escape the "low wages" and "lack of a career path" in the "pink ghetto" of traditionally female jobs, including nursing and teaching, and move into "demanding," "professional" careers like law and accounting.[49] The author and the consultant who was her main source, Jonamay Lambert, seemed unaware that a world without skilled nurses and teachers would also lack the lawyers and accountants they value so highly. If nurses do have too little money or power, is the solution to urge them all to flee, or to improve their wages and working conditions? Obviously, many nurses *have* fled the bedside. It seemed that those responsible for this piece would be thrilled if they could help even more women escape. Of course, fewer nurses means more death.

But as the noted employment consultant Ebenezer Scrooge once observed, death is a good way to "decrease the surplus population."[50]

In the July 2004 *New Yorker* piece "To Hell with All That," Caitlin Flanagan compared her mother's return to her career in nursing during the author's childhood to the career-versus-home dilemma that many mothers face today.[51] The article showed a general appreciation for what Flanagan's mother's work meant to her, and the piece even gave some sense that her mother's success at nursing school meant something. But it also seemed to reflect a lack of respect for nursing as a profession.

> It's even harder today than it was in my mother's era, because the modern professional-class mother is not pursuing the kind of women's work for which my mother and her friends had been trained, and to which they eventually returned: nursing and elementary-school teaching and secretarial work and the like. These were posts that could be abandoned and returned to without a significant loss of stature, and were usually predictable in terms of both hours and workload. . . . Today's career moms are often trying to make partner or become regional sales manager or executive editor, jobs that require a tremendous number of hours and a willingness to allow urgent appeals, via BlackBerry or cell phone, to interrupt even the best-laid plans for family time.

Strictly speaking, Flanagan is comparing jobs decades ago with women's current career options. But readers are likely to come away with their ugliest present-day stereotypes confirmed. In fact, graduate-prepared nurses, including scholars, policy makers, executives, and advanced practice nurses, typically do lose status if they "abandon" their careers, even if they are not aiming for "regional sales manager." In addition, the nurses who struggle with short-staffing and mandatory overtime would be surprised to hear that their jobs are "predictable" in hours and workload. Flanagan's implication is that truly able women today do not do traditional "women's work" like nursing, which is not a "modern professional-class" career, but a "post" that now rests in the dustbin of smart-girl history.

Even pieces that aim to show respect for nursing may confuse the profession with generic femininity. In September 2009 the *Salon* website ran an item by *Prairie Home Companion* radio host Garrison Keillor about his stay at the Mayo Clinic following a minor stroke. Keillor said his nurses were "smart" and "utterly capable," with the psychosocial skills to get patients through tough times. But the female nurses also had "the caring gene most men don't," and in one Keillor sensed "some human tenderness . . . as if she thought, I could be the last woman to hold that dude's hand." Keillor referred to a "dark-haired beauty named Sarah" who not only "coache[d] him on self-administered shots of heparin," but also inspired him to plunge the needle in without hesitation, since "no man is a coward in the presence of women." Keillor saw that his nurses had skills, but he seemed to respond at least as much to their gender and physical attributes. The piece also mentioned Keillor's physicians, including at least one female, but oddly, we heard nothing about their appearance![52]

Nursing also suffers by omission in reports about careers for women. Since the notorious 2005 remarks by former Harvard president Lawrence Summers (no relation) about women in science,[53] the media has been full of stories about women's status in "science and engineering" fields. For instance, a long December 2006 piece by Cornelia Dean in the *New York Times* discussed the progress women have made in such fields. This article was more concerned with those who have become university professors in fields like molecular biophysics than it was with the applied sciences or health care. But the piece did note that half of US medical students are now women. One of the women quoted at length was a New York psychologist. Yet there was not a word about nursing, or the thousands of women with nursing doctorates who are now teaching and conducting scientific nursing research at US universities.[54] In a July 2008 interview with the *Baltimore Sun*, National Organization for Women President Kim Gandy lamented the continuing gender segregation in jobs: "Why are so few women in STEM careers—science, technology, engineering and mathematics? Those are the careers of the future, where the real money is." In other words, nursing is not a science. What matters is getting more women into traditionally male fields where the "money" is, not revaluing traditionally female ones like nursing which are not, evidently, the "careers of the future."

The Male Nurse Action Figure: The Media Confronts Men in Nursing

Men have provided health care to others for thousands of years, but today fewer than 10 percent of US nurses are male, and that generally appears to be the case worldwide.[55] Only one in ten US men has even contemplated nursing as a career.[56] Still, the percentage of US men in nursing has risen from 2.7 percent in 1970 to 9.6 percent in 2011, according to US Census data.[57] Increasing the number of male nurses is a critical part of helping the profession gain the power and diversity it needs to overcome the current global shortage. In 2011 the American Assembly for Men in Nursing launched the "20 X 20 Choose Nursing Campaign," a public relations effort to increase the enrollment of men in US nursing programs to 20 percent by the year 2020.[58]

The social view that nursing is "women's work" has particular importance for men in the profession. Even the English language reflects that traditional view. People still use "nursing" to mean breastfeeding. The terms "matron" and "sister" remain common ones for nurses in some nations, including the United Kingdom. In 2002 Johns Hopkins University School of Nursing changed its pink student identification cards to green to make men more comfortable wearing them. Many people wrongly believe that all male nurses are gay, or that they're not smart or motivated enough to be physicians, as the research discussed above showed.

These attitudes have a real impact. Roslyn Weaver led the 2013 study of Hollywood's portrayals of male nurses published in the *Journal of Advanced Nursing*. She told Reuters that "when men in nursing are almost invisible in popular culture or are stereotyped as incompetent or somehow 'unmasculine,' then men who choose to enter nursing can find it difficult to combat," and "perhaps reflecting this, there are often higher attrition rates for male students than female students in nursing."[59] A 2003 *NurseWeek* study found that nearly a third of male nurses said they had experienced "sexual harassment or a hostile work environment related to the conduct of physicians."[60]

Fictional media creators clearly have had trouble resisting the male nurse as object of ridicule. Some portrayals have used male nurses for their novelty value, notably for the feminist role reversal described previously: nothing makes the new breed of female professionals look more powerful than having a cute male nurse to order around. In Hollywood and advertising products, the sexual identity of male nurses is often an issue in a way it simply would not be for other characters. But even Hollywood has generally resisted the worst stereotypes. There have been portrayals of strong male nurses, although rarely prominent or long-lasting ones. The news media has also reported effectively about men practicing nursing and about efforts to recruit men to help resolve the shortage. These efforts do often stress that "real men" can be nurses, arguably reinforcing exclusionary gender stereotyping, as Thomas Schwarz suggested in his 2006 piece in the *American Journal of Nursing*, "I Am Not a Male Nurse: Recruiting Efforts May Reinforce a Stereotype."[61]

A video advertisement for the "jerky snack" Slim Jim that ran in 2013 was a striking illustration of the fictional media's apparent ambivalence toward men in nursing. The advertisement featured a self-identified "murse" distributing the product in a hospital waiting room to men suffering from different forms of "male spice loss." That malady was the subject of a broader advertising campaign ostensibly aimed at helping men who had abandoned accepted macho pursuits in favor of weird, vaguely feminine activities. The nurse mocked the "patients" by publicly labeling them (e.g., "tantric yoga guy") and throwing their prescribed snacks to them (naturally, they couldn't catch). Still, he projected traditional masculinity, with his authoritative voice and military fatigue pants, and he did things that were supposed to amuse the young male target audience.[62] On the whole, the advertisement was laughing with the nurse, not at him. Traditionally male health workers, including physicians, played similar roles in other "spice loss" campaign spots. So, despite the "murse" term and the gender-role intolerance, the advertisement could be seen as a small step toward normalizing the idea of men in nursing with the campaign's target audience.

Some recruiting materials have struck a good balance. A clever, irreverent rap recruiting video created in 2004 by nurse Craig Barton and other staff at the University of Alabama at Birmingham showed emergency department nurses of all genders grinning and strutting toward the camera, as Barton rapped about specific and at times technical aspects of the nurses' work.[63] Gender did not seem to be an issue. Another interesting item was Archie McPhee's Male Nurse Action Figure, which was sold from 2004 to 2011. Of course it would have been better to simply call him a "nurse:" we can tell he's male. And there was a tongue-in-cheek element, as in other McPhee items. But the product said nothing directly about sexual identity. Instead, the package noted that men who become nurses "are blazing the trail as role models and mentors for generations to come. Thank a male nurse today!"

Nurses and Murses: Men in Hollywood Nursing

Hollywood has paid considerable attention to men in nursing given that these nurses still make up fewer than 10 percent of the total. Some portrayals have been good, although even some generally helpful ones have had fun with the male nurse stereotype. That has often occurred through juvenile wordplay, like calling someone a "murse" or giving the nurse character a name that suggests a lack of conventional manliness.

Belize, the tough, skilled, imperfect nurse in the film *Angels in America*, is perhaps the best recent Hollywood portrayal of a man in nursing.[64] As explained in Chapters 3 and 4, Belize was a 1980s AIDS nurse caring for dying power broker Roy Cohn. The closeted Cohn noted that Belize was his "negation," an openly gay black nurse who would "escort me to the underworld." Cohn lashed out at Belize from the first moment. Yet when Cohn admitted to his own need for human contact, Belize was honest with him about his likely fate. He advised Cohn to avoid the radiation the physicians would push on him. When Cohn wondered why he should trust a nurse instead of his "very expensive, very qualified WASP doctor," Belize snapped, "He's not queer. I am." With luck viewers won't think that is the sole reason for Belize's expertise. Belize also advised Cohn, who had pulled strings to get into an early AZT drug trial, to beware of the "double blind," which might result in his getting a placebo instead of the real drug. Belize was convinced, as many AIDS activists were, that things were moving far too slowly, while thousands died. In his view, he was protecting his patient from a dysfunctional health-care and political system. Belize was gay, but not stereotypical.

Perhaps the best-known film portrayals of a man in nursing have been the hugely popular romantic comedies *Meet the Parents* (2000), *Meet the Fockers* (2004), and *Little Fockers* (2010). In these films, the lead character was Chicago "male nurse" Gaylord Focker. First off, of course, there was his name, which included the word "gay." What a laugh riot!

In *Meet the Parents*, Gaylord, who preferred to be called Greg, first faced off with prospective father-in-law-from-hell Jack Byrnes in an attempt to win Jack's blessing for a marriage proposal to his daughter Pam. Jack, an intense, WASPy retired CIA agent, turned a family visit into an interrogation and son-in-law fitness test for the easygoing, Jewish Greg. Since part of Jack's skepticism about Greg related to his career choice, common misperceptions of nursing were a recurring theme. Despite condescending challenges to Greg's intellect and manhood from Jack and others, including the physician who was about to marry Jack's other daughter, Greg stood his ground. He refused to quit nursing despite pressure from Jack. He explained why he became a nurse despite high MCAT scores, why he found nursing more fulfilling than he would have found medicine, and that nursing is in fact a paid profession, not volunteer work, as Pam's ex-fiancé implied. The character might have done more to rebut the stereotypes, but at least the film rejected them. Greg's tormentors were generally presented as ignorant and status-obsessed. So although the film was built around Greg's misadventures, he was a smart, resourceful nurse who endured real adversity to win the woman he loved.[65]

Unfortunately, *Meet the Fockers* took several steps backward for nursing. Greg had finally earned a place within Jack's "circle of trust," and he would soon be able to marry Jack's daughter Pam, provided that all went well at a weekend get-together at the home of Greg's touchy-feely parents. Greg remained a positive character. However, the film implied that nursing is for people who are good-hearted but not very ambitious. Greg's father proudly displayed a "Wall of Gaylord," which celebrated his son's past achievements—mainly certificates of completion and awards for ninth-place finishes. Greg's parents said they never pushed him too hard, because it was more important that he become a good, loving person. Jack sneered at this celebration of Greg's "mediocrity," noting that competition has been a critical element in keeping America strong. The film was not endorsing Jack's views, but it did regard nursing as a good vehicle to show that the heart matters as much as, or more than, the mind.[66] The stereotype that nursing is for people who are nice but kind of slow is particularly damaging for men, who (like Greg) must often explain what they are doing in nursing.

Little Fockers was far better. Greg again overcame misunderstandings and small failures to show Jack why he was the right man for Pam and the two kids they now had. By this time Greg had become a nursing manager who directed a medical-surgical unit, wrote articles for the "*AMA Journal*," and dealt with drug representatives, including an attractive, articulate nurse who persuaded Greg to moonlight by promoting an erectile dysfunction drug to physicians. That nurse turned out to be a glib party girl who tried to seduce Greg. The film did remind viewers of society's preconceptions about men in nursing; the director of a private school assumed that Greg and Jack were life partners partly because Greg was a nurse. But no one really questioned Greg's choice of nursing. Indeed, he showed real healthcare skill on more than one occasion in the film. In the end, Greg Focker was a regular guy and a talented health professional who was, yes, prone to comic misfortune.[67]

Television portrayals of men in nursing are similarly mixed. Most of the major Hollywood healthcare shows have occasionally included male nurse characters. Sometimes those nurses have been bitter lackeys with no significant clinical role. That was certainly the case with *Grey's Anatomy* nurse Tyler, the smug, petty bureaucrat who appeared in a number of episodes in the show's early years and who, as in 2009–2010 episodes, viewed his role as doing as little as possible to help the physicians.[68] Tyler did return in an April 2014 episode as an apparent nurse manager who claimed to be "in charge of" a critical care unit. But he was still doing his best to obstruct heroic young surgeons, refusing to lock down the unit during a flu outbreak or to provide any nurses for a surgeon's three patients (in Hollywood, as we have seen, nurses are optional).[69] At least the show made no issue of his gender, which was not true with *House*'s Nurse Jeffrey, the effeminate nurse who tried to push back a bit against House's toxic commentary, notably in a November 2009 episode in which House told him that he could not remember if "I mocked you yet for being a male nurse."[70]

Other characters in this category have been more substantial and more clinically involved, with no real questioning of their gender, but they have still acted essentially as aides-de-camp. On *Miami Medical*, which aired in spring 2010, Tuck Brody was a "head nurse" who projected some authority and skill, although he was ultimately an assistant to the surgeons.[71] Similarly, on the summer 2011 show *Combat Hospital*, Commander Will Royal was an unusually assertive nurse manager, but to a large extent he was a logistics manager for the trauma physician stars.[72]

Among the more significant portrayals on hospital shows, arguably the most interesting have been the hunky straight nurses who report to authoritative female physicians in apparent feminist role reversals. *Grey's* had the 2010–2011 episodes with Nurse Eli. He was a swaggerer who did display some strength and skill in advocating for patients, but as discussed in Chapter 4, he ultimately admitted to his girlfriend, surgeon Miranda Bailey, that "inside the hospital, you're the man."[73]

Other nurses in the role reversal category have been more evolved. The only regular nurse character on *Strong Medicine* was nurse midwife Peter Riggs, who acted as a foil to the two female physicians who dominated the show. Riggs was gorgeous, sensitive, holistic, übersexual—check his motorcycle! At times he seemed to operate with some autonomy, counseling and treating patients, but his subservience to the show's physicians was clear. In one episode Riggs confronted a powerful OB/GYN who had performed an unnecessary C-section, resulting in a hysterectomy. But she threatened to have Riggs fired, and Riggs's boss, physician Luisa Delgado, had to save him from the OB/GYN's wrath. In the February 2006 series finale, Riggs did affirm that he would rather be a nurse than a physician, resisting pressure from his girlfriend, physician Kayla Thornton, to go to medical school. She called it his "way out of nursing." The show acknowledged other male nurse stereotypes; Riggs's own mother thought he was gay. But his main role seemed to be to invert the paradigm of the powerful male physician surrounded by pretty female nurses.[74]

With the cute receptionist and eventual midwife Dell Parker, *Private Practice* discarded most of what was good about the Peter Riggs formula.[75] The show initially presented Dell as a nurse with some aptitude but without serious skill or experience, and it also mocked his midwifery studies. Like Riggs, Dell was the evolved yet junior male who served the powerful female professionals. Unlike Riggs, Dell was mostly an empty vessel until near the end of his time on the show. There are few male midwives in real life, but both significant Hollywood midwife characters have been men—because they had little to do with reality and everything to do with the superficial "feminist" vision of the media creators. Dell's admission to medical school just before his death, although obviously empowering in Hollywood terms, still reinforced the wannabe physician stereotype that real male nurses face.

Even *The Mindy Project* has included male midwives, specifically two New Agey men who run a holistic midwifery practice that competes with Mindy's traditional OB/GYN practice. It is not clear if the midwives are nurses. A December 2012 episode presented them as "stealing" Mindy's patients, but she got the patients back by telling them that midwives have no significant health training or skill, lies the show presented as hard but inescapable truths. Still, the lead midwife was the strong, quick-witted Brendan, who pointedly noted that midwifery predated obstetrics, and in later episodes he dated Mindy. It is telling that the show, like *Strong Medicine* and *Private Practice*, chose male midwives. Female midwives would not have furthered the show's gender goals, which here involved getting the Mindy character the respect of male physicians—and viewers. And let's not forget *Mindy*'s Morgan Tookers, a good-hearted but odd and pathetic nurse with little apparent health knowledge who instinctively defers to the physicians.[76]

The nurse-focused shows premiering in 2009 introduced many male nurse characters, but they were minor and virtually all of the real expertise and advocacy came from the females. The best of the men was *Nurse Jackie*'s Mohammed (Mo-Mo) de la Cruz, a strong, witty, and skilled gay man who seemed to be Jackie's best friend in nursing during the first season. In one June 2009 episode, Mo-Mo provided adroit psychosocial care to a boy who had been badly injured in a playground fall, at one point singing softly to him. But sadly the character left after the first season. In the 2011 season, the show included nurse Kelly, a tough, savvy African-American man with serious skills, but in light of his use of drugs, he was a threat to Jackie's sobriety and she eventually got rid of him.[77] The show's most prominent male nurse character has been Thor, a large, amusing, effeminate gay man who is intensely loyal to Jackie—almost a lapdog—but who rarely displays much clinical expertise or strength. Recent seasons have also included the straight, cool South Asian nurse Sam, a man who, like Jackie, is a recovering drug addict (yes, the show has perhaps leaned a little too hard on the drugs-in-nursing theme). In a May–June 2010 plotline, Sam broke physician Fitch Cooper's nose after Cooper slept with Sam's girlfriend, who broke up with Sam because he was a nurse. That suggested Sam was no pushover at least in his personal life. But since then he has been mostly a Jackie sidekick, displaying no great skill.[78]

Mercy had Angel Lopez, a gay man who made witty remarks about the action around him and seemed to have some health knowledge. But he was very deferential and generally amounted to a less developed version of Thor. In a May 2010 episode Angel did provide some good technical and psychosocial care to an old friend who had been badly beaten by a local gang, defibrillating and even spotting a clot in the chest tube that was preventing her lung from expanding. But his advocacy with the emergency department physician wasn't very strong, and the same plotline suggested that the physician controlled which cases Angel worked on. It was rare that Angel played even this limited clinical role.[79]

HawthoRNe's Ray Stein was straight, he showed some skill, and he made a couple spirited defenses of nursing, but in general he was pretty pathetic. In the June 2009 premiere, Ray tried to protect a diabetic patient from the nasty physician Marshall's incorrect insulin prescription. But Ray ended up giving the dose anyway, lamenting that he had to "follow doctors' orders" because "that's what nurses do." The patient crashed. So Ray was not much of a patient advocate. He was also insecure because he really wanted to be a physician, but his test scores were too low—reinforcing the damaging stereotype that male nurses want to be physicians but are not smart enough. At times Ray also seemed hapless; he was outmaneuvered by everyone from manipulative patients to Larry in accounting, and during the second season, he actually had an affair with Marshall. Ray did not appear in the show's last season, but that was no great loss for men in nursing.[80]

One of the most troubling recent portrayals of a man in nursing has been Patsy De La Serda, the nursing supervisor of the marginalized geriatric care unit where the HBO sitcom *Getting On* is set. Virtually all of the show's main characters are deeply flawed, but some of Patsy's flaws feed stereotypes about the strength and sexuality of men in nursing. Patsy seems to think he is a serious professional. But the show suggests that he is bogus, full of the latest corporate talk about customer service and workplace sensitivity, yet grossly insensitive himself, weak and self-pitying, and not great with patients. His obesity receives derision. Patsy has also used his pathetic subordinate, nurse Dawn, for drunken sex. Yet Patsy is, or is pretending to be, confused about his sexual orientation.[81] In one December 2013 episode, Dawn reported that she and Patsy had gone to a gay bar to find out if he was gay. Results were inconclusive.[82]

ER included some fairly good portrayals of men as staff nurses. The show always included at least one male as a recurring minor nurse character, the straight Malik McGrath and, for a time, the gay Yoshi Takata. Both were presented as competent.[83] *ER* episodes in late 2006 and early 2007 included traveling nurse Ben Parker, as discussed in Chapter 4.[84] Parker was a love interest for major nurse character Sam(antha) Taggart, which at least suggested that nurses are not just potential physician appendages. We found that plotline refreshing because nurses have rarely even talked to each other, much less dated, on Hollywood shows other than the recent nurse-focused ones. But Parker also seemed designed to present a tough, secure, skilled man in nursing. In a November 2006 episode, he controlled a violent patient, while nearby male physicians admitted they had been, as one said, "shown up by a murse."[85]

Scrubs illustrated the range of Hollywood portrayals of male nurses. Early 2003 episodes featured confident, witty nurse Paul Flowers (yes, a male nurse named Flowers). Female physician Elliot dated Paul, but she struggled with her self-esteem when she belatedly learned that he was a nurse, not a physician. Paul also faced anti-male nurse bigotry from other physicians; they called him a "murse" who did "women's work," possibly the earliest prominent use of the term "murse." But Paul easily rose above the slurs, and the show made sure viewers knew the stereotypes were stupid.[86] On the other hand, the ridiculous February 2007 *Scrubs* plotline in which chief of medicine Bob Kelso became a substitute nurse manager while nurse Carla was on maternity leave effectively endorsed the same kind of stereotypes. The show mocked Kelso for engaging in girly nurse activities, like gossiping with other nurses. Attending physician Perry Cox ordered Kelso to fetch fresh scrubs and to "put on a bra, [because he was] distracting some of the other doctors."[87]

Appearances by male nurse characters on nonhealthcare dramas range from pretty good to atrocious. Early 2014 episodes of ABC Family's *Switched at Birth* included the confident, skilled nurse practitioner Jorge as a romantic interest of Daphne, one of the main characters. Daphne met Jorge while doing community service at a Kansas City clinic, where he was her direct supervisor. In one February episode, Jorge explained to Daphne that he had chosen nursing because of his mother's experience while dying of cancer. Jorge said that physicians had "put her through hell, trying to fix her," but the nurses had "treated her like a person," taking care of her mind, body, and spirit.[88] Daphne responded that Jorge had "the same gift" with patients.

From 2010–2012 the legendary UK science fiction series *Doctor Who* included nurse Rory Williams, a companion of the alien Time Lord. Rory was perhaps overshadowed by his wife, the more important companion Amy Pond, but he was a competent, steady character who displayed wit and resilience in the face of mind-bending challenges.[89]

However, other male nurse characters have reinforced the worst stereotypes. In a December 2011 episode of ABC's *Desperate Housewives*, major character Gaby tried to get into the rehabilitation facility where her husband was a resident by flirting with the man who controlled access. But she failed when the man simply pointed to his chest and said "male nurse"—meaning that he was of course gay and so not interested in Gaby. The nurse was articulate, but he did nothing a layperson could not do, and the first thing he did when Gaby approached was to complain that she was keeping him from reading *The Help*.[90]

An August 2010 episode of TNT's drama *Rizzoli & Isles* set a standard for male nurse mockery that would be hard to surpass.[91] The show is about an odd couple of Boston crime fighters: the swaggering, deep-voiced homicide detective Jane Rizzoli and her super-smart, girly-girl medical examiner friend Maura Isles. In the episode, Isles set Rizzoli up with a handsome yoga classmate named Jorge whom Isles said was in "medicine." To Rizzoli's chagrin, he turned out to be a *nurse*, and a man who was determined to play a stereotypically female role in the relationship and to be a "stay-at-home daddy"—all of which was the target of an episode's worth of jeering from Rizzoli, despite Isles's half-hearted pleas that maybe a nice, supportive guy was what the somewhat abrasive detective needed. The episode mocked nursing as only "technically" a part of "medicine," but it was more concerned with exploring gender roles. The plot involved the murder of a woman outside a lesbian bar. Viewers were invited to compare same-sex relationships to the Rizzoli-Isles friendship, including its possible romantic overtones, and to Rizzoli's relation with Jorge, which Isles finally ended by telling him that Rizzoli actually was a lesbian. Jorge was an ugly caricature of a traditional woman: submissive, touchy-feely, chirpy, picky, smothering. Rizzoli's traditionally male traits have drawn affectionate ribbing, but they have been a source of power, a force for good. By contrast, Jorge's "feminine" traits were shown to be silly and annoying, and his work was dismissed.

Men who actually are nurses have occasionally appeared on entertainment television, although their roles have been limited. One of the nurses who received some attention in the 2010 ABC documentary *Boston Med* was Mike O'Donnell, an articulate Massachusetts General emergency nurse who was shown providing supportive care and vacationing with his fellow "murses" (really). But viewers did not see O'Donnell display a great deal of health expertise.[92] Three of the nine nurses on MTV's reality show *Scrubbing In* were men. Of course, the show was almost entirely about personal conflicts and romantic misadventures. But a December 2013 episode did include a short segment in which nurse Adrian displayed technical knowledge in providing skilled patient education—partly in Spanish!—to a woman with diabetes.[93]

I Want to Be a Macho Man: Male Nurses in the News

The news media's recent coverage of men in nursing is perhaps the least bad aspect of the media's overall treatment of nursing. Some pieces have candidly discussed the "male nurse" stigma. In October 2013, the *Los Angeles Times* published an in-depth profile by Ari Bloomekatz about new nurse David Fuentes, who went from a very tough childhood to practicing in the intensive care unit at UCLA Santa Monica. The piece focused on Fuentes's personal background. But it also addressed the growing number of men in the profession, as well as the stereotypes they confront, quoting UCLA Dean Courtney Lyder: "Nursing doesn't have a gender. Society and media have portrayed nursing as feminine. It's not." There were indications of Fuentes' skill in addressing patients' needs, such as checking blood and oxygen flow, monitoring pain, speaking softly but directly to the patients, and spending "the whole night standing guard." The article even included Mel Melcon's photograph of Fuentes working with an intensive care unit patient's arm while looking at the monitor, doing something technologically challenging, a rare example of a still image that conveys something of the skill involved in nursing.[94]

Similarly, in July 2013 *USA Today* published an article by Lexy Gross entitled "More men join nursing field as stigma starts to fade," featuring a profile of Tennessee nurse Ryan McFarland. The piece, originally from The *Tennessean*, included the standard data about nursing's slowly changing demographics, some valuable historical perspectives, a general description of how nursing differs from medicine, and, of course, a discussion of the stereotypes. Ryan said his friends thought that since he "played sports in high school," he would "take on a more manly job. But this is a manly job. There are so many things in this field that aren't easy—most people don't have the stomach for it."[95] That's fine as far as it goes; having what the piece called the "fortitude" to confront "bedpans" and "moving patients from bed-to-bed" matters. But it would have been better to stress that the work is appropriate for anyone because it involves life-saving skills and professional autonomy.

A July 2007 profile by Christina Chin in the *Star* (Malaysia) described the reaction of nursing student Irwin Choo's parents on learning that he wanted to pursue nursing: "His mother wept and his engineer father was dead against it. But their reaction is not uncommon—not many parents would be thrilled that their son has chosen to enter the medical profession as a male nurse!" The reporter asked other male nursing students about the "general perception that male nurses are 'soft' (effeminate)" and that " 'male nurse' doesn't exactly reek of the 'cool factor.' " In each case, she elicited confident and rational rebuttals from the students.[96]

Press items that describe the work of men in nursing can be helpful whether or not they stress gender. The April 2013 CNN piece by Elizabeth Cohen about the efforts of two experienced nurses who provided emergency care after the Boston Marathon bombing, discussed in Chapter 3, made no mention of their gender—they were plainly "nurses," not "male nurses."[97] In June 2006 the *Belfast Telegraph* published Jane Bell's portrait of "alcohol liaison nurse" Gary Doherty. "I'm Not a 'Male Nurse'—I'm a Nurse and Proud of It" did use gender as a hook, but it generally kept the focus on Doherty's pioneering work handling endemic alcohol-related problems at a north Belfast hospital.[98]

In May 2004 Garry Trudeau's comic strip *Doonesbury* featured US military nurse Lieutenant Chance Lebon. Lebon cared for tough regular character B.D., a soldier who had lost part of his leg to a rocket-propelled grenade in Iraq. Lebon handled B.D.'s initial chagrin at having a male "night nurse" by steamrolling through it, guiding B.D. through hospital life, skillfully coordinating B.D.'s interactions with loved ones, and making irreverent comments that reminded B.D. that he remained part of the human community. Lebon told his patient that he would not be much of a challenge, since he had lost "only one limb." The nurse was hoping for a "basket case." B.D. said he was hoping for Ashley Judd as his nurse. When B.D. declined to be set up as a celebrity for the nearby press, despite his civilian status as a college football coach, Lebon marveled that he must put "his pants on one leg at a time." B.D. wondered if that was from "the nurse's joke manual." Lebon: "Number 14."[99]

Still other pieces discuss affirmative efforts to attract more men to the profession to help resolve the shortage. In June 2006 the *Southeast Missourian* ran a revealing story by Scott Moyers reporting that Southeast Missouri Hospital had held a "guys-only nursing camp" to interest male high school students in the profession. The nurse recruiter who organized the camp said participants were "brave enough to say 'I'm interested in nursing.' "[100] The students shadowed "male nurses" at work. Jared Lacy, seventeen, said he had gotten "a little" grief about wanting to be a nurse, but his "insecurities" faded when he learned about the salary. He added, "To see somebody come in here sick and to help them get healthy again . . . well, I want to be a part of that." Of course, given peer pressure, few men have gone to nursing school right out of high school. A nurse anesthetist who participated in the camp said he "doesn't worry about telling people what he does." How does he handle it? "I muster my deepest voice and say: 'I'm a nurse.'" However, female nurses don't have to dramatically alter their voice pitch when telling people what they do.

An August 2005 piece on the New Kerala website implicitly suggested that transnational migration stemming from the nursing shortage itself might help close the gender gap. The story discussed the apparent surge in interest in nursing among the men in the Indian state of Kerala, noting that local males were being lured by the "lucrative nursing options" overseas, with 20 percent of current Indian nursing school graduates going abroad.[101]

Some areas may face even deeper issues in recruiting men. In August 2009 the *Times of India* reported that a female judge in Madras had upheld the Tamil Nadu state government's decision to bar men from the state's nursing diploma program on the grounds that the new course syllabus included midwifery (in which men can evidently play no role) and that there were already enough "male nurses" in the few practice areas where they were needed, such as jails and orthopedics. The underlying assumption seemed to be that nursing is essentially a female profession.[102]

A May 2007 Gulfnews.com piece by Nina Muslim discussed efforts to increase the number of men in nursing in the United Arab Emirates, which appeared to rely heavily on foreign nurses. The report said that getting more men into nursing was especially important because they do not face the "taboo" on women having physical contact with men in "conservative Muslim" societies. The article reported that there were almost no male nurses in civilian hospitals because there were few nursing programs "for men." Emirates Nursing Association president Saeed Fadhel said that there was "no stigma" in men becoming nurses, although the piece suggested there was a broader stigma—for anyone with other options.[103]

A September 2004 piece by Colleen Kenney in the Nebraska *Lincoln Journal Star* described one of the more inventive efforts to recruit men to nursing. "Hunky Nurses Pose for Pin-up Calendar" reported that twelve men who were nurses appeared (clothed) in a 2005 calendar published by the Nebraska Hospital Association. The goal was "to help get more men into nursing and to show it's a job for a regular guy." The article emphasized the calendar guys' "male" activities, such as playing football, lifting weights, and shooting turkeys with arrows. One nurse noted that people tend to assume that he is doing a woman's job, that he is gay (a word it seems he can't quite bring himself to utter), or that he is or soon will be a physician. But the piece did not suggest that it's wrong to look down on male nurses who *are* gay or effeminate. Just don't confuse *us* with *them*.[104]

These stories point to a dilemma in nursing's issues with gender. There is a huge incentive to address the shortage by any means necessary, even if that means cutting some corners, including in how we promote the profession. We might hope that nurse recruiting efforts would tell people it's OK for men to be nurses, whether or not they fit traditional notions of masculinity. For example:

FIRST MALE NURSE: Some of us are gay.
SECOND MALE NURSE: Some of us aren't.
FEMALE NURSE: Whatever . . . What we all have in common—
FIRST MALE NURSE: Is that we save lives and improve public health every day—
SECOND MALE NURSE: In a challenging modern scientific career. So—
FEMALE NURSE: Do you have what it takes to be a nurse?

Can nursing persuade the public to reconsider its assumptions not only about what work matters, but about who men and women are? Maybe it can—if we put our pants on one leg at a time and muster our deepest voice.

Notes

1. TAN, "Ms. Goldberg Needs Some Helpers" (June 16, 2009), http://tinyurl.com/jwaf3hs.
2. The Women's Museum, Dallas, exhibit audio (visited April 2011).
3. Leslie Wagner, "Find Heroines in Texas History Thanks to Ruthe Winegarten and Ann Richards," *Dallas History Examiner* (March 16, 2013), http://tinyurl.com/muhprqp.
4. National Women's History Museum, "About Us," accessed March 26, 2014, http://www.nwhm.org/about-nwhm/.
5. International Council of Nurses, "Position Statement: Socio-Economic Welfare of Nurses" (2009), http://tinyurl.com/kvl2dkp.
6. Mireille Kingma, "Nurses on the Move," in *Nurses—Past, Present, and Future: The Making of Modern Nursing*, ed. Kate Trant and Susan Usher (London: Black Dog Publishing, 2010), 61.
7. Union Aid Abroad—APHEDA, "Global Nursing Industry Comparative," accessed March 26, 2014, http://tinyurl.com/mbe8lp7.

8. Mireille Kingma, "Nurses on the Move," in *Nurses—Past, Present, and Future: The Making of Modern Nursing*, ed. Kate Trant and Susan Usher (London: Black Dog Publishing, 2010), 81.
9. TAN, "Just How Undervalued and Underfunded *Is* Nursing?," accessed March 26, 2014, http://tinyurl.com/k7m4wep.
10. Anne Busch and Elke Holst, "Gender-Specific Occupational Segregation, Glass Ceiling Effects, and Earnings in Managerial Positions," Deutsches Institut für Wirtschaftsforschung (January 2011), http://tinyurl.com/kax6ek6; Paula England, *Comparable Worth: Theories and Evidence* (Aldine Transaction, 1992), http://tinyurl.com/mlcaas5; Ronnie Steinberg, "Social Construction of Skill: Gender, Power and Comparable Worth," *Work and Occupations* 17, no. 4 (1990): 449–482, http://tinyurl.com/m4al298; Liebeskind, U., "Arbeitsmarktsegregation und Einkommen: Vom Wert "weiblicher" Arbeit," *Kölner Zeitschrift für Soziologie und Sozialpsychologie* 56, no. 4 (2004): 630–652.
11. Trond Peterson and Ishak Saporta, "The Opportunity Structure for Discrimination," *American Journal of Sociology* 13 (2004): 852–901, http://tinyurl.com/nqvrjb3; Juliane Achatz, Hermann Gartner, and Timea Glück, "Bonus oder Bias? Mechanismen Geschlechtsspezifischer Entlohnung," *Kölner Zeitschrift für Soziologie und Sozialpsychologie* 57, no. 3 (2005): 466–493, http://tinyurl.com/lzph7e6.
12. Karen A. Hart, "Study: Who Are the Men in Nursing?" *Imprint* (November/December 2005): 32–34, http://tinyurl.com/ygua27x.
13. JWT Communications, "Memo to Nurses for a Healthier Tomorrow Coalition Members on Focus Group Studies of 1,800 School Children in 10 U.S. Cities" (2000), http://tinyurl.com/l2q5mma.
14. Robert Zavuga, "Uganda: Check Bias Against Male Nurses," *New Vision* (November 25, 2008), http://tinyurl.com/ktz56zs.
15. Roslyn Weaver and Ian Wilson, "Australian Medical Students' Perceptions of Professionalism and Ethics in Medical Television Programs," *BMC Medical Education* 11 (2011): 50, http://tinyurl.com/l3z8ss2.
16. TAN, "*Private Practice* Episode Analyses" (2013), http://tinyurl.com/lecehka.
17. CBS News, "Heroic Nurse, Shot 27 Times, Saved Lives" (March 30, 2009), http://tinyurl.com/kqv2bs6.
18. Tony Kushner, writer, Mike Nichols, director, *Angels in America*, HBO Films (2003); CFNA, "Angels in America," TAN (April 4, 2004), http://tinyurl.com/mqcbd3l.
19. TAN, "*Nurse Jackie* Episode Reviews," accessed March 24, 2014, http://tinyurl.com/kqm3k6b.
20. TAN, "Commander" (September 2011), http://tinyurl.com/n8z5zum.
21. Karen A. Hart, "Breakthrough to Nursing National Survey Results," *Imprint* (February / March 2006): 29–33, http://tinyurl.com/yhc3qep.

22. CFNA, "*New Zealand Herald*: 'Nursing in Terminal Decline,'" TAN (December 3, 2005), http://tinyurl.com/lvohzdw.
23. American Association of Colleges of Nurses, "Nursing Faculty Shortage," accessed March 26, 2014, http://tinyurl.com/ky5qbaj.
24. Suzanne Gordon and Ruth Johnson, "How Hollywood Portrays Nurses," *Revolution: The Journal for RNs & Patient Advocacy* 5, no. 2 (March–April 2004): 14–21, http://tinyurl.com/q2mwbal.
25. Ellen D. Baer, "The Feminist Disdain for Nursing," *New York Times* (February 23, 1991): 25.
26. Holly Hobbie, *Fanny* (New York: Little, Brown and Company, 2008); TAN, "Fanny" (June 4, 2010), http://tinyurl.com/klpmcpv.
27. TAN, "*Call the Midwife* Episode Reviews," accessed March 24, 2014, http://tinyurl.com/m3bf4lw.
28. Christopher Hampton, screenplay based on the novel by Ian McEwan, Joe Wright, director, *Atonement*, Working Title Films/Relativity Media (2007); CFNA, "Atonement" (film review), TAN (January 13, 2008), http://tinyurl.com/ooxmyvm.
29. Kenton Allen, Dan Cheesbrough, Matthew Justice, Jon Hamm, Saskia Schuster, Lucy Lumsden, executive producers, *A Young Doctor's Notebook*, Sky Arts/Ovation, accessed March 25, 2014, http://tinyurl.com/k8ghrlf.
30. Anne Perry, *The Sins of the Wolf* (New York: Random House Publishing Group, 1994); CFNA, "The Sins of the Wolf," TAN (September 27, 2007), http://tinyurl.com/n5nyjmv.
31. TAN, "*Grey's Anatomy* Analyses and Action," accessed January 29, 2014, http://tinyurl.com/pgayg7h.
32. TAN, "*The Mindy Project* Reviews," accessed March 24, 2014, http://tinyurl.com/pu8wxuv.
33. Mary Murphy, "The Women Who Revived 'ER,'" *TV Guide* (February 14, 2004), http://tinyurl.com/lvtmaqh.
34. Lydia Woodward and Lisa Zwerling, writers, Paul McCrane, director, "Ruby Redux," *ER*, NBC (April 28, 2005); CFNA, "Judas in a Lab Coat: 'ER' Takes on That Whole 'Female-Physician-Mistaken-for-a-Nurse' Thing," TAN (April 28, 2005), http://tinyurl.com/ksyumg7.
35. Greg Daniels and Michael Schur, creators, *Parks and Recreation*, NBC, accessed June 24, 2014, http://tinyurl.com/pmy4zqz; Neil Drumming, "Goodbye to Ann Perkins: Can *Parks and Recreation* Still End on a High Note?," *Salon* (January 29, 2014), http://tinyurl.com/mf4k9as.
36. TAN, "*HawthoRNe* Episode Reviews" (2011), http://tinyurl.com/jwd7neg.
37. TAN, "*Mercy* Episode Reviews" (2010), http://tinyurl.com/kj3t63s.
38. TAN, "*Nurse Jackie* Episode Reviews," accessed March 25, 2014, http://tinyurl.com/kqm3k6b.

39. Liz Heldens, writer, Adam Bernstein, director, "Can We Get That Drink Now?," *Mercy*, NBC (September 23, 2009); TAN, "Traffic Is Backed up in the Tunnel Heading into Respect" (September 23, 2009), http://tinyurl.com/kaqvmo7.
40. Carly Mensch and Heidi Schreck, writers, Seith Mann, director, "Sidecars and Spermicide," *Nurse Jackie*, Showtime (June 15, 2014).
41. Ginia Bellafante, "From Iraq Hellfire to Hospital Halls, TV Nurses Wage a Battle for Respect," *New York Times* (September 23, 3009), http://www.nytimes.com/2009/09/23/arts/television/23mercy.html; TAN, "Did You Just Call Me a Nurse?" (October 21, 2009), http://tinyurl.com/kj2onpb.
42. Heather Havrilesky, "The Best and the Worst of the New TV Season," *Salon* (October 21, 2009), http://tinyurl.com/lhwbtxe; TAN, "Did You Just Call Me a Nurse?" (October 21, 2009), http://tinyurl.com/k77ybxe.
43. Suzanne Gordon and Ruth Johnson, "How Hollywood Portrays Nurses," *Revolution: The Journal for RNs & Patient Advocacy* 5, no. 2 (March-April 2004): 14–21, http://tinyurl.com/q2mwbal.
44. Richard LaGravenese, writer and director, *Living Out Loud*, Jersey Films/New Line Cinema (1998).
45. Linda Lopez McAlister, "Living Out Loud" Review (1998), http://tinyurl.com/q22ve89.
46. Doug Atchison, writer and director, *Akeelah and the Bee*, 2929 Entertainment/Lionsgate (2006); CFNA, "Akeelah and the Bee," TAN (June 7, 2006), http://tinyurl.com/kmhqced.
47. Lisa Marie Petersen and Karen Janszen, writers, Davis Guggenheim, director, *Gracie*, Picturehouse/Elevation Filmworks (2007); CFNA, "Gracie," TAN (June 29, 2007), http://tinyurl.com/luhzk8a.
48. Cynthis Fuchs, "Gracie," *PopMatters* (June 1, 2007), http://tinyurl.com/lf8jyry.
49. Carol Kleiman, "Pink-Collar Workers Have Own Barriers to Break," *Chicago Tribune* (December 6, 2005), http://tinyurl.com/kwa3o5u; CFNA, "Pink Ghetto Unfabulous," TAN (December 6, 2005), http://tinyurl.com/lja57ty.
50. Charles Dickens, "A Christmas Carol," Literature.org (December 19, 1843), http://tinyurl.com/yevsrpm.
51. Caitlin Flanagan, "Domestic Life: To Hell with All That," *New Yorker* (July 5, 2004), http://tinyurl.com/khultv8; CFNA, "You've Come a Long Way, Nurse's Baby," TAN (July 5, 2004), http://tinyurl.com/k57b584.
52. Garrison Keillor, "Nice 67 Y.O. Male Has Brush with Mortality," *Salon* (September 16, 2009), http://tinyurl.com/kmrfcn5; TAN, "Staying Awake and Alert" (September 16, 2009), http://tinyurl.com/m5mppru.
53. Sam Dillon, "Harvard Chief Defends His Talk on Women," *New York Times* (January 18, 2005), http://tinyurl.com/mq6pxts.
54. CFNA, "You Want a Career in Science? Then Why Are You Applying to Nursing School?," TAN (July 1, 2007), http://tinyurl.com/m6wa2b9.

55. US Census Bureau, "Men in Nursing Occupations: American Community Survey Highlight Report" (February 2013), http://tinyurl.com/mjxgvue.
56. Cathryn Domrose, "Mending Our Image," *NurseWeek* (June 26, 2002), http://tinyurl.com/l6j486c.
57. US Census Bureau, "Men in Nursing Occupations: American Community Survey Highlight Report" (February 2013), http://tinyurl.com/mjxgvue.
58. Don Anderson, "Man Enough: The 20 X 20 Choose Nursing Campaign," *Minority Nurse* (2011), http://tinyurl.com/k2jy8uc.
59. Roslyn Weaver, Caleb Ferguson, Mark Wilbourn, and Yenna Salamonson, "Men in Nursing on Television: Exposing and Reinforcing Stereotypes," *Journal of Advanced Nursing* 70, no. 4 (April 2014): 833–842, http://tinyurl.com/mjz8qmy.
60. Joan Sosin, "Indecent Proposals: Nurses Experiencing Harassment, Discrimination in the Workplace Are Reminded That the Law Is on Their Side," *NurseWeek* (February 28, 2003), http://tinyurl.com/mnz7xnf.
61. Thomas Schwartz, "I Am Not a Male Nurse: Recruiting Efforts May Reinforce a Stereotype," *American Journal of Nursing* 106, no. 2 (February 2006): 13, http://tinyurl.com/k9nplkm.
62. TAN, "Jerky" (August 2013), http://tinyurl.com/kquykha.
63. CFNA, "Rap Recruiting Video," TAN (2004), http://tinyurl.com/l7oo4tf.
64. Tony Kushner, writer, Mike Nichols, director, *Angels in America*, HBO Films (2003); CFNA, "Angels in America," TAN (April 4, 2004), http://tinyurl.com/mqcbd3l.
65. John Hamburg and Jim Herzfeld, writers, Jay Roach, director, *Meet the Parents*, Dreamworks SKG/Universal Studios (2000); CFNA, "Meet the Parents," TAN (December 30, 2002), http://tinyurl.com/mtp2qqq.
66. Jim Herzfeld and Marc Hyman, writers, Jay Roach, director, *Meet the Fockers*, Tribeca Productions (2004); CFNA, "Meet the Fockers" (January 12, 2005), http://tinyurl.com/mf6sdpf.
67. John Hamburg and Larry Stuckey, writers, Paul Weitz, director, *Little Fockers*, Tribeca/Everyman Pictures (2010); TAN, "Little Fockers" (August 4, 2011), http://tinyurl.com/oko5yzw.
68. TAN, "*Grey's Anatomy*: Have Fun Playing Nurse!" (August 10, 2010), http://tinyurl.com/kg4cumk.
69. Zoanne Clack, writer, Nicole Cummins, director, "You Be Illin'," *Grey's Anatomy*, ABC (April 3, 2014).
70. David Shore and David Hoselton, writers, Greg Yaitanes, director, "Ignorance is Bliss," *House*, Fox (November 23, 2009).
71. TAN, "*Miami Medical* Episode Reviews" (2010), http://tinyurl.com/pveg9xt.
72. Jinder Chalmers, Daniel Petrie Jr., and Douglas Steinberg, *Combat Hospital*, Global/ABC (2011); TAN, "Commander" (September 2011), http://tinyurl.com/n8z5zum.
73. TAN, "Who's the Man?" (October 13, 2011), http://tinyurl.com/onha8uc.

74. TAN, "*Strong Medicine* Single Episode Analyses" (2006), http://tinyurl.com/o5q2awp.
75. TAN, "*Private Practice* Individual Episode Analyses" (2013), http://tinyurl.com/lecehka.
76. TAN, "*The Mindy Project* Reviews," accessed March 24, 2014, http://tinyurl.com/pu8wxuv.
77. TAN, "Thank You Nurses!" (May 2012), http://tinyurl.com/kp5kder.
78. TAN, "All the Work, None of the Pay, Zero Glory" (June 7, 2010), http://tinyurl.com/kesj4x7.
79. TAN, "*Mercy* Episode Reviews" (2010), http://tinyurl.com/kj3t63s.
80. TAN, "*HawthoRNe* Episode Reviews" (2011), http://tinyurl.com/jwd7neg.
81. Jo Brand, Vicki Pepperdine, Joanna Scanlan, Mark V. Olsen and Will Scheffer, creators, *Getting On*, HBO, accessed March 24, 2014, http://www.hbo.com/getting-on.
82. Mark Olsen and Will Scheffer, writers, Howard Deutch, director, "The Concert," *Getting On*, HBO (December 29, 2013).
83. TAN, "*ER* Episode Analyses" (2009), http://tinyurl.com/odsbmqw.
84. Lisa Zwerling and Karen Maser, writers, Steve Shill, director, "Crisis of Conscience," *ER*, NBC (February 15, 2007); CFNA, "Midnight in the Garden of Nurses and Murses: Crisis of Conscience," TAN (February 2007), http://tinyurl.com/m6bq5ou.
85. Karen Maser, writer, Laura Innes, director, "Tell Me No Secrets . . . " *ER*, NBC (November 30, 2006); CFNA, "Midnight in the Garden of Nurses and Murses: Tell Me No Secrets," TAN (February 2007), http://tinyurl.com/q43xt9l.
86. Bonnie Sikowitz and Hadley Davis, writers, Ken Whittingham, "His Story," *Scrubs*, NBC (January 30, 2003); CFNA, "Men at Work: Is 'Scrubs' Hurting or Helping Male Nurses?," TAN (January 30, 2003), http://tinyurl.com/mzdgt2o; Janae Bakken and Debra Fordham, writers, Marc Buckland, director, "My Karma," *Scrubs*, NBC (February 20, 2003); CFNA, "Second 'Scrubs' Episode with Rick Schroder Continues Positive Depiction of Male Nurse," TAN (February 21, 2003), http://tinyurl.com/lkgngn5.
87. Mike Schwartz, writer, Linda Mendoza, director, "His Story IV," *Scrubs*, NBC (February 1, 2007); CFNA, " 'Scrubs,' Lift Us up Where We Belong," TAN (February 1, 2007), http://tinyurl.com/nh2t6a5.
88. Linda Gase and Henry Robles, writers, Melanie Mayron, director, "It Hurts to Wait with Love If Love Is Somewhere Else," *Switched at Birth*, ABC Family (February 3, 2014).
89. Tardis Data Core, "Rory Williams," accessed March 25, 2014, http://tinyurl.com/2wurtwa.
90. Sheila R. Lawrence, writer, David Warren, director, "Putting It Together," *Desperate Housewives*, ABC (December 4, 2011); TAN, "Seriously? Male Nurse." (December 4, 2011), http://tinyurl.com/ko46osz.

91. Alison Cross, writer, Michael Zinberg, director, "I Kissed a Girl," *Rizzoli & Isles*, TNT (August 16, 2010); TAN, "I Kissed a Male Nurse Girl" (August 16, 2010), http://tinyurl.com/kt7zf5u.
92. Terence Wrong, executive producer, *Boston Med*, ABC (2010); TAN, "Physicians Are Awesome" (July 22, 2010), http://tinyurl.com/o7m9olh.
93. Dave Caplan, Mark Cronin, and Shannon Fitzgerald, executive producers, "God Save the Queen," *Scrubbing In*, MTV (December 13, 2013).
94. Ari Bloomekatz, "A Nurse Who Is Healing Patients and Himself," *Los Angeles Times* (October 9, 2013), http://tinyurl.com/okjkle2.
95. Lexy Gross, "More Men Join Nursing Field as Stigma Starts to Fade," *Tennessean*, republished in *USA Today* (July 10, 2013), http://tinyurl.com/k8ade96.
96. Christina Chin, "Nursing a Dream," *The Star* (July 9, 2007), http://tinyurl.com/pmd6kou.
97. Elizabeth Cohen, "Nurses Relied on Trauma Experience to Help Bombing Wounded," CNN (April 16, 2013), http://tinyurl.com/kxy4wns; TAN, "Everyone Worked in Tandem" (April 17, 2013), http://tinyurl.com/k4mun2n.
98. Jane Bell, "I'm Not a 'Male Nurse'—I'm a Nurse and Proud of It," *Belfast Telegraph* (June 28, 2006), http://tinyurl.com/lzg2huk; CFNA, "A Time to Dance, A Time to Mourn," TAN (June 28, 2006), http://tinyurl.com/nye8pe7.
99. Garry Trudeau, "Doonesbury" (May 21, 2004), http://tinyurl.com/lxtgeyb; CFNA, "Chance the Good," TAN (May 29, 2004), http://tinyurl.com/m5mhjgn.
100. Scott Moyers, "Camp Urges Males to Consider Career in Nursing," *Southeast Missourian* (June 28, 2006), http://tinyurl.com/k6xyv8q.
101. *New Kerala*, "Kerala Male Nurses Storm Traditional Female Bastion" (August 23, 2005), http://tinyurl.com/n8oxeh6; CFNA, "Could Shortage-Driven Migration Change Nursing's Gender Gap?," TAN (August 23, 2005), http://tinyurl.com/kq69n44.
102. *The Times of India*, "HC Upholds Govt's Decision Not to Admit Boys in Nursing Course" (August 20, 2009), http://tinyurl.com/k8fajum; TAN, "Boys Don't Nurse" (August 20, 2009), http://tinyurl.com/knoa5bv.
103. Nina Muslim, "Emirati Men Urged to Become Nurses," *Gulf News* (May 14, 2007), http://tinyurl.com/mqnpgdf; CFNA, "Stigma," TAN (May 14, 2007), http://tinyurl.com/pp4yb3n.
104. Colleen Kenney, "Hunky Nurses Pose for Pin-Up Calendar," *Lincoln Journal Star* (September 18, 2004), http://tinyurl.com/l4ltqda; CFNA, "Nursing that Pesky Y Chromosome," TAN (September 18, 2004), http://tinyurl.com/moqfdj5.

7 YOU ARE MY ANGEL

One night in the late 1980s, we were at a party on DC's Capitol Hill. A female law student, meeting a nurse friend of ours for the first time, asked what the nurse did for a living. Upon learning the answer, the law student brightened and replied, "Isn't that sweet! That's what I wanted to be when I was in kindergarten!"

The nurse—who had worked all the previous night using her bachelor of science degree to save sick children's lives—was amused.

Two decades later, nurses are still widely regarded as angels of mercy, noble spiritual beings, or loving mothers. The *New York Times*' annual "Tribute to Nurses" has included real stories of nursing achievement, but the advertising supplement has promoted them with a focus on touching, feeling, and warming hearts.[1] When television psychologist Dr. Phil tried to make amends for his nurse-as-gold-digger comments, his praise for nursing relied largely on soft helping imagery.

Compassion and caring are important parts of nursing. But the extreme emphasis on "angel" qualities reinforces the prevailing sense that nurses are all about touching and feeling rather than thinking or using advanced skills. It suggests that nurses, as virtuous spiritual beings, have little need for clinical resources, education, rest, or security. The angel stereotype deters men and women (consider that law student) from entering the profession. It implies that nurses should meet certain moral and sexual standards that are not a proper part of the modern workplace. It is another in the matched set of feminine stereotypes that plague nursing, along with the naughty nurse and the battle-axe. Collect them all! Nursing has.

The angel image is not just something society has forced on nurses. Many nurses and their supporters continue to embrace and perpetuate it. Johnson & Johnson's (J&J) long-running Campaign for Nursing's Future, which aims to address the nursing shortage, has run sentimental television advertisements about "the importance of a nurse's touch" and similar concepts.[2] However, it is unlikely the nursing crisis has occurred because the public forgot those aspects of nursing. Nurses have had input on the advertisements, and many nurses have defended them. Similarly, many stories that nurses present to the public about their work rely heavily on emotional themes, as in popular books like *Chicken Soup for the Nurse's Soul* (2001).[3] In Lee Gutkind's introduction to *I Wasn't Strong Like This When I Started Out: True Stories of Becoming a Nurse* (2013),[4] the respected *Creative Nonfiction* editor described the book's stories this way:

> [A]ll of the essays have a common theme: No matter how difficult nurses' lives or how secret their suffering, becoming a nurse entails movement into another dimension of strength and character and persistence; it is a path of irreplaceable and often unacknowledged service to society and humanity. All nurses will understand the message inherent in the title of this book. It is the theme of survival, the theme of maturity, the theme of selflessly treating and healing all patients in any way possible, whether the credit that is due is forthcoming or not.

Those themes have value. But extolling nurses' "service," their "secret suffering," and their working "selflessly" even without getting the "credit" they are due reflects another "common theme": the angel stereotype.

Of course, the angel image has deep roots. Nursing was traditionally seen as a religious vocation, and the perception of moral purity gave women social license to provide the intimate care nursing involves. That care requires great strength and inspires genuine appreciation. But the angel image operates not only to exclude nursing from consideration as a serious modern profession but also to discourage nurses from advocating for themselves—and their patients. Like Jacob in the Bible, nurses must wrestle and overcome the angel.[5]

What's Wrong, Angel?

The angel image of nursing pleases some, but it has fatal flaws.

The image fails to convey the college-level knowledge base, critical thinking skills, and hard work required to be a nurse. If nurses are angels, then perhaps they can care for an unlimited number of patients, although research shows fewer nurses means higher patient mortality.[6] Maybe nurses can endure inordinate levels of workplace stress and abuse from patients and colleagues, as recent research suggests they do.[7] Maybe nurses can work mandatory overtime, because they don't have children at home who need care, food, or clothing. Angels don't need rent money; they live in heaven. Angels don't eat or go to the bathroom, so they can work thirteen-hour shifts without even a moment's break, as many nurses must do today. Angels don't even need manna from heaven, which is a good thing, because many nurses don't have time to eat it! The stereotype suggests that nurses are loving nurturers who need no say in healthcare decision-making or policy. If nurses suffer in such conditions, some may view it only as evidence of nurses' virtue, not a reason to alter the conditions. Likewise, it may be unclear why angels need well-paid professors or years of college-level education: after all, they're mostly just holding hands and lifting spirits.

In everyday conversation, it is more common for women than men to be described as angels. This fact may discourage men from entering nursing. The angel and related maternal stereotypes also complement the "naughty nurse" and the repressed battle-axe images. All define nurses by dubious visions of female sexual extremes, from Madonna to whore, rather than by nurses' professional skills or effort. Indeed, some feel that putting nurses in these boxes is a way for vulnerable male patients to reassert their traditional power over the females who now appear to control their lives in the hospital.

In the popular imagination, angels are pure and gentle. But patient advocacy may require that nurses assertively challenge an established system or proposed course of action. Florence Nightingale was no "angel." The common image of Nightingale holding a lamp may suggest faithful virtue at the bedside, but in fact she was a bright, aggressive, flawed human being who made lasting scientific and social contributions.[8] That lamp was not just a beacon of hope, but a tool and symbol of the relentless 24/7 surveillance and intervention that is the nursing practice model, as we explained in Chapter 1. Monitoring patients and rescuing them when needed is one way nurses keep people alive.

In Buresh and Gordon's *From Silence to Voice* (2013) and in Gordon's *Nursing Against the Odds* (2005), the authors document the roots, nature, and effects of what they call the "virtue script" of nursing, as we also discussed in Chapter 1.[9] The authors show how nineteenth-century reformers created a respectable job for women by using that moral script and assuring physicians that nurses were no threat to them. Indeed, nurses' historic oppression by physicians parallels the oppression of women by men. The authors argue that because of nurses' socialization in the virtue script and the imperative to "say little and do much," most nurses still display a bone-deep self-effacement and fear of controversy. Even many nursing scholars, Buresh and Gordon note, define the profession mainly in bland relational terms. Angel imagery buries nurses' real knowledge and skill, and that may suit some physicians, who receive the credit and resources nursing would otherwise claim. But the authors contend that nurses must overcome their fears and stop disrupting their own "definitional claims" by reinforcing stereotypes. Similarly, in the 2006 essay collection *The Complexities of Care: Nursing Reconsidered* (edited by Sioban Nelson and Suzanne Gordon), nursing scholars argue persuasively that the prevalence of "caring discourse" within nursing is a key factor in society's failure to value nurses' knowledge and skills.[10] The unsurprising result is that the beleaguered profession often does not get the resources it needs to provide good patient care or protect the well-being of nurses themselves.

We sometimes hear that leaving the angel behind would mean abandoning compassion in nursing, and that that special quality is what sets nurses apart. We agree that nurses must be compassionate. But when nursing is described mainly in terms of female love and devotion, the public views nursing in the same way—not as the work of highly skilled professionals of both genders, but as the work of nuns, or a kind of paid mothering service. Of course, the emotional support nurses give is actually psychosocial care shaped by their training and experience. It does have real health benefits, and it is not something that just any nice person could do.

We think what sets nursing apart is the *combination* of technical prowess, psychosocial skills, and mental toughness that good nurses have. But the media tends to ignore the "harder" aspects of nursing, such as nurses' advanced skills and the stress they endure. Gordon notes that while she values nurses' emotional support, if given a choice between a compassionate nurse and one who could save her life, she would take the life saver. The public must understand that side of nursing in order for the current crisis to be resolved.

Nursing has topped the Gallup public opinion poll measuring the "honesty and ethical standards" of different professions every year since nursing was added to the poll in 1999, except in 2001 when firefighters led the list following the 9/11 tragedy.[11] Those results go hand in hand with the prevailing vision of nurses as devoted and angelic. But if everyone loves nurses so much, why has a global shortage rooted in a lack of resources and understanding been taking lives worldwide since 1998? Because, we think, what those polls measure has little to do with the real respect that determines how scarce economic and social resources are allocated. Yet even some nursing leaders have embraced the "honest and ethical" label as a reason that policy makers should address nurses' concerns. It seems to us that patients trust nurses to hold their wallets while they're in surgery but not to save their lives. Some professions near the bottom of the Gallup list—such as law and advertising—do not seem to lack willing workers, good working conditions, or social status. We wonder how many of the people who trust nurses so much would react if their child announced that he or she wanted to be a nurse.

In July 2004 the *American Journal of Nursing* published an op-ed by Margaret Belcher entitled "I'm No Angel: I Am a Nurse—and That's Enough."[12] Belcher wrote that while nurses liked imagery focusing on compassion, such imagery did not make her proud. She argued that the emphasis on self-sacrifice has led to burnout and compassion fatigue. With unusual courage and insight, Belcher got to the heart of the "angel myth":

> I have the education and experience to do for others what they cannot do for themselves. But it's the intimacy of the work that feeds the angel myth. I listen to patients, touch them, reassure them, help them eat and drink, assist them with bodily functions. They are often ashamed of their need for help, and they're grateful to be treated with respect. . . . I don't exist on a higher plane because I work at the bedside. . . . But to call nursing a job rather than a calling isn't to diminish it. I will not stop touching lives if I refuse to call the work magic. I will not be a failure if I give up self-sacrifice for self-care. Nurses have not learned this lesson well. If we indeed were to put ourselves first, perhaps there wouldn't be a nursing shortage.

As we often hear on airplane flights, we must put on our own oxygen masks before we can help others.

Many "angel" comments from patients and families seem to result from the nurse's cleaning up poop in a way that preserves the patient's dignity. Responding to unpleasant tasks and patient abuse with control and respect may encourage people to call nurses angels. But attributing this difficult work to spiritual grace does the humans who actually perform it a disservice. At the same time, nurses are rarely called angels for detecting a deadly symptom or advocating for a life-saving intervention.

As we explained in Chapters 2 and 4, studies from around the world have confirmed that nurses face a high level of abuse from colleagues and patients. Research often points to institutional reluctance to address such abuse. Nurses commonly receive inadequate support. Of course, abuse of women is often discounted. But nurses in particular may be expected to simply "get over it" because they are spiritual beings with a vocation who do not suffer like others do. Angels don't get posttraumatic stress disorder.

As Belcher noted, there remains plenty of support for the angel within nursing. In fact, a December 2007 editorial in the popular *RN* magazine urged nurses to "put an end to angel bashing."[13] The author asserted that the image arose from nurses' helpful behavior with patients and that getting rid of the image would require nurses to stop being helpful. Some responding letters suggested that the angel is better than some of the alternatives and that jettisoning the image would entail moving to the other extreme. Nurses would lose their focus on "caring" and become harsh technicians. However, neither the image nor the reality of nursing must be confined to stereotypical extremes. We believe that the public is capable of seeing nurses as the three-dimensional beings they are: strong, skilled professionals of both genders who excel at both technical tasks and the psychosocial work often described as "caring" and "compassion."

'Bless This Angel of Mercy' Nurse Collectible Figurine!

Angel imagery continues to infect the media's treatment of nursing. These images range from casual references to in-depth portrayals, from daytime television to the print press. Let's look at some notable examples.

Angels Everywhere

For some in the media, the word "angel" is interchangeable with "nurse." In January 2007 the *Scotsman* ran Angus Howarth's "Robot Nurses Could Be on the Wards in Three Years, Say Scientists."[14] The piece reported that the "mechanised 'angels' " would "perform basic tasks such as mopping up spillages, taking messages and guiding visitors to hospital beds." These "angels" aren't exactly working at the core of patient care, are they? In January 2005 the *Guardian* (UK) website posted Jamie Doward's "Row Erupts over Secret Filming of Hospital Filth," about a television documentary for which two nurses used hidden cameras to document "appalling conditions" at two British hospitals. The documentary was named *Dispatches: Undercover Angels*.[15]

When it comes to nursing, angel imagery remains a staple for a wide variety of media creators. Television personality Dr. Phil tried several times to make amends for his 2004 comments suggesting that many nurses were out to marry physicians in order to avoid "having to work as a nurse," which we discussed in Chapters 3 and 5. In a December 2004 statement he assured viewers that the "men and women" in nursing are "dedicated," "devoted," "extremely well-trained," and "the backbone of the medical profession." He also noted that no matter "how much technological advance we make with machines to monitor patients, machines can't do the loving, nurturing care that a nurse can do, can't have the judgment, can't have the wisdom and can't be replaced by machines." Machines do help nurses assess patients and plan care. But Dr. Phil's statement suggests that maybe technology really does do everything except for nurses' "devoted" "loving" and "nurturing." Most of his comments paint nursing as a physically demanding support vocation focused on emotional care.[16]

In April 2005 the *Dr. Phil* show aired "Stories of Survival," which featured two victims of violence who were living with permanent facial disfigurement.[17] They were a former deputy sheriff named Jason and Dr. Phil's sister-in-law Cindi Broaddus. The idea was to help Jason and his family, using Cindi as an inspirational example. Another guest was nursing assistant Daphne, who had helped Cindi during her recovery. Dr. Phil, Cindi, and Clarice Marsh, director of pediatric nursing at UCLA, offered brief testimonials for nursing as the underappreciated "backbone" of health care, as Dr. Phil again put it. In fact, the media commonly describes nurses as the "backbone" of the health system, as NPR *Morning Edition* host Renee Montaigne did in a May 2012 report on nurse understaffing.[18] But we're still waiting to hear a media reference to nurses as the "brains" of the system.

The 2005 *Dr. Phil* episode mostly suggested that nurses are virtuous, hard-working hand-holders. Clarice Marsh did say that nurses are "incredibly intelligent" and that their work is "multi-faceted." She also said that in nursing "the art is the relationship" and that nurses form a "bond" that can't be found anywhere else. Dr. Phil said Daphne was a "wonderful example" of that. Yet nursing assistants, who have minimal training, are not nurses. Dr. Phil said he did not think Cindi would have made it without the "tremendously inspired and dedicated" nursing staff. Cindi agreed that nurses were "wonderful, wonderful." But no one explained specifically what nurses *do* for patients. During her four minutes on screen, Daphne did not utter *one word* that was audible to viewers. The last shot in the segment was a close-up of the nursing assistant and Cindi holding hands.[19]

The print press is hardly immune to that kind of imagery. In June 2010 the *Seattle Times* published a piece by Sharon Randall, a nationally syndicated columnist, that was built around the comic idea that Randall was acting as a "home nurse" in caring for her child when he was a newborn as well as for her husband after a recent operation.[20] Randall threw in positive accounts of the care she and her child had received from real nurses, those "compassionate" "angels" whose work is apparently defined by "loving kindness" and "tender mercy," phrases she used *twice*. Randall made clear that she was a very imperfect "nurse." But it was evident that the reason she fell so short was temperament, rather than education. So her equating of her unskilled care with actual nursing reinforced the idea that nursing requires little skill. The subtext—which no one would take as a joke—was that what makes a real nurse is kindness, patience, and endurance.

For years the *New York Times* has published an annual "Tribute to Nurses" advertising supplement and it has given related awards, in recent years for achievement in areas including research and leadership. But to gather the stories it includes, the paper has also used language like this, from April 2007:

> *The New York Times* invites you to share your personal story in The Nursing Diaries. Whether heartwarming or humorous, we want to know your inspirations, challenges, lessons learned and experiences that have left a footprint on your heart forever.[21]

A *footprint*? Despite that (presumably unintentional) nod to the stress of nursing, the stories that the *Times* has collected with that kind of language have tended to reinforce the sense of nurses as virtuous angels rather than life savers. Note the paper's use of the word "heart" twice in a single sentence.

In September 2006 the *Liberty Times* (Taiwan) profiled Chuan Ya-lan, a young nurse who had "become lauded by the Taichung Hospital as an angel for her service."[22] Chuan showed "an extraordinary degree of patience with the patients, and everyone comment[ed] how nice she [wa]s." Indeed, Chuan was "a model in terms of having the compassion and expertise required of a nurse." A manager said many new graduates could not cope with the "heavy workload and stress" of handling at least eight patients at a time, and most resigned "after a relatively short period." But Chuan "never complained about the workload." This piece's "angel" focus (despite the passing reference to "expertise") suggested that nurses are relatively unskilled spiritual beings who can be expected to make inhuman sacrifices. We might see a willingness to assume an enormous patient load without complaint as laudable devotion—or as a sign that nursing is too weak to stand up for itself or its patients. A nurse may be able to endure a patient load of eight or more, but as research shows, her patients cannot.[23]

Even generally helpful press pieces may not be able to resist the angel. In January 2014, the NL News Now site of St. John's (Newfoundland and Labrador) posted an article by Wesley Harris about protests over the elimination of a local clinic nurse position. The piece was headlined "She Was Like Our Guardian Angel." A local official reportedly justified the move with "statistics to show that the skill set of the registered nurse in the Hermitage Clinic wasn't always the best use of resources—in other words Tammy Hollett often did clerical duties (taking appointments, filing, etc)." The official also suggested that the clinic's physician might now do some of the things Hollett had done, "like EKG's and blood pressure." Protester Melita Goods said she had often visited the clinic with her diabetic husband, noting that "Tammy was like a guardian angel to us." Even where, as here, the angel imagery seems to have been drawn from a comment from a news source, the media should consider whether amplifying such comments is fair—especially when other information makes clear that nurses have a valuable "skill set" that enables them to do things like EKGs and blood pressure. As we have noted, celebrating nurses as "angels" rather than cost-effective professionals who improve outcomes has not proved sufficient to protect them from the kind of cost-cutting described in the piece itself.[24]

In March 2009, the Kampala-based magazine *The Independent* published an article by Mubatsi Asinja Habati about the challenges of nursing in Uganda, and in particular, the good work of veteran midwife Irene Nabukeera.[25] The article said that nursing could be "very stressful," the pay was not high, and there was a risk of contracting deadly diseases. However, Ugandan nurses who decline to go abroad to work "find that saving lives makes up for the stress." Despite a lack of many specifics, the piece did give a sense of how important and difficult nursing work is in a nation without many clinical or educational resources. Unfortunately, the title of the article, "Nurses—Uganda's Angels," reinforced the idea that nurses are spiritual beings that may not really need those resources.

Of course, some pieces revel in the idea that nurses are pure spiritual beings. In June 2005 the *Age* (Melbourne) ran "Saint Be Praised," Brian Courtis's profile of actress Georgie Parker and her television character, a nursing manager on the popular Australian hospital drama *All Saints*.[26] One good passage suggested that television's heroic health worker narrative may actually undermine efforts to ensure adequate health care funding, but the piece reinforced stereotypes that have the same effect. Parker, the "saintly practitioner of the blessed art of medical melodrama," was leaving *All Saints* after years of "compassionate caring" as "much-loved nurse Terri Sullivan."

The character's "enigmatic, soulful and spiritual bedside manner produced miracles" for patients. "Critics loved her, and now network beatification must surely follow." (In fact, beatification is one step toward sainthood; canonization is the actual making of the saint. There's a whole course on this in nursing school.) The report concluded that "St. Terri" had earned her place in the "stained-glass windows of soap opera."

Be that as it may, overt angel imagery has not played a significant role in recent television dramas. Maybe producers just don't think it would make for compelling, persuasive drama for key viewer demographics today. The recent nurse-focused shows have not focused on handholding, instead showing that nurses have advanced technical skills and that they can push back against poor physician care. Granted, one *Mercy* nurse was named Angel Lopez.[27] In the June 2009 premiere of *Nurse Jackie*, nurse Zoey Barkow told Jackie she was an "angel," startling the normally unflappable veteran.[28] One reviewer actually found the crusading lead character in *HawthoRNe* too "saintly," despite the prickly manager's endless conflicts with everyone from physicians to nurses to her teenage daughter.[29] The nurse midwives of *Call the Midwife*, some of whom are nuns, have at times been surrounded by a sort of holy glow as they rescue poor mothers in distress.[30] But aside from the endlessly wise Sister Julienne, the midwives also argue, snipe, make mistakes, struggle with a lack of resources, date men, and most importantly, display healthcare expertise and autonomy. On the whole, the flawed, street-smart characters in recent nurse-focused dramas have been no more "angelic" than the physician heroes of other shows.

But commercial media sources still rely on angel imagery. In February 2005 Tickle, then the "leading interpersonal media company," offered an online test called "Who's Your Inner Nurse?"[31] The lighthearted test offered respondents a series of stereotypes. One question invited nurses to report that patients found them gentle, cheerful, dependable, or selfless. We guess there wasn't quite enough room for "expert" or "savvy." Another question gave test takers the chance to specify that they wouldn't "make [their] rounds without" their "stickers and lollipops."

Speaking of lollipops, starting in 2008 and continuing until at least early 2014, an Angela Moore jewelry catalog featured Nurse Nancy bracelets composed of four different types of balls strung together.[32] The balls showed a smiling nurse in a white uniform giving a balloon to a girl, a ladybug next to a stethoscope, a nurse's cap with a thermometer, and a stuffed bear holding flowers next to a lollipop. In 2008, the promotional text asked readers to buy the jewelry to "celebrate the ladies who give lollipops and band aids a whole new meaning." We contacted Angela Moore about this imagery, and by 2014 the text had improved somewhat: "Here's a special theme to celebrate the wonderful nurses who promote health and do such valuable work. Talented, terrific and leaders to love!" However, the bracelet's soft and fuzzy images remained the same.

But that's nothing. For years, companies like Precious Moments have offered figurines that present nurses as noble, selfless, sweet, tender, loving, wonderful, maternal, faithful, special, devoted, cuddly, comforting, gentle, delicate, blessed, adorable saints—and those are the edgy ones. In 2004 the marketing copy for Precious Moments' Bless This Angel of Mercy Nurse Collectible Figurine noted that it would be just the thing for the "special nurse" who gives you "comforting attention and care."[33] As for the Special Delivery Nurse Figurine, a teddy bear nurse holding a teddy bear newborn:

> Faithful Fuzzies Nurse is "Beary" Special . . . No matter how long her shift is, you won't hear this faithful nurse complain, because cradling this little miracle in her arms is reward enough for her sincere devotion. That's because her job requires the "gentle art of caring"—it's more than hard work, it's "heart" work![34]

This virtuous "nurse" had no complaints no matter how bad conditions were! The Sending Love from Above Figurine nurse dispensed a "dose of 'loving, caring and sharing'" wherever she went, from her "delicate angel wings" to her "adorable nurse's bag filled with pink pearlized heart-shaped messages of faith and love."[35] In 2013 Precious Moments was still selling products along these lines, including the Loving Touch Nurse[36] and, of course, the You're an Angel nurse.[37]

Don't get us wrong: we don't object to this imagery in isolation any more than we do to sexual imagery. Fusing it with the profession of nursing is the problem.

Nurse or Mom?

Some press items present the nurse as professional mother, no matter how skilled or authoritative she may be, or how good the story may otherwise be. In October 2007 *Time* magazine profiled US Navy Commander Maureen Pennington, the "first nurse to lead a surgical company during combat operations." Caroline Kennedy's "Beyond the Call of Duty" highlighted Pennington's leadership, communication, and cross-cultural skills. But even so, the piece focused on vague helping imagery. A physician's assistant said Pennington was "like a mom to all of us." Pennington herself said she understands Marines: "Being a mother, I know you also have to be willing to be hated in order to be loved. I knew it was up to me to make sure that there were rules and structures in place because people need those too when the world is falling apart."[38] OK, but even a tough, able mother would not necessarily have Pennington's advanced science training and clinical skills. Although we heard all about what kind of mom she was, there was nothing in the story about her education. In fact, she had a master's degree in nursing.[39]

Similarly, in January 2006 the *Detroit Free Press* ran a generally good story by Patricia Anstett about Wayne State University nurse practitioner Mary White. Although the piece focused on White's innovative methods, which included health-oriented *Jeopardy!* contests and "condom bingo" in the dormitories, it unfortunately also noted that White is "a nurse first and foremost, with all the loving compassion the term typically conveys." Yuck. Later, readers were told that White was "all pro, plus surrogate mom." One sophomore referred to White as "like a mom to me now." White herself described her appeal to the students this way: "I'm the mom image, but I'm safe because I don't lecture them." But Mom does not know how to titrate life-saving medications. And Mom is not hosting condom bingo.

The Fallen Angels

The media also takes an intense interest when nurses *fail* to be noble angels, when they are seen as too demanding or uppity, when they're promiscuous or irreverent, or when they're malevolent "angels of death." Despite the obvious differences, in all of these cases nurses have failed to follow the virtue script.

The Strivers Who Have Forgotten Their Place

Some nurses seem to misplace their heart-shaped messages of faith and love. In August 2009 the UK press carried many items about a recent report detailing cruelty and neglect by some nurses. A *Times* column by Minette Marrin argued that the problems stemmed not from a lack of resources but from a "cultural collapse" within nursing.[40] Marrin attributed that decline partly to efforts to increase nurses' "professional status with a university degree," which had led them away from "old-fashioned bedside" care. The headline was "Fallen Angels: The Nightmare Nurses Protected by Silence."[41] Marrin returned to the theme with a November 2009 piece in the *Sunday Times* attacking a government plan to require that all nurses have a three- or four-year university degree by 2013. Marrin argued that the plan would have "disastrous" effects primarily because it would exclude those who would make "excellent" nurses even though they were "not particularly academic" or "not particularly bright."[42]

Similarly, in August 2011 the *Telegraph* published "Nursing Is No Longer the Caring Profession." Christina Odone's piece argued that a controversial UK program in which nurses were to wear "do not disturb" tabards while on drug rounds to reduce errors was emblematic of a system in which nurses saw patients as a "nuisance" to be "ignored" as the nurses worked their way up to a "desk job."[43] Odone, like Marrin, could tell that the real culprit was nurses' aspirations to higher education. In particular, compulsory university degrees "professionalised" what had been a "vocation," so that the former "angel[s] of the ward" became too uppity for "soothing fevered brows and administering TLC." In fact, compassion and diligence are essential qualities for nurses, and allegations of abuse and neglect must be addressed. But nurses are not angels giving simple custodial care. They need university education because they need advanced skills to save lives and improve outcomes.

In mid-2006 anonymous UK physicians published op-eds designed to discourage the government from allowing nurses to move into clinical roles that have traditionally been the province of physicians. "Are Nurses Angels? I Don't Think So"[44] ran in the *Daily Mail*, and "Why Nurses Are No Angels"[45] appeared in the *Independent* and the *Belfast Telegraph*. These paternalistic essays urged the National Health Service to stop assigning nurses new roles, a practice that had supposedly produced nurses who were stupid, uncaring, lazy, and eager to dump everything on physicians while wrongly seeking the same high status. Instead, the pieces argued, nurses should focus on the basic caring and hygiene tasks the physicians thought defined nursing. Maybe their halos would reappear.

Christie Blatchford's column "Militant Angels of Mercy," in a June 2003 edition of Canada's *National Post*, yearned for the days when nurses were "kind" and "loved, if not always respected."[46] Blatchford claimed nurses had not received much public support for their work battling SARS because too many had become "outright shiftless or worse, just plain mean." One problem was that nursing had "come to be deemed a capital-P profession, as opposed to a calling," so that people became nurses as much for "opportunities or pay or perquisites" as to help the ill. Maybe Blatchford would prefer a system in which patients perished because the nurses were angelic but unskilled volunteers: at least we'd die smiling! Blatchford linked the alleged decline in nursing care to nursing militancy. But she failed to reconcile this self-seeking militancy with the ongoing nursing crisis, which has included a global shortage and often atrocious working conditions.

Promiscuous Girls

Needless to say, nurses may also fall from grace through sex and drugs. Thus, if someone were to create a television series about hot young female nurses hooking up, it might be called *No Angels.*

Oh wait—that actually happened. In February 2004 the *Times* (UK) published nurse Vici Hoban's piece about a new Channel 4 drama called *No Angels*. The show had aimed to "explode the myth of angels by the bedside" and provide "a witty and truthful exposé of nursing" in the modern National Health System.[47] But the first episode showed the nurses "laughing over a corpse that they have warmed up in the bath to disguise the fact that the patient died, unnoticed, hours earlier," as well as "tricking colleagues into taking drugs, showing off visible panty lines to doctors and having sex in cupboards."[48] The show lasted three seasons. In September 2004 Reuters reported that *No Angels* was "up for translation into a Stateside version."[49] But that show did not appear, and we heard no more until September 2013, when *Variety* reported that ABC had landed a version of the show to be run by several US sitcom veterans. The item noted that the "laffer centers on a raucous group of female nurses who work together and live in the same house."[50] Let the laffs begin!

The Angel of Death

Sadly, as in any profession of millions, there are a very small number of dangerously troubled nurses. Not surprisingly, coverage of their bad acts tends to highlight their deviation from the virtue script.

In November 2004 *Reader's Digest* ran Max Alexander's generally fair cover story on Charles Cullen, a nurse who had pled guilty in New Jersey to having killed thirteen patients with drug overdoses, and who by his own account may have killed twenty-seven more. Cullen was shown to have a history of troubled relationships, mental illness, and substance abuse. The headline was "The Killer Nurse," and the internal subhead was "Why No One Stopped the Angel of Death." Of course, the contrast between the usual angel stereotype and Cullen's actions made for a great story. Similarly, in April 2013, CBS's *60 Minutes* aired the first televised interview with Cullen. Even the legendary news show could not resist the angel, titling its report "Angel of Death: Killer Nurse Stopped, but Not Soon Enough."[51] Because the interview was news, it got coverage in places like *The Daily Mail*, whose headline quoted the phrase " 'Angel of Death.' "[52]

The Cullen story appears to have inspired a December 2004 episode of NBC's short-lived prime-time show *Medical Investigation*, a drama that followed a team led by heroic National Institutes of Health physicians. The show generally presented nurses as peripheral handmaidens, but they finally got some attention in "The Unclean." In that episode, after suspicious deaths at a Baltimore hospital, the investigators searched for infection control problems. They finally realized that some "angel of death" had been infecting patients with a bloody sheet. Although the physicians were initially suspicious of a weasely nurse, he turned out to have been the whistle-blower (although he got no credit). The team ultimately found that the "angel of death" was in fact a meek, helpful nurse who had gained access to experimental bacteria and, like the real-life Cullen, had left a trail of suspicious patient deaths at her prior jobs. The show did not explore why she might have done it.[53]

That reticence was missing from an astonishing April 2004 op-ed in the *Philadelphia Inquirer*. In "Nursing Compassion to Health," NYU forensic psychiatrist Michael Welner actually argued that Cullen's murders were the result of the modern emphasis on "material" benefits in the training and hiring of hospital workers.[54] To reverse this trend, healthcare facilities should "focus on hiring those with the most compassionate personalities." Apparently Cullen was not an aberrant sociopath, but just an extreme example of what nurses have become.

> Employment ads solicit health-care workers based on material benefits. Whom, then, will such ads aim to attract? Not the nuns of yesteryear. . . . So we need to integrate vigorous empathy training and stress management into medical and nursing education. . . . Tomorrow's professionals need to be prepared for the adverse climate of providing health-care services within institutional frameworks that are insensitive by design.

So the answer to "insensitive" care systems lies not in restructuring healthcare financing or better oversight, but simply in hiring nicer people with better stress management skills! Nurses are spiritual beings that don't need the substantive training and resources on which other professions rely to ensure high performance. It was not clear if Welner's emphasis on selflessness and compassion in health care extended to his own lucrative New York consulting practice, the Forensic Panel. Since the time of the *Inquirer* piece the Panel's website has extolled the advanced credentials of Welner and the other consultants at "the preeminent consultation practice in America." One of its FAQs gives a nuanced answer to the vexing question "Are the services of the Forensic Panel costly?"[55]

The Angel Within

Arguably the most striking angel imagery appears in statements by nurses and their advocates. Consider that each year on May 12, the anniversary of Florence Nightingale's birth, nurses around the world celebrate Nurses Day; in the United States, there is a whole Nurses Week![56] Of course, this is the classic form of sentimental recognition for groups that don't get enough real respect or resources the rest of the year. As one might expect, on these occasions there is a flood of angel stereotyping.

Perhaps it's not surprising that nonnurses who want to express support for nurses conceive of nursing in terms of divine virtue, given the profession's history. It seems to be the first thing that occurs to many patients. In a widely reported June 2013 speech about mental health awareness, US Vice President Joe Biden mentioned his personal experience with neurosurgery and opined that "if there's any angels in heaven, by the way, they're all nurses."[57] When the Cincinnati Children's Hospital invited people to thank its nurses during Nurses Week 2013 by posting Facebook messages, there was a predictable gush of angel commentary from parents (e.g., "They really are Gods Angels!!!!").[58] In that same week, *Huffington Post* blogger Lisa Lori thanked her son's pediatric intensive care unit nurses for providing "comfort" and "love," holding hands, hugging, crying, and enduring verbal abuse—but not for their life-saving skills.[59] In a February 2008 article in the *Chronicle Herald* (Nova Scotia), "Let 'Angels' Spend More Time Nursing," a grateful cancer patient said his nurses were "the closest I have ever met to angels."[60] And in a June 2007 piece from Boston's State House News Service, "Nurses Demand Stronger Protections Against On-the-Job Violence," the husband of a nurse who had been assaulted referred to nurses as "angels in scrubs."[61]

Hospitals often use angel imagery, stressing the emotional, nontechnical aspects of nursing. Maine Coast Memorial Hospital's Nurses Week page informs us that "Nursing is the gentle art of caring" and "Nurses are Angels in comfortable shoes."[62] For Nurses Week 2012, Saint Peter's University Hospital in New Brunswick, Canada, launched a program called "Angels of Caring," in which patients and their families nominate nurses or other staff to be recognized through a donation to the hospital."[63] Each December New Jersey's Shore Medical Center honors members of its staff (overwhelmingly nurses) with "Guardian Angel" awards—a name that at least hints at nurses' real role as sentinels for patients.[64] The University of Texas Medical Branch celebrated Nurses Week 2012 by giving out "Silent Angel Awards," with the "silent" element seeming to reinforce the longstanding imperative for nurses to remain docile and not seek further recognition or resources.[65]

Nurses themselves continue to embrace this kind of imagery. The 2012 feature film *Nurses: If Florence Could See Us Now*, directed by nurse Kathy Douglas, offered some helpful information about the diversity and rewards of nursing practice. But it was dominated by vague, emotional imagery, with little about what nurses do specifically to improve patient outcomes. The movie featured footage from interviews with more than one hundred US nurses, but what the director chose to include in the film focused on passive handholding. Interviewees emphasized what a "privilege" it is to be a nurse, noting that the profession involves "bearing witness" to pain and suffering, without much indication that nurses are key players in averting that suffering. The film seems unlikely to teach laypersons much about nursing that they do not already know.[66]

Some nursing groups have had themes for Nurses Day that emphasize nurses' substantive achievements, but even those groups have not been consistent. In 2010 the Geneva-based International Council of Nurses (ICN) used "Delivering Quality, Serving Communities: Nurses Leading Chronic Care." In recent years, ICN themes have been based on United Nations health development goals, such as "Closing the Gap: Millennium Development Goals 8, 7, 6, 5, 4, 3, 2, 1" (2013)[67]—no one could find the angel in there. However, from 2000 to 2002, each ICN theme included the emotional phrase "Always there for you."[68] ICN also sells the "Florence Nightingale Teddy Bear" to raise funds for its worthy Girl Child Education Fund, which pays for the education of orphaned daughters of nurses in the developing world.[69] "Florence" the teddy bear is better than Precious Moments products—at least she has a lamp, bag, and bandages, like she actually does something useful—but she still associates professional nursing with cuddly children's dolls.

The American Nurses Association (ANA) adopted as its 2003 Nurses Week theme the angel-tastic "Nurses: Lifting Spirits, Touching Lives."[70] In 2000 the ANA's "Nurses: Keeping the Care in Health Care"[71] implied that nurses focus on "care" while someone else (guess who!) takes the lead on "health." The group's 2011 theme, "Nurses Trusted to Care," was emotional and vague.[72] Fortunately, more recent ANA themes have been much better: "Nurses: Advocating, Leading, Caring" (2012),[73] "Nurses: Delivering Quality and Innovation in Patient Care" (2013),[74] and "Nurses: Leading the Way" (2014).[75]

The angel also appears in nursing specialty groups' promotional efforts. In October 2013, the International Association of Forensic Nurses (IAFN) unveiled a new logo and tagline. The tagline was all right ("Leadership. Care. Expertise."). So was the image of a magnifying glass (science!). But the magnifying glass was focusing on a Greek cross and a heart. IAFN explained in a press release that the redesign project was led by Shoestring, a "nonprofit branding and public relations agency," and that "the heart inside the magnifying glass represents the care and compassion of the dedicated nurses in the field."[76] Many IAFN members felt that some rebranding was in order.[77]

Perhaps most ironic is the tendency of media aimed directly at resolving the nursing shortage or recruiting nurses to use angel imagery, particularly when that seems to serve a different institutional agenda. In 2002 J&J initiated the massive Campaign for Nursing's Future to address the nursing shortage and increase interest in nursing careers. The company financed an extensive nursing website, raised funds for faculty fellowships and student scholarships, and sponsored the helpful 2004 recruiting video *Nurse Scientists: Committed to the Public Trust.*[78]

But the J&J campaign project with the greatest influence was undoubtedly the television advertisements. The theme of the early advertisements was "the importance of a nurse's touch."[79] The spots included a few elements suggesting that nurses had some skill, and the young nurses who appeared were diverse. But the soft-focus advertisements relied mainly on angel and maternal imagery. The three spots that began airing in 2005 all featured the same semi-cooing female narrator, the kind of voice used to advertise cuddly products for babies. The opening: "At Johnson & Johnson, we understand the importance of a nurse's touch." The closing: "Nurses: we need you more than ever. A message of caring from Johnson & Johnson." One advertisement used the word "touch" five times in thirty seconds.

The focus on "caring" and "touching" in such images clearly serves the business interests of a major pharmaceutical company. J&J has long tried to project a baby-soft image to consumers, even as the company has made headlines for things like suing the American Red Cross for trademark infringement,[80] and in 2013, paying billions in fines for illegally marketing drugs[81] and billions more to settle claims that it had knowingly sold defective hip implants,[82] among other serious publicity problems.[83] In April 2013, the *New York Times* reported that J&J had launched an emotional new "branding campaign" called "For All You Love"—with an advertisement featuring family scenes and voiceover about what "love is"[84]—"perhaps to distance itself from the bad press of product recalls and pending litigation."[85] Similarly, fusing the J&J brand with the angel stereotype of nursing reinforces the idea that the company is as honest and ethical as nurses are seen to be.[86] But that convergence does nursing no favors.

In 2007 J&J unveiled two new spots.[87] Those advertisements did not abandon angel imagery, particularly in the use of gooey music with lyrics about being "born to care," which suggested that nursing is more of a divine vocation than a profession requiring intensive training. But both spots did emphasize that nurses are not just angelic hand-holders. They made clear that nurses save lives and improve outcomes, even offering specific examples, like defibrillation. One advertisement paid tribute to nurse educators, showing the impact they have through their students.

Three more J&J advertisements appeared in 2011.[88] These spots, like those released in 2005 and 2007, conveyed something helpful about nursing skill. But each advertisement focused mainly on the emotional support nurses give patients, and each concluded with the vaguely uplifting message "NURSES HEAL." One featured an authoritative emergency nurse reacting quickly to a trauma case, but even that one was dominated by the nurse's returning of a lucky charm to the patient. The other two advertisements, in which a hospice nurse and a pediatric nurse used good psychosocial skills to help patients through hard times, were also likely to strike viewers as being mostly about hand-holding.

More recently, the J&J Campaign sponsored a program called "Amazing Nurse 2013" that aimed to identify and show the public exceptional nurses. But despite passing references to knowledge and skill, the main themes were angel-oriented. The program website explained:

> In celebration of [nurses'] dedication, we want to highlight Amazing Nurses who make a difference in your life and the lives of those around you. Nurses take care of and heal so many of us - now let your Amazing Nurse know how much you care.[89]

In June 2013, the J&J Campaign's "Nursing Notes" Facebook page promoted the Amazing Nurse program with a poster that read: "Nursing is not just an *art*, it has a he*art*. Nursing is not just a *science*, but it has a con*science*." Oh, right, and is nursing not just about *caring*, but also teddy *bearing*?[90] In January 2014, the Campaign's Facebook page featured a poster telling us that nursing is "truly about caring hearts in action."[91]

In 2007 the University of Michigan ran radio advertisements featuring men describing why they became nurses at the university.[92] The spots seemed to be directed at recruiting nurses and nursing students, although they may also have been part of the university's capital campaign. The nurses came off as substantial people whose work has real meaning. Sadly, the advertisements relied on generalized, emotional angel imagery. We heard about the nurses setting up a summer camp for disabled kids, getting smiles, loving what they did and not looking at it as a "job," "helping" kids fight cancer, inspiring and being inspired. But nowhere did listeners hear what nurses *actually do for patients*.

In March 2009 the National Organisation of Nurses and Midwives of Malawi began a campaign to persuade the nation to provide the funds needed to train and retain more nurses and midwives. The campaign was launched to try to help a profession hobbled by low pay and workplace abuse, as well as a critically high level of nurse migration and the resulting "brain drain." Unfortunately, the campaign was called "Soon There Will Be No Angels on Earth."[93]

For Nurses Week in May 2011, the major US managed healthcare group Kaiser Permanente ran a sixty-second radio advertisement that may have been the most extreme presentation of angel imagery that we have ever seen. The spot called nurses "noble" and "selfless," then went on about their "colossal" "capacity to care," their "superhuman" "sympathy," their "heart" of "compassion," their "love," and how the self-effacing givers endure their exhausting, disgusting jobs without complaint. There was a passing reference to being "tough," but the advertisement also stressed that "mothers nurse their children." The angel imagery here was so undiluted by any hint that nurses are educated professional humans that it arguably worked to undermine the claims of Kaiser's 45,000 nurses to adequate resources, to persuade them that their obligation was to endure the unendurable. Some nurses loved the advertisement; maybe it's hard to see what's wrong with a series of gushing compliments, especially when they play into what society has long told nurses sets them apart. But as long as nurses are defined solely by their "gargantuan heart all squishy with compassion thumping away"—yes, the Kaiser advertisement script really said that—nurses will not get the respect or resources they need.[94]

Transcending the Angel: What Can Be Done?

Because angel imagery is so deeply embedded both in the public consciousness and nursing culture, overcoming it will be a challenge. But it can be done. Nurses can have a public image that acknowledges the value of caring and compassion, but that also shows respect for nursing as a skilled modern profession. Any of the media items discussed elsewhere in this book that present nurses as educated, life-saving professionals counter the angel stereotype.

The recent nurse-focused television dramas have subverted the angel to some extent, particularly the flawed but virtuosic lead character in *Nurse Jackie*. In an April 2013 episode, Jackie intubated a head trauma patient when no physician was available.[95] Despite that display of technical skill, the patient's family member called Jackie an "angel." In response Jackie gave a tiny, polite smile and quickly turned away, muttering "Far from it," an apparent reference to her own ongoing struggle with drug abuse.

In May 2005 the California Nurses Association (CNA) vowed to celebrate Florence Nightingale's birthday by staging a protest at the San Francisco offices of J&J.[96] CNA's press release argued that the company had supported recent efforts to limit the political participation of nurses and other public employees, and asserted that it had donated huge sums to defeat measures designed to lower drug prices in California. The union said its protest honored the "legacy of the original nurse activist." Whatever the merits of CNA's specific position, its protest contradicted the inaccurate image of Nightingale and the nurses who have followed her as cuddly saints.

In October 2006 the *Boston Globe* posted a poll on its website after a successful nurses' strike in Worcester. As we noted in Chapter 3, the text described contracts under which the "average nurse . . . working a 40-hour week makes $107,000 a year," and the poll asked whether the nurses "deserve this six-figure salary for what they do."[97] The nurses' union, the Massachusetts Nurses Association, urged nurses to respond to the poll by explaining why they were worth the money. The union reminded nurses, "You work in one of the most dangerous professions (you're injured as much as construction workers, you're assaulted more than prison guards), you deal with deadly infectious diseases; you hold life and death in your hands every minute of every shift."

The Los Angeles poetry magazine *Rattle* placed a "Tribute to Nurses" in its Winter 2007 issue.[98] The forty-five–page section included only nurses' own work. You might think the "tribute" approach would lead editors right to the angel image, but *Rattle* offered insightful essays and well-crafted, irreverent poems that captured modern lives and deaths without sentiment. The poems suggested the scope of patients' lives through their physicality, their frailties, their suffering. To some extent we also saw nurses' complex, difficult inner lives. The tribute presented nurses not as angels but as keen observers and courageous workers who help us in our darkest hours.

In 2004 nurse Craig Barton and other emergency department staff at the University of Alabama at Birmingham created an irreverent one-minute rap recruiting video.[99] The video was a clever and infectious slice of the life of an urban emergency department nurse. In the video, nurses moved toward the camera, strutting and grinning, as Barton rapped about their work. We heard about starting intravenous lines and handling a heart patient with a "positive history" who needs "a twelve-lead EKG." More lyrics: "Ka-boom! We're the UAB emergency room! And we treat every single patient from the womb to the tomb!;" "We're ER nurses! Medications we disburses!;" "We expect the unexpected! That's why we're well-respected!;" and "Yo, we're savin' lives up in here!" Barton's engaging focus on nurses' life-saving, technical skill, and team spirit was a welcome alternative to the sentimental imagery in many recruiting efforts. This one kept it real.

In the third season of the BBC Sherlock Holmes adaptation *Sherlock*, broadcast in early 2014, the godlike genius's sidekick Dr. John Watson married nurse Mary Morstan, with whom Watson worked at a clinic. (Spoiler alert!) Morstan did not get the chance to do too much clinically. But she was a clever, savvy woman who seemed to display a confident knowledge of patient conditions—not to mention being finally revealed as a formidable ex-CIA assassin who nearly killed Holmes yet ultimately remained an ally of the Baker Street duo. Nothing says "no angel" quite like that sort of plotline.[100]

Notes

1. *New York Times* & Monster, "Tribute to Nurses" (2006), http://tinyurl.com/kptwyej.
2. TAN, "Johnson & Johnson Nurse Television Commercials" (2011), http://tinyurl.com/pc42jyt.
3. Jack Canfield, Mark Victor Hansen, Nancy Mitchell-Autio, and LeAnn Thieman, *Chicken Soup for the Nurse's Soul: Stories to Celebrate, Honor and Inspire the Nursing Profession* (Deerfield Beach: Health Communications, Inc., 2001).
4. Lee Gutkind, *I Wasn't Strong Like This When I Started Out: True Stories of Becoming a Nurse* (Pittsburgh: In Fact Books, 2013), http://tinyurl.com/bpmzb9f.
5. Genesis 32:22–32, *The Bible*, English Standard Version, accessed March 28, 2014, http://tinyurl.com/kdamkrc.
6. TAN, "What Happens to Patients When Nurses Are Short-Staffed?," accessed March 26, 2014, http://tinyurl.com/ancmo7r.
7. Dianne M. Felblinger, "The Impact of Violence in the Nursing Workplace and Women's Lives," *Journal of Obstetric, Gynecologic, & Neonatal Nursing* 37, no. 2

(March/April 2008): 218, http://tinyurl.com/l9rtt63; Dianne M. Felblinger, "Incivility and Bullying in the Workplace and Nurses' Shame Responses," *Journal of Obstetric, Gynecologic, & Neonatal Nursing* 37, no. 2 (March/April 2008): 234–242, http://tinyurl.com/lsehhn4; John S. Murray, "On Bullying in the Nursing Workplace," *Journal of Obstetric, Gynecologic, & Neonatal Nursing* 37, no. 4 (July/August 2008): 393, http://tinyurl.com/mpqaddf.

8. Victoria Sweet, "Far More Than a Lady With a Lamp," *New York Times* (March 3, 2014), http://tinyurl.com/l6rbu8l; Florence Nightingale Museum, "Florence's Biography," accessed June 17, 2014, http://tinyurl.com/mppnene.
9. Bernice Buresh and Suzanne Gordon, *From Silence to Voice*, 3rd ed. (Ithaca: Cornell University Press, 2013); Suzanne Gordon, *Nursing Against the Odds: How Health Care Cost-Cutting, Media Stereotypes, and Medical Hubris Undermine Nursing and Patient Care* (Ithaca: Cornell University Press, 2005).
10. Sioban Nelson and Suzanne Gordon, eds., *The Complexities of Care: Nursing Reconsidered* (Ithaca: ILR Press, 2006).
11. Gallup, "Honesty/Ethics in Professions," Poll of December 5–8, 2013, accessed March 26, 2014, http://tinyurl.com/lcer8a; TAN, "Are Nurses Angels of Mercy?," accessed March 26, 2014, http://tinyurl.com/l96jpyb.
12. Margaret Belcher, "I'm No Angel: I Am a Nurse—and That's Enough," *American Journal of Nursing* 104, no. 7 (July 2004), http://tinyurl.com/q2tr7lc.
13. Terri Metules, "Let's Put an End to Angel Bashing: It's Far Scarier to Think of What We Would Have to Do to Get Rid of the Angel Image," *Modern Medicine* (December 1, 2007), http://tinyurl.com/lvslpug.
14. Angus Howarth, "Robot Nurses Could Be on the Wards in Three Years, Say Scientists," *The Scotsman* (January 22, 2007), http://tinyurl.com/lrxd4rg; CFNA, "Interaction and Intelligence," TAN (January 22, 2007), http://tinyurl.com/mln6lp6.
15. Jamie Doward, "Row Erupts Over Secret Filming of Hospital Filth," *The Guardian* (January 30, 2005), http://tinyurl.com/jw2oe8p; CFNA, "Undercover Angels!," TAN (January 30, 2005), http://tinyurl.com/nxpzszc.
16. CFNA, "Dr. Phil Expresses Appreciation for Nurses and Their Image Problems on the Air, Still Struggles with Apology and Stereotypes," TAN (December 20, 2004), http://tinyurl.com/jwbsc4z.
17. "Stories of Survival," *Dr. Phil* (July 14, 2005), http://tinyurl.com/mc4w796; CFNA, "Feel Good, Inc.," TAN (July 14, 2005), http://tinyurl.com/n6opthx.
18. Patti Neighmond, "Need a Nurse? You May Have to Wait," National Public Radio (May 25, 2012), http://tinyurl.com/7kf9eab; TAN, "Are Your Knuckles White?" (May 25, 2012), http://tinyurl.com/nhdpoas.
19. "Stories of Survival," *Dr. Phil* (July 14, 2005), http://tinyurl.com/mc4w796; CFNA, "Feel Good, Inc.," TAN (July 14, 2005), http://tinyurl.com/n6opthx.

20. Sharon Randall, "Confessions of a Home Nurse," Scripps Howard News Service/*Seattle Times* (June 10, 2010), http://tinyurl.com/mhuodzw; TAN, "Confessions of a Non-Nurse" (June 10, 2010), http://tinyurl.com/mog8eua.
21. *The New York Times*, "Nursing Diaries," accessed February 8, 2014, http://tinyurl.com/kqd8qc3.
22. *Liberty Times*, "Young Nurse at Taichung Hospital Cares for Patients" (September 5, 2006); CFNA, "The Deadly Virtues," TAN (September 5, 2006), http://tinyurl.com/k32jlsv.
23. TAN, "What Happens to Patients When Nurses Are Short-Staffed?," accessed January 29, 2014, http://tinyurl.com/ancmo7r.
24. Wesley Harris, "She Was Like Our Guardian Angel," *NL News Now* (January 23, 2014), http://tinyurl.com/mefdj3m.
25. Mubatsi Asinja Habati, "Nurses—Uganda's Angels," *The Independent* (March 11, 2009), http://tinyurl.com/pecllhe; TAN, "To Everyone We Are Just Tools" (June 1, 2009), http://tinyurl.com/mv9kdl8.
26. Brian Courtis, "Saint Be Praised," *The Age* (June 19, 2005), http://tinyurl.com/lodhucn; CFNA, "Saintly Saints and the Canonizers Who Canonize Them," TAN (June 19, 2005), http://tinyurl.com/mdpj4sd.
27. Liz Heldens, creator, *Mercy*, NBC (2009–2010), http://tinyurl.com/qzmwxvr; TAN, "*Mercy* Episode Reviews" (2010), http://tinyurl.com/kj3t63s.
28. Liz Brixius, Linda Wallem, and Evan Dunsky, Pilot, *Nurse Jackie*, Showtime (June 8, 2009); TAN, "The Henchman of God" (June 8, 2009), http://tinyurl.com/m8lo9kk.
29. Joanne Ostrow, "'Dark Blue' Promising as TNT's Summer Hit," *Denver Post* (July 3, 2009), http://tinyurl.com/ksze6cq.
30. TAN, "*Call the Midwife* Episode Reviews," accessed March 24, 2014, http://tinyurl.com/m3bf4lw.
31. CFNA, "Tickle: Is the Best Thing About Nursing 'Meeting Hot Doctors?' Ha Ha! Just Joking!," TAN (February 8, 2005), http://tinyurl.com/n3k56bo.
32. Angela Moore, "Nurse Nancy Classic Bracelet w/ Gold," accessed February 9, 2014, http://tinyurl.com/kabv3ls.
33. Collectibles-4u, "Bless This Angel of Mercy Nurse Collectible Figurine," accessed March 26, 2014, http://tinyurl.com/kg7brjo.
34. Bradford Exchange, "Special Delivery Figurine," accessed March 26, 2014, http://tinyurl.com/oyblydl.
35. Bradford Exchange, "Precious Moments Angels of Mercy Nurse Figurine Collection," accessed March 26, 2014, http://tinyurl.com/m54b5fu.
36. Precious Moments, "Loving Touch Nurse – Blonde," accessed March 26, 2014, http://tinyurl.com/kyt7pmk.
37. Precious Moments, "You're an Angel," accessed March 26, 2014, http://tinyurl.com/o4c6alf.

38. Caroline Kennedy, "Power of One: Beyond the Call of Duty," *Time* (October 25, 2007), http://tinyurl.com/k6ao7qv; CFNA, "The Commander," TAN (October 25, 2007), http://tinyurl.com/kos766y.
39. Naval Hospital Bremerton, "Command Leadership," US Navy, accessed March 26, 2014, http://tinyurl.com/k8jb4q4.
40. Minette Marrin, "Oh Nurse, Your Degree Is a Symptom of Equality Disease," *The Sunday Times* (November 15, 2009), http://tinyurl.com/pdkgd5g; TAN, "Fighting Equality Disease" (November 15, 2009), http://tinyurl.com/m239pxv.
41. Minette Marrin, "Fallen Angels: The Nightmare Nurses Protected by Silence," *The Sunday Times* (August 30, 2009), http://tinyurl.com/q3khrhu; TAN, "Fighting Equality Disease" (November 15, 2009), http://tinyurl.com/lxx32t5.
42. Minette Marrin, "Oh Nurse, Your Degree is a Symptom of Equality Disease," *The Sunday Times* (November 15, 2009), http://tinyurl.com/pdkgd5g; TAN, "Fighting Equality Disease" (November 15, 2009), http://tinyurl.com/m239pxv.
43. Cristina Odone, "Nursing Is No Longer the Caring Profession," *The Telegraph* (August 28, 2011), http://tinyurl.com/3e73la9.
44. *The Daily Mail*, "Are Nurses Angels? I Don't Think So" (July 18, 2006), http://tinyurl.com/n7vzq3x; CFNA, "These Days There's Far Too Much Emphasis on Academia and an Overwhelming Desire to Achieve an Equal Status with Doctors," TAN (July 25, 2006), http://tinyurl.com/mgw3chm.
45. *The Independent*, "Why Nurses Are No Angels" (June 20, 2006), http://tinyurl.com/lmj2r2f; CFNA, "These Days There's Far Too Much Emphasis on Academia and an Overwhelming Desire to Achieve an Equal Status with Doctors," TAN (July 25, 2006), http://tinyurl.com/mgw3chm.
46. Christie Blatchford, "Militant Angels of Mercy," *The National Post* (June 7, 2003), http://tinyurl.com/m4sdajc; CFNA, "National Post's Blatchford: Bring Back the Handmaidens," TAN (June 26, 2003), http://tinyurl.com/mf6vu6e.
47. Vici Hoban, "A New Nursing Drama Leaves Former Nurse Vici Hoban Ill at Ease," *The Times* (February 28, 2004), http://tinyurl.com/m4sld5v.
48. Simon Heath, Helen Gregory, executive producers, *No Angels*, Channel 4 (2004–2006), http://tinyurl.com/mkyeukh.
49. *Hollywood Reporter*, "'No Angels' Set to Nurse U.S. Viewers" (September 21, 2004), http://tinyurl.com/msw78wb.
50. AJ Marechal, "'My Name Is Earl' Alums Set Nurse Comedy at ABC," *Variety* (September 26, 2013), http://tinyurl.com/ldx5pmm.
51. Tom Anderson, Graham Messick, and Michelle St. John, producers, "Angel of Death: Killer Nurse Stopped, but Not Soon Enough," *60 Minutes*, CBS (April 29, 2013), http://tinyurl.com/kz4egqa.
52. *Daily Mail*, "'Angel of Death' Nurse Who Murdered at Least 40 Patients to Become One of America's Worst Serial Killers Speaks from Prison for the First Time to Chillingly Claim: 'I Thought I Was Helping'" (April 29, 2013), http://tinyurl.com/cngeylo.

53. Mark Dodson, writer, Elodie Keene, director, "The Unclean," *Medical Investigation*, NBC (December 3, 2004); CFNA, "Hungry Ghosts," TAN (December 3, 2004), http://tinyurl.com/k67f4w8.
54. Michael Welner, "Nursing Compassion to Health," *Philadelphia Inquirer* (April 30, 2004), http://tinyurl.com/n5yrzq8; CFNA, "NYU Physician – Charles Cullen Killing Result of Widespread Materialism, No Compassion," TAN (April 30, 2004), http://tinyurl.com/nxh6z3p.
55. The Forensic Panel, "Frequently Asked Questions: Are the Services of The Forensic Panel Costly?," accessed February 16, 2014, http://tinyurl.com/kpkee3s.
56. American Nurses Association, "National Nurses Week," accessed March 27, 2014, http://tinyurl.com/crzyprh.
57. US Vice President Joseph Biden, Remarks at the National Conference on Mental Health, The White House (June 3, 2013), http://tinyurl.com/m4otmbc; TAN, "Come with Me If You Want to Live" (June 3, 2013), http://tinyurl.com/kqqkov9.
58. Cincinnati Children's Hospital Medical Center, "In Celebration of National Nurses Week" (May 9, 2013), http://tinyurl.com/m5p9o34.
59. Lisa Lori, "Happy Nurses Week," *Huffington Post* (May 10, 2013), http://tinyurl.com/kv4fh4h.
60. Cancer Advocacy Coalition of Canada, "Not Just About Money: The Cancer Advocacy Coalition's 2007 Report," businesshealth (July 2008), http://tinyurl.com/odf5yoq.
61. "Nurses Demand Stronger Protection Against On-the-Job Violence," *Seachange Bulletin* (June 27, 2007), http://tinyurl.com/qzq42yf.
62. Maine Coast Memorial Hospital, "National Nurses' Week May 6th–May 12th," accessed March 27, 2014, http://tinyurl.com/kejmcz3.
63. Jennifer Bradshaw, "Saint Peter's University Hospital Celebrates National Nurses Week," *New Brunswick Patch* (May 9, 2012), http://tinyurl.com/mw5qye8.
64. Shore Medical Center, "Shore Medical Center Honors Guardian Angels at Annual Pinning Ceremony" (December 18, 2013), http://tinyurl.com/lhr3vvq.
65. The University of Texas Medical Branch, "Celebrating Nurses and Hospital Week" (May 23, 2012), http://tinyurl.com/kht7n2q.
66. Kathy Douglas, director, *If Florence Could See Us Now*, First Run Features (2012), http://tinyurl.com/lk6baox.
67. International Council of Nurses, "Closing the Gap: Millennium Development Goals 8, 7, 6, 5, 4, 3, 2, 1" (May 10, 2013), http://tinyurl.com/mw9n25f.
68. International Council of Nurses, "2002 - Nurses Always There for You: Caring for Families" (2002), http://tinyurl.com/ke28fqn.
69. Florence Nightingale International Foundation, International Council of Nurses, "The Florence Nightingale Teddy Bear," accessed March 27, 2014, http://tinyurl.com/mwwsdja.
70. *The Capital-Journal*, "Celebrate Nurses Week" (May 10, 2003), http://tinyurl.com/md7uoby.

71. Debbie Hatmaker, "Nurses Keeping the Care in Healthcare," *ADVANCE for Nurses* (May 1, 2000), http://tinyurl.com/meenoud.
72. American Nurses Association, "National Nurses Week 2011 Theme" (January 14, 2011), http://tinyurl.com/kxl3hxf.
73. Gretchen Barrett, "Nurses: Advocating, Leading, Caring," phillyBurbs.com (May 8, 2012), http://tinyurl.com/q4h7oty.
74. Karen Daley, "Reflect on and Celebrate Your Contributions to Quality and Innovation," American Nurses Association, accessed March 28, 2014, http://tinyurl.com/ltktgur.
75. Adam Sachs, "Nurses Leading the Way," *The American Nurse* (May 1, 2014), http://tinyurl.com/l7xgdct.
76. International Association of Forensic Nurses, "International Association of Forensic Nurses Unveils New Logo at Annual Conference," PRWeb (October 25, 2013), http://tinyurl.com/lns5aqj.
77. Norah Sullivan, personal communication (November 4, 2013).
78. Friends of the National Institute for Nursing Research, "Nurse Scientists: Committed to the Public Trust" (October 2004); CFNA, "Johnson & Johnson-Sponsored 'Nurse Scientists' Video," TAN (May 2006), http://tinyurl.com/krrplkw.
79. CFNA, "Touching the World," TAN, accessed March 27, 2014, http://tinyurl.com/lmvgd4y.
80. Associated Press, "Johnson and Johnson Sees Red, Sues Red Cross," NBC (August 9, 2007), http://tinyurl.com/mpgtj85.
81. Katie Thomas, "J.&J. to Pay $2.2 Billion in Risperdal Settlement," *New York Times* (November 4, 2013), http://tinyurl.com/ksjmv9b.
82. Barry Meier, "Johnson & Johnson in Deal to Settle Hip Implant Lawsuits," *New York Times* (November 19, 2013), http://tinyurl.com/ldxluxn; Barry Meier, "J.&J. Loses First Case Over Faulty Hip Implant," *New York Times* (March 8, 2013), http://tinyurl.com/bz54sbq.
83. Amrita Nair-Ghaswalla, "J&J's Licence to Make Baby Powder Cancelled," *Business Line* (April 25, 2013), http://tinyurl.com/kglzplj.
84. Johnson & Johnson, "For All You Love" (2013), http://tinyurl.com/muahfjb.
85. Tanzina Vega, "Trying to Burnish Its Image, J.&J. Turns to Emotions," *New York Times* (April 24, 2013), http://tinyurl.com/lbr783r.
86. TAN, "Why Aren't You More Excited That Public Opinion Polls Often Put Nurses at the Top of the List of 'Most Trusted' and 'Most Ethical' Professions?" (December 17, 2013), http://tinyurl.com/79yx6pa.
87. CFNA, "Baby We Were Born to Care," TAN (November 2007), http://tinyurl.com/oysyl4t.
88. TAN, "Lucky Charms" (June 2011), http://tinyurl.com/q7xtf2t.
89. Johnson & Johnson, "About Amazing Nurses 2013" (2013), http://tinyurl.com/larnahg.

90. Johnson & Johnson, "Journal Photos - Nursing Notes by Johnson & Johnson," accessed March 27, 2014, http://tinyurl.com/kqfelft.
91. Johnson & Johnson, "Nursing Notes by Johnson & Johnson," accessed March 27, 2014, http://tinyurl.com/m6jegfx.
92. CFNA, "To Inspire and Be Inspired," TAN (August 2007), http://tinyurl.com/kvm9jpu.
93. National Organisation of Nurses and Midwives of Malawi, "Soon There Will Be No Angels on Earth" (March 2, 2009), http://tinyurl.com/mfcxh6k.
94. TAN, "That Gargantuan Heart All Squishy with Compassion Thumping Away!" (May 2011), http://tinyurl.com/k44qxt9.
95. Clyde Phillips, writer, Randall Einhorn, director, "Happy F**king Birthday," *Nurse Jackie*, Showtime (April 14, 2013); TAN, "Cunning, Baffling, Powerful" (April 14, 2013), http://tinyurl.com/kgrdrne.
96. San Francisco Bay Area Independent Media Center (Indybay), "May 12 S.F. Nurses' Day Protest against Johnson & Johnson" (May 16, 2005), http://tinyurl.com/kh65gj9.
97. CFNA, "'Do They Deserve This Six-Figure Salary for What They Do?'," TAN (October 26, 2006), http://tinyurl.com/p5y7bml.
98. *RATTLE* #28: Tribute to Nurses (Winter 2007), Timothy Green, editor, http://tinyurl.com/n6o3sy7; CFNA, "Rattle: Tribute to Nurses (Winter 2007)," TAN (May 16, 2008), http://tinyurl.com/m284jar.
99. Craig Barton and Company, University of Alabama at Birmingham Recruiting Video (2004); CFNA, "Rap Recruiting Video," TAN (May 2006), http://tinyurl.com/l7oo4tf.
100. Steven Moffat and Mark Gatiss, creators, *Sherlock*, BBC, accessed May 9, 2014, http://tinyurl.com/7gdtv26.

8 WINNING THE BATTLE-AXE, LOSING THE WAR

Nurse Linda S. Smith once entered the room of a young male inpatient to give him his medications. The patient "grinned and naughtily paraphrased the words he had just read on one of his [get-well] cards: 'Nurse, are you coming in to give me one of those famous sponge baths? If you are, I'm ready!'" On his nightstand, one card showed a sexy young nurse offering sponge services. That much is hardly news—just another hostile work environment linked to the naughty nurse image.

But when Professor Smith and her students at Oregon Health and Science University later conducted a study of such greeting cards, they found more than the expected naughty nurse themes. There was also a focus on what an August 2003 Oregon Public Broadcasting piece about the study called the "sadistic shot giver." As Smith wrote in *Nursing Spectrum*:

> Patients may believe the greeting card image that [the nurse] will cause fear and anxiety, often threatening to inflict pain while using devices such as syringes, thermometers, or whips. . . . Disguised as humor, this disrespect and lack of understanding echoes back to the hard, commanding, uncaring image of Nurse Ratched in the movie *One Flew Over the Cuckoo's Nest.*[1]

Nurse Mildred Ratched is indeed the modern archetype of the nurse as battle-axe. Milos Forman's classic 1975 film adaptation of Ken Kesey's novel captured the antiauthoritarian spirit of the 1960s counterculture. In the movie, Randle McMurphy was a charismatic roughneck who engineered a transfer from a work farm, where he had been serving a sentence for assault, to an Oregon state mental health facility he thought would be easier. He joined a unit of men with psychiatric problems. Ratched dominated the unit, leading the patients in what at first seemed like actual group therapy and offering calm, rational explanations for an array of rules. But McMurphy gradually realized that Ratched was a cunning sociopath who psychologically tortured those she was ostensibly helping, aided by the meek Nurse Pilbow. Ratched manipulated the young patient Billy through his fear of his mother, making Billy feel that his interest in sex was evil. Meanwhile, as absentee male physicians debated whether McMurphy was really ill, McMurphy worked to undermine Ratched's authority. He led the patients on forbidden adventures involving wine, women, and song, which plainly promoted more healing than Ratched's joyless regime. As McMurphy's refusal to conform instilled a sense of independence in the other patients, Ratched resorted to increasingly harsh measures to maintain control, with tragic results.

Nurse Ratched was a repressive soul killer. Even her name evokes words like "rat," "wretched," and "hatchet." The film offered no positive counterexample or explanation for her behavior, such as burnout after years in a difficult care setting. Ratched could be a warning about the potential for abuse in the nursing profession, but she can't be separated from the film's views of women generally. They were either emasculating, antisex mother figures like Ratched; spineless mice like Pilbow; or easy, giggling facilitators like McMurphy's girlfriend, whose name was Candy. The movie indicted establishment power structures, suggesting that real men must reclaim their power and freedom from the oppressive modern state. But the film seemed to place the blame mostly on Mom, who just won't let boys be boys. Of course it doesn't make much sense: women were not the main creators of those power structures. But no one said misogyny was rational. Evidently, Ratched is what happens when you *do* give women control. What kind of place is it where a *nurse* has more power than the *physicians*? A twisted, unnatural place, dominated by the Other.

The other important modern battle-axe was the Margaret "Hot Lips" Houlihan character who first appeared in the film *M*A*S*H.* Robert Altman's innovative 1970 movie about a US Army surgical unit in the Korean War, based on the 1968 novel by Richard Hooker, mockingly dissected those involved in the military's effort there. The dark comedy was another anti-authoritarian classic with a viscerally misogynistic approach. The nurses who appeared fell into the categories of naughty, handmaiden, and/or battle-axe. Major Houlihan, the unit's new chief nurse, was a martinet aghast at the unmilitary conduct she found. She and the inept surgeon Frank Burns tattled to the military brass in Seoul, and they began a cringe-inducing affair, although he was married. In response, the film's heroes, the cynical surgeons

Hawkeye and Trapper, engineered a nasty invasion of privacy that humiliated Burns and Houlihan. Then our heroes implemented a plan to determine Houlihan's true hair color that the film found hilarious, but which has something in common with gang rape. After that, "Hot Lips" was more docile, Trapper praised her nursing, and she seemed to earn some redemption by joining the surgeons' boyish fun.

In the popular *M*A*S*H* television series that followed (1972–1983), the depiction of nursing was better. The show's nurses were still mostly assistants and easy romantic foils for the surgeons, who received virtually all the credit or blame for patient outcomes. But the series showed some actual nursing, and there was little doubt about Houlihan's authority over the nurses, her nursing skills, or her commitment to the patients. As the series went on, she grew increasingly sympathetic. Unlike Ratched, Houlihan made a clear positive difference for patients. However, especially in the early years, she was still a fairly pathetic figure, grasping at power and petty discipline—and a man to fill the void in her career-dominated life, a struggle that was the subject of endless mockery. Houlihan was far more than a battle-axe, but the influential character still suggested that strong nurses are control freaks driven by half-repressed romantic urges.

Ratched and Houlihan set the standards for a certain type of fictional nursing image in later decades: the older female nurse as bitter crone and vindictive bureaucrat, often with at least a hint of sexual frustration or even aggression. In general, the battle-axe inverts both the maternal/angel image and the naughty image, as Figure 8.1 illustrates. She is yet another one-dimensional female extreme, a way to put women in their place if they are doing something you don't like. It may be that this image has resonated because of patients' feelings of vulnerability and anxiety at being at the mercy of female caregivers who would normally be in a subservient social position. The classic battle-axe has appeared in many Hollywood products, often as the nasty enforcer of hospital rules that are presented as oppressive or trivial, even though some are actually vital to the patient's recovery.

A recent variation on the classic battle-axe is the malevolent hottie, a sexually aggressive young "nurse" who poses a real or mock threat to patients or others, as we noted in Chapter 5. This fictional image, which we might call the "naughty-axe," has appeared in connection with films, advertisements, and video games. Perhaps foreshadowed by the naughty elements of "Hot Lips" Houlihan, the naughty-axe seems to invert only the maternal stereotype. The naughty-axe does not oppose sex. But because the image does associate sexuality with danger, it is true to the underlying spirit of the classic battle-axe.

Nursing's Sex-Related Stereotypes:
A Bermuda Triangle of Professional Imagery

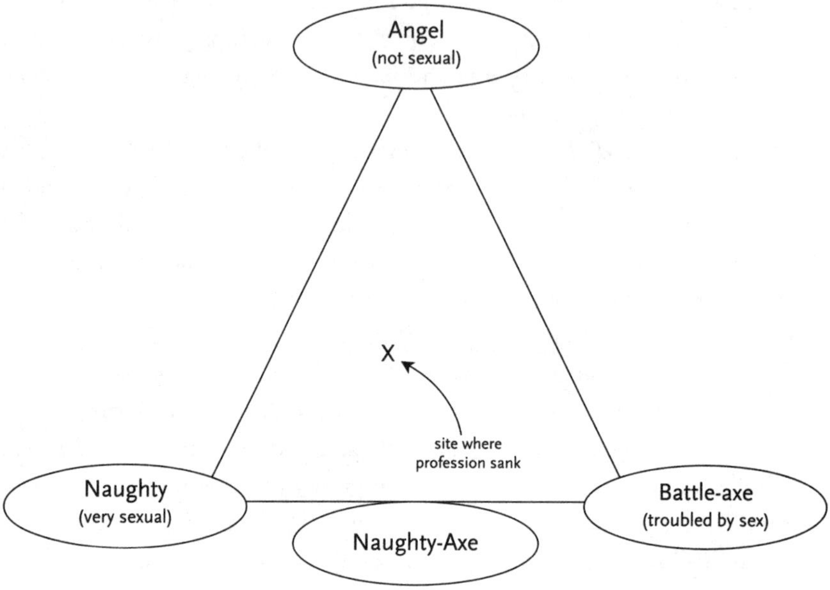

FIGURE 8.1 Nursing's Sex-Related Stereotypes: A Bermuda Triangle of Professional Imagery.

In 2012, part of the Oregon State Hospital where *One Flew Over the Cuckoo's Nest* was filmed became a Museum of Mental Health that provides a forum to reconsider past treatment of psychiatric patients.[2] But nurse battle-axe imagery has persisted in the media, largely unquestioned. Why is that, since women have far more power in the workplace now? Do some nurses really act like vindictive martinets? Of course some do, as in any profession. That is especially unsurprising for an underpowered profession in the midst of a long staffing crisis. But battle-axe portrayals typically provide little balance or context to explain why some nurses might act that way. By contrast, there are many admiring depictions of powerful female physicians. And portrayals that do question female physicians' use of power often make clear how hard it still is for women to assert authority without being seen as "bitches."

So although modern society may be at least ambivalent about punishing women *generally* for exercising power, it remains acceptable to punish women for being powerful *nurses*—a practice even "feminists" engage in, as explained in Chapter 6. So the nurse battle-axe image is a safe outlet for feel-good regressive values. Enjoy that misogyny responsibly!

Tyrants, Bureaucrats, Monsters: Hollywood Celebrates Nursing Authority

Prime-time US television has rarely shown a positive nurse character with genuine authority. The recent nurse-focused shows have, at least, generally avoided battle-axe imagery. Nurse Evangelina on *Call the Midwife* is an authoritative senior nurse who has displayed what might be seen as battle-axe traits, harshly seizing upon flaws in some of those around her.[3] But in contrast to classic battle-axes, Evangelina is fiercely devoted to her patients. Her toughness seems to be rooted in her high standards for care and her own history of fighting her way out of poverty. She is eventually revealed to be good-hearted. In addition, the actual midwife supervisor, Sister Julienne, is strong and skilled but also wise and gentle, if anything an idealized vision of a nursing manager. Sister Julienne expertly manages senior midwives like Sister Monica Joan, who has periods of dementia, while mentoring junior ones, like lead character Jenny Lee, who may be struggling in their practice. At the same time, Sister Julienne ensures that patients receive the best care possible under difficult circumstances.[4]

The lead character in *HawthoRNe* was a commanding and even combative chief nursing officer, and at times she alienated administrators and physicians. But like Sister Evangelina, Hawthorne ruffled feathers in fighting for the well-being of patients and staff, and she did not display the battle-axe qualities of bureaucratic vindictiveness and hostility toward patients.[5]

Ironically, the only real battle-axe imagery on the recent nurse shows has appeared on *Nurse Jackie*, despite its generally strong portrayal of nursing. In the first season, Jackie Peyton's emergency department nurse manager, Gloria Akalitus, was a seemingly heartless killjoy obsessed with enforcing rules regardless of their effect on patients. In one July 2009 episode, she prevented a responsible 10-year-old girl from sitting with her mother, who had lupus, because of a hospital age limit.[6] The show often punished Akalitus. In that same episode, while yelling about a Taser someone had left on the floor, Akalitus accidentally Tasered herself. In a June 2009 episode, she drank Jackie's coffee, not realizing it had been spiked with Jackie's painkillers; Akalitus spent the rest of the episode slurring and embarrassing herself. Some managers are harsh and bureaucratic, and these staff nurse revenge fantasies may be amusing. But they reinforce the damaging notions that nurses can't wield administrative authority and that managers are not real nurses. In another June 2009 episode, Jackie invited Akalitus to be a "nurse again for one second" in assessing a patient, as if the manager was no longer a nurse.[7]

Fortunately, Akalitus became far more nuanced in later seasons, revealing genuine concern for others beneath the gruff exterior. She repeatedly supported Jackie in her struggles with drug abuse and even acted to protect patients, as in a May 2013 episode in which she caught a patient's condition that the chief emergency physician had missed.[8] Jackie herself countered the battle-axe image in projecting sensitive clinical authority, and in June 2012 episodes, actually running the emergency department with impressive skill.[9]

But the initial Akalitus portrayal is more typical. In the April 2013 finale of TNT's *Monday Mornings*, one of the heroic surgeon characters was critically ill in the intensive care unit (ICU) following an operation. When she awoke, all her surgeon colleagues naturally rushed to her bedside. Leave it to an older ICU nurse named Gladys—the only nurse named in the episode—to try to limit visitors to two at a time! An authoritative senior surgeon calmly overruled Gladys, telling her to pick her battles. He might as well as have told her not to be such a battle-axe.[10]

Grey's Anatomy has also presented senior nurses as vindictive bureaucrats who are working against the young surgical heroes. In one November 2005 episode discussed in Chapter 3, hotshot intern Cristina Yang stole an interesting case from the psychiatric ward. But cranky veteran nurse Debbie questioned Cristina: "This room is supposed to be unoccupied. Whose patient is this? . . . Who transferred him? I don't have any paperwork, any transfer documents." Yang dismissed Debbie by noting that the physicians would let her know if a bedpan needed changing. The nurses retaliated by paging Yang to do disgusting scut work.[11]

This absurd fantasy about workplace roles was likely a misguided effort to show nurses respect. But it did not suggest that disrespecting nurses is wrong or unsafe, merely that, as chief resident Miranda Bailey noted, it's "stupid" to antagonize the nurses. Debbie might have been shown humiliating Cristina by catching the intern's error and saving a patient's life. Or she might have simply explained what nursing really is. Instead, Debbie's revenge was that of a petty bureaucrat who really *is* all about bedpans. And Cristina had the last laugh. Recall Winston Churchill's response to Bessie Braddock, a Member of the UK Parliament who reportedly once told him, "Winston, you are drunk, and what's more you are disgustingly drunk." According to his bodyguard, Churchill replied, "Bessie, my dear, you are ugly, and what's more, you are disgustingly ugly. But tomorrow I shall be sober and you will still be disgustingly ugly."[12] Cristina may have been a little drunk on ego and ambition, but in the morning of future episodes, she remained a pretty, esteemed surgeon. Debbie was still a disagreeable battle-axe who cleaned up the mess.

As we saw in Chapters 3 and 4, several late 2005 *ER* episodes did feature the strong nurse manager Eve Peyton, a clinical expert with a doctorate who seemed to care about patients. But Peyton was a strict micromanager; one staff nurse suggested that she was a "bitch."[13] Peyton's departure marked a crude and implausible swerve into extreme battle-axe territory. In one December 2005 episode, Peyton got dumped by her boyfriend; decked an offensive patient dressed as Santa Claus and poured urine on him, with no physical provocation and no regret; was fired on Christmas Eve; and bid farewell to the staff with standard PhD-type phrases, such as "bite me," "screw yourselves," and "you all suck."[14] Maybe this all seemed funny because many still consider nurses to be "angels." But the episode is a bit less amusing when you consider that emergency nurses are many times more likely to be the victims than the causes of workplace violence[15]—something *ER* rarely showed.

There was no significant *ER* nurse character to balance Peyton. Major nurse character Sam Taggart was expert, but she was not that senior and had no obvious authority. By comparison, *ER*'s depictions of harsh physician managers Kerry Weaver and Robert Romano were countered with many portraits of wise, humane ones, such as Susan Lewis, Mark Greene, and Elizabeth Corday. On her way out, Peyton ranted that she "tried to elevate this stupid ER." But she was less a frustrated reformer than a nurse who had the temerity to push back against her *ER*-assigned role as physician subordinate. Apparently it's fine for women to be assertive in traditionally male professions like medicine. But aggressive nurses are too much of a threat to the natural order, it seems, and perhaps to the "feminist" doctrine that able women who choose healthcare careers must become physicians. So any assertive woman who chooses *nursing* must be a bitter, dangerous loon, frustrated in love—a battle-axe.

A memorable battle-axe also appeared in a January 2004 *ER*, when medical student Abby Lockhart did a rotation in the neonatal ICU (NICU). This unit seemed to be staffed mainly by physicians and medical students, rather than the nurses who would staff it in real life. In this physician-intensive care unit, one of the two nurses who emerged from the wallpaper left the impression that veteran NICU nurses are fussy tyrants bent on terrorizing medical students. A NICU attending physician introduced nurse Virgie as a twenty-year veteran whose mission was to protect the babies from medical students. That is one thing NICU nurses do, but Virgie was hostile, rule-bound, and—contrary to the attending's introduction—apparently not concerned about the patients. Virgie refused Lockhart's request that she give, without advance physician authorization, medication to a deteriorating infant to stop his full-body seizures. When Lockhart (who was also a nurse) did it herself, Virgie whined that she would report Lockhart to the attending physician. Virgie made no effort to intervene and stop the patient's seizures. Instead she stood by, focused on her charting as her patient teetered in crisis. Virgie also confronted Lockhart for having changed a diaper without weighing it, ruining her count of "ins and outs." Lockhart apologized but noted that the diaper was now in the trash. Virgie snapped "Not good enough!" and insisted that Lockhart find and weigh it. We got no explanation that ins and outs are critical measures of a newborn's health. The episode also included Tom, a kind, cooperative nurse who deferred to the students: so much for protecting the babies. In any case, Virgie dominated the episode's vision of nursing.[16] Not good enough!

Another notable battle-axe appeared on ABC's short-lived *MDs*, which aired in 2002. The drama tried to transplant the basic premise of *M*A*S*H*—two renegade surgeons thwarting a bad system to save lives—to a twenty-first century San Francisco hospital. Physicians provided all important care, but the show did not ignore nurses: one major character was "Nurse 'Doctor' Poole," who used her PhD—in management—to act as a heartless enforcer for the evil HMO that controlled the hospital. Poole was a Frankenstein made from the worst parts of Nurse Ratched and Margaret Houlihan, a bean-counting monster who relished denying patients needed care. Like Ratched, Poole used her training to control patients and undermine their health. Like Houlihan at her worst, Poole was obsessed with enforcing rules and frustrated by subversive surgeons who wouldn't conform. Poole, like Houlihan, even had a pathetic affair with a married cohort. Of course, some real nurses have been co-opted by the managed care system, but far more fight constantly to protect their patients from it. The crowning touch was Poole's "Doctor" label, which the show itself put in quotes. *MDs* mocked the very idea of a nurse with a doctorate and linked it with the perceived backwardness of managed care.[17] What kind of system allows a *nurse* to pretend to be a doctor?

The nurse battle-axe also pops up on nonhealthcare shows. The September 2011 premiere of NBC's *Whitney* included the lead character's misadventures in a naughty nurse costume, as discussed in Chapter 5. But Whitney and her boyfriend also encountered a "real" nurse when they arrived at the emergency department to see about the minor injury he sustained while trying to get with his sexy girlfriend. The real nurse mocked Whitney as a "stripper," which was actually good considering her outfit, but the nurse also barred Whitney from staying with her boyfriend because they were not married. Thus, to the extent the nurse showed authority, she did so as a petty hospital bureaucrat, preventing a loved one from seeing a patient.[18]

The September 2005 season premiere of CBS's *Cold Case* focused on an investigation involving a pro-life school nurse. Nurse Laura manipulated a high school couple into having their baby—lying to them about the effects of and legal requirements for abortion—and set in motion forces that destroyed their lives. Nurse Laura also had a record of arrests for assaulting clinic workers, and the show presented her as a moralizing hypocrite, herself having an affair with a married teacher (recall Houlihan and Poole).[19]

Two months later an episode of NBC's *Law and Order* focused on the death of an abusive mother who had been jailed for allegedly killing a man who reported her to child protective services. The mother's death was caused by a reaction to an intrauterine device given to her by nurse Gloria, who was secretly sterilizing women she deemed unworthy of having children. The show's district attorneys prosecuted Gloria. Both shows included strong female law enforcement characters.[20]

These crime shows retooled Nurse Ratched for the modern era. Neo-Ratched still embodied institutional oppression and sexual intolerance: both nurses in these plots used their authority to deny troubled women the right to make their own reproductive choices. Unlike Ratched, the nurses were motivated by understandable goals. But far beyond merely taking a principled stand against abortion or child abuse, these nurses abdicated their ethical duties and actually hurt *women*—something Ratched did not do. Nursing seemed to be a backwater populated by zealots with no use for the lawful avenues democracies offer to effect social change. Neo-Ratched was a throwback dragging other women back with her, doing a job that enlightened women like our law enforcement heroes had left behind. Once again, only women who pursue traditionally male professions are worthy of real power.

A March 2006 episode of HBO's *The Sopranos* found Mafia boss Tony Soprano gravely wounded and in a coma on a hospital ventilator. Tony's family and subordinates kept watch. Nurses appeared from time to time, but Tony's wife Carmela and daughter Meadow took a far more active role in his care. They talked to the unconscious Tony, they touched him, and Meadow even climbed into bed next to him. Because none of the episode's nurses got a name, we'll assign them numbers.

At one point Nurse 1 chastised Silvio, Tony's consigliere, at the nurse's station: "Sir, it's family only in the unit." Silvio said he would be out of her hair in a minute. Nurse 1: "I keep telling you people—I'm gonna have to call the hospital administrator." At another point, we saw Nurse 1 working at the bedside, emptying blood out of a drain. She exited, looking bitter and eyeing Meadow and mob guy Paulie: "Only one person at a time, please." After she left, Meadow confirmed, "She's a ball buster." At another point Carmela entered the comatose Tony's room as Nurse 2 was adjusting his tubes. Nurse 2 snapped, "Don't get in bed with him again—you dislodged his drains." Carmela: "That was my daughter, and I can't help but think that physical affection means something." Nurse 2 shook her head as if Carmela was deranged. Later, after Tony had been out of the coma for some time, Carmela entered his room to find him sitting propped up in a chair. She asked Nurse 3, "You've got him up?" Nurse 3: "I know how it looks, but he should be upright as much as possible." Nurse 3 did not explain why. Instead, she checked something and left quickly.[21]

Nurse 3 was not too bad, but on the whole, the episode portrayed ICU nurses as nasty, rule-bound bureaucrats who actually impede psychosocial care. There was no context to explain why that might be, no indication of poor workplace conditions, no indication even that the nurses found that dealing with a group of mass murderers made them a little edgy. Viewers were unlikely to see the importance of any of the rules the nurses enforced. No one explained. Of course, pulling out drains could result in serious complications, but nurses should and do still help families find ways to provide physical affection to patients. In fact, however realistic it was, this episode suggested that Tony was brought back from the edge of death by awareness of his loved ones' presence. In effect, the message was that nurses could learn something about psychosocial care and family presence from the Mafia family. Maybe Carmela and Meadow could have given the nurses some clinical training! One nurse who would not need such training is the expert Jackie Peyton, who is played, like Carmela, by actress Edie Falco. Did this 2006 *Sopranos* episode inspire Falco to pursue nursing full time?

The battle-axe has also haunted other great shows. For example, the classic science-fiction series *The X-Files* adapted Ratched for its own purposes in a May 1997 episode. In that one, after the typical set-up of mysterious deaths and paranormal visitations, it turned out that a bitter, older psychiatric facility nurse had murdered several young women one of her patients had doted on. Apparently the nurse killed the women in order to punish the patient for feeling a love the nurse never could.[22] The Ratched reference underlined one of the show's own well-known mantras: trust no one![23]

Nor are serious films above deploying the battle-axe. One striking example is Nurse Noakes, a minor character in *Cloud Atlas* (2012), directed by the Wachowski siblings and Tom Tykwer based on a novel by David Mitchell.

The film had several related plotlines that took place over different time periods in Earth's past, present, and future. Nurse Noakes was the oppressive, unattractive supervisor of the nursing home Aurora House, a sinister present-day facility that confined aged "loved ones" who were no longer wanted by their unscrupulous relatives. In one plotline, the hapless book editor Timothy Cavendish was tricked into the facility by his devious brother as revenge for an affair Timothy had had with the brother's wife. Noakes menaced Timothy, hitting him and threatening to make him eat soap. At one point, Tim pleads with his brother to be released and apologizes for the affair, but his brother says there is no need for that, his exile is enough, "although I do have my fingers crossed for a scenario involving you, Nurse Noakes, and a broom handle." Timothy and a few other resident-inmates finally managed to escape to a local pub, where they got away from Noakes in the confusion of a huge brawl in which Noakes got the thumping she evidently deserved.[24]

Noakes was female, but she was played by actor Hugo Weaving. That reflected the directors' decision to have their actors play multiple roles across gender, racial, and time lines, which seemed to emphasize both the unity and the divergence in the course of human events. However, it also underlined the Otherness of the Noakes character, arguably suggesting that the nurse was sexually frustrated or at least confused, and perhaps that was at the root of his/her evil. Of course, the "broom handle" comment made the potential sexual assault more immediate and explicit. But the character was similar enough to Ratched that it still worked as a useful shorthand. Viewers could be counted on to get the idea quickly: "Oh yeah, Ratched-type nurse who delights in torturing those she is supposedly helping in an involuntary institutional setting—poor Timothy must escape." He isn't the only one.

On a related note, recall that recent horror films have relied on naughty-axe imagery, which in one neat package provides the fear and sexuality that often drive those films, as discussed in Chapter 5. As we noted, nurse characters of this type figured in the recent *Silent Hill* films. Those nurses were at times presented sexually, but they were also deformed monsters who manifested human fears—not a bad definition of a battle-axe.[25] A more recognizably human naughty-axe appeared in *Nurse 3D*, which was released in mainstream US theatres in 2014.[26] That film was a violent thriller about a vengeful nurse who, as the film's promotion coyly noted, used her sexuality to lure "dishonest" men for "severe" punishment. To be more specific, she was a hospital nurse manager *and* a sadistic, sexually aggressive serial killer who targeted men for cheating on their wives, in addition to murdering pretty much anyone who got in her way (tag line: "your pain is her pleasure"). That plotline seems to tap into male fears of female sexuality, doesn't it? Characters like these differ from the classic battle-axe in that they are presented as sexually active and attractive, of course, but they achieve a similar effect: to link nurses who actually have power with malevolence.

Hovering Like Ghouls: Battle-Axes in Other Media

The battle-axe appears in a variety of recent media, in both her classic and naughty-axe forms. For instance, in 2014 the online Spirit Halloween store was selling a "Nurse Mercy" costume that really did not seem to involve a lot of mercy. The malevolent-looking model wielded a big syringe as she displayed the costume's "blood-spattered apron" and jagged dress hem.[27] In 2005 the Kentucky company Diversified Designs ran an advertisement for its CompuCaddy computer stands in such magazines as *Health Data Management*. In the advertisement, a furious nurse pointed her finger and bared her teeth. She wore a severe, traditional white uniform, and her name tag read "HELEN WHEELS, R.N." The caption: "The morning shift would like a word with you!" Helen was mad because her computer stand battery was dead: the idea was that CompuCaddy would help prevent that crisis because its batteries last longer.[28] Of course, any nurse in Helen's situation might be displeased, but the character's "hell on wheels" name and general presentation suggested that she was an ogre to be avoided under any circumstances.

But that's nothing. In T. Coraghessan Boyle's short story "Chicxulub," nurses are cold functionaries who represent the mindless brutality of the universe. No, really. The story appeared in *The New Yorker* in March 2004 and in Boyle's 2005 collection *Tooth and Claw*. It compares the potential loss of a couple's beloved teenage daughter to the ever-present possibility that a big rock will strike the Earth and end civilization. The father/narrator describes the night he and his wife are called to the hospital following a serious car accident. Arriving at what appears to be the emergency department, the couple approaches the "admittance desk." The young "Filipina" nurse there greets the distraught parents by demanding, "Name?" She has "opaque eyes and the bone structure of a cadaver; every day she sees death and it blinds her. She doesn't see us." Retrieving information from her computer with her "fleshless fingers," the nurse refuses to tell them anything more than that their daughter is still in surgery. The father wonders why he "despise[s] this nurse more than any human being [he's] ever encountered"—this woman "with her hair pulled back in a bun and a white cap like a party favor perched atop it, *who is just doing her job*?" Why does he want to "reach across the counter that separates us and awaken her to a swift, sure knowledge of hate and fear and pain? Why?"

The desperate couple proceeds to surgery, "and here is another nurse, grimmer, older, with lines like the strings of a tobacco pouch pulled tight around her lips." The couple asks if their daughter will be all right. " 'I don't have that information,' the nurse says, and her voice is neutral, robotic even. This is not her daughter." The father can't handle this "maddening clinical neutrality" and he explodes, suggesting that it's the nurse's job to know what's going on after the couple has been dragged in and told their daughter has been hurt. The nurse "drills" the father with a look. She steps away from her desk, revealing herself to be "short," "dumpy," and "almost a dwarf." She leads the couple to a room, saying, "Wait here. . . . The doctor will be in in a minute." Then she disappears, leaving them alone there for "a good hour or more." Won't someone rescue this poor couple from the clutches of modern nursing? Someone will, as a young surgeon finally appears and offers the only decent words the parents have heard at this hospital. Then he leads them through what sounds like an ICU, where patients are surrounded by machines with "nurses hovering over them like ghouls."[29]

Of course, nurses who work in stressful conditions can behave badly, but the extreme battle-axe vision that this sympathetic narrator presents is hard to miss, and Boyle gives us no real reason to question it. Yes, the father is upset. But consider the dramatic ascent from the ugly, hateful nurses to the sensitive physician who will actually give the parents information and who has apparently been trying to save the couple's daughter all by himself. The nurses guard their computers or hover like "ghouls," protecting themselves by brutalizing distraught family members. They are inhuman bookkeepers of death.

The naughty-axe image also figures in various pop culture products. In particular, the hottie as "sadistic shot giver" wielding an enormous phallic syringe seems to be a cool way for pop musicians to move product. As we explained in Chapter 5, a 2004 Skechers advertising campaign featured naughty nurse Christina Aguilera brandishing an enormous syringe connected to a big needle.[30] The band blink-182 used a porn star as a naughty nurse flaunting another huge syringe in the artwork of a 1999 album.[31]

But naughty-axes don't just look threatening, they also kick ass. Two popular recent wrestling video games have featured sexy "nurse" images. In Yuke's *WWE SmackDown! vs. Raw 2006,* gamers competing in barely-dressed female "nurse" and other modes could slap, kick, and grapple, toss each other on a bouncy bed, rip each other's clothes off, and spank each other. Yeah, baby.[32]

Konami's *Rumble Roses* games, released in 2004 and 2006, featured an evil naughty nurse character named Anesthesia. She had devastating moves and was also, needless to say, using the body parts of her victims to create a malevolent cyborg to help her rule the world.[33] Of course, as we've noted, real nurses are the health workers most likely to be the victims of workplace violence.[34]

At the risk of being labeled battle-axes, we have to say that the continuing appearance of battle-axe imagery suggests that, for many, nursing remains caught in an ugly cultural time warp. Female nurses with any power must be threatening, sexually frustrated, and/or disagreeable. Yes, the media tells us, some women today can handle real authority—women with the brains and education to pursue a traditionally male profession. But a good nurse's role is submission.

Notes

1. Linda S. Smith, "Image Counts: Greeting Cards Mail It in When It Comes to Accurately Portraying Nurses," *Nursing Spectrum*, Southern ed. (October 1, 2003), http://tinyurl.com/ye38eqg.
2. Kirk Johnson, "Once a 'Cuckoo's Nest,' Now a Museum," *New York Times* (March 31, 2013), http://tinyurl.com/k765vqd.
3. TAN, "*Call the Midwife* Episode Reviews," accessed March 24, 2014, http://tinyurl.com/m3bf4lw.
4. TAN, "*Call the Midwife* Episode Reviews."
5. TAN, "*HawthoRNe* Episode Reviews" (2011), http://tinyurl.com/jwd7neg.
6. Taii K. Austin, writer, Steve Buscemi, director, "Daffodil," *Nurse Jackie*, Showtime (July 6, 2009); TAN, "Take the Blue Pill" (July 6, 2009), http://tinyurl.com/o9e4m2h.
7. Mark Hudis, writer, Craig Zisk, director, "Chicken Soup," *Nurse Jackie*, Showtime (June 22, 2009); TAN, "The Good, the Bad and Zoey's Stethoscope," http://tinyurl.com/m7zzgt.
8. Cindy Caponera, writer, Randall Einhorn, director, "Good Thing," *Nurse Jackie*, Showtime (May 12, 2013).
9. TAN, "Cunning, Baffling, Powerful" (April 14, 2013), http://tinyurl.com/kgrdrne.
10. Amanda Johns, David E. Kelley, Karen Struck, writers, based on the novel of Sanjay Gupta, Bill D'Elia, director, "Family Ties," *Monday Mornings*, TNT (April 8, 2013); TAN, "Picking Battles" (April 2013), http://tinyurl.com/n65ovcn.
11. Stacy McKee, writer, Adam Davidson, director, "Something to Talk About," *Grey's Anatomy*, ABC (November 6, 2005); CFNA, "The Drunk and the Ugly," TAN (November 6, 2005), http://tinyurl.com/o7ob6nt.

12. Richard M. Langworth, "Drunk and Ugly: The Rumor Mill," The Churchill Centre (January 31, 2011), http://tinyurl.com/l9ektwf.
13. CFNA, "Peyton Place," TAN (October 20, 2005), http://tinyurl.com/p8239cy.
14. CFNA, "A Lump of Coal," TAN (December 8, 2005), http://tinyurl.com/kk2h69z.
15. Deborah D. May and Laurie M. Grubbs, "The Extent, Nature, and Precipitating Factors of Nurse Assault among Three Groups of Registered Nurses in a Regional Medical Center," *Journal of Emergency Nursing* 28, no. 1 (2002): 11–17, http://tinyurl.com/ks7cdj9 and http://tinyurl.com/l9rruax.
16. Lisa Zwerling, writer, Laura Innes, director, "NICU," *ER*, NBC (January 15, 2004); CFNA, "Physician-Intensive Care Unit," TAN (January 15, 2004), http://tinyurl.com/obgpkk8.
17. Gary Tieche, creator, *MDs*, ABC (2002–2003); CFNA, "MDs," TAN (February 8, 2003), http://tinyurl.com/qxqf8e3.
18. Whitney Cummings, writer, Andy Ackerman, director, "Pilot," *Whitney*, NBC (September 22, 2011); TAN, "Whitless" (July 2011), http://tinyurl.com/cmt47df.
19. Meredith Steihm, writer, Mark Pellington, director, "Family," *Cold Case*, CBS (September 25, 2005); CFNA, "Ratched Redux: Family," TAN (December 4, 2005), http://tinyurl.com/lzx72az.
20. David Slack, writer, Constantine Makris, director, "Birthright," *Law and Order*, NBC (November 2, 2005); CFNA, "Ratched Redux," TAN (December 4, 2005), http://tinyurl.com/mvqx59f.
21. Matthew Weiner, writer, Jack Bender, director, "Mayham," *The Sopranos*, HBO (March 26, 2006); CFNA, "Family Presence and Psychosocial Care of the Comatose ICU Patient, Cont. Nursing Ed. HBO-068, Instructors: Carmela and Meadow Soprano," TAN (March 26, 2006), http://tinyurl.com/nzj8x7h.
22. John Shiban, writer, Jim Charleston, director, "Elegy," *The X-Files*, Fox (May 4, 1997); Todd VanDerWerff, "The X-Files: 'Elegy,'" A.V. Club (March 5, 2011), http://tinyurl.com/lh957d4.
23. TV.com, "The X-Files," accessed February 16, 2014, http://tinyurl.com/6rfxc77.
24. Lana Wachowski, Tom Tykwer, and Andy Wachowski, writers, based on the novel by David Mitchell, Tom Tykwer and Andy Wachowski, directors, *Cloud Atlas*, Warner Bros. (2012); Wikia, "Nurse Noakes," accessed February 16, 2014, http://tinyurl.com/kt9bzs9.
25. Roger Avary, writer, Christophe Gans, director, *Silent Hill*, TriStar Pictures (2006), http://tinyurl.com/2s3ne5; Jill Garson and Kate Robbins, writers, Kate Robbins, director, *Candy Stripers*, Screen Gems (2006), http://tinyurl.com/l3xywv4; Piraphan Laoyont and Thodsapol Siriwiwat, directors, *Sick Nurses* (Suay Laak Sai), Magnolia Home Entertainment (2007), http://tinyurl.com/lxvsf2r.
26. Douglas Aarniokoski and David Loughery, writers, Douglas Aarniokoski, director, *Nurse 3D*, Lionsgate (2014), http://tinyurl.com/m4tvzu6; TAN, "Nurse 0D: *Nurse 3D* Finally Released" (January 2014), http://tinyurl.com/mg4kqqa; TAN,

"Sexy Killer Nurse Movie *Nurse 3D* Starts Filming" (August 2011), http://tinyurl.com/44cryfc.

27. "Nurse Mercy Adult Women's Costume," Spirit Halloween, accessed May 9, 2014, http://tinyurl.com/kyy3225.
28. CFNA, "'Helen Wheels, R.N.'—CompuCaddy Pulls Battle-Axe Ad," TAN (July 25, 2005), http://tinyurl.com/l2jqaom.
29. T. Coraghessan Boyle, "Chicxulub," *The New Yorker* (2004), http://tinyurl.com/yhocdov; CFNA, "Chicxulub," TAN (September 18, 2005), http://tinyurl.com/k5yr6t4.
30. CFNA, "Inject Me," TAN (August 2004), http://tinyurl.com/konqwjc.
31. blink-182, *Enema of the State*, MCA Records (1999); CFNA, "blink-182, 'Enema of the State,'" TAN (July 11, 2003), http://tinyurl.com/kay9bgp.
32. CFNA, "Not Sure If You'd Rather Hit Nurses or Have Sex with Them? Do Both!," TAN (December 1, 2005), http://tinyurl.com/ottdl8x.
33. CFNA, "Not Sure If You'd Rather Hit Nurses. . ."
34. Rose Chapman, I. Styles, L. Perry, and Shane Combs, "Examining the Characteristics of Workplace Violence in One Non-Tertiary Hospital," *Journal of Clinical Nursing* 19 (2010): 479–488, http://tinyurl.com/m77bhcx; Fran Lowry, "Nurses Are Frequent Targets of Workplace Violence," Medscape (February 4, 2010), http://tinyurl.com/ksfow8d.

9 ADVANCED PRACTICE NURSES

SKILLED PROFESSIONALS OR CUT-RATE "PHYSICIAN EXTENDERS"?

In late 2005 Mattel, the world's leading toy maker, released a small collectible duck doll called the Nurse Quacktitioner.[1] Dressed in a white laboratory coat and a white cap with a red heart on it, the doll sold at Target, Walmart, and other major toy retailers. Whatever Mattel's intent, the name suggested that nurse practitioners (NPs) are "quacks," untrained persons who pretend to be physicians.[2] Mattel said it had no idea that this doll would be taken as an attack on NPs, whose main professional stereotype has been that they are, uh, untrained persons who pretend to be physicians. The company explained that the name included the word "quack" because ducks quack, a point that had *completely* eluded the more than 2,000 nurses who objected to the doll. Mattel refused to remove the doll before the end of its planned run, even after we convinced Walmart to sell the dolls back to Mattel.[3]

Meanwhile, physicians in the United Kingdom learned of the controversy, and many sent letters of support—to Mattel, urging the company to keep selling the doll because it *would* foster contempt for NPs. The physicians argued that NPs are indeed unqualified practitioners (well, quacks) used to cut costs at the expense of quality care.[4]

Not to be outdone, Disney later weighed in with its own anti-NP insult in a product aimed at impressionable children. Disney XD's tween television series *Lab Rats* focuses on a trio of bionic teenagers who live incognito with their brilliant inventor father and fight Evil. In an August 2013 episode, the father's exiled brother and former business partner returned to take revenge and use the teenagers for nefarious ends. At one point, the father mocked his brother by noting that he had turned into "Dr. Evil . . . or should I say Nurse Practitioner Evil, since you flunked out of med school!" No one on the show disputed the idea that NPs are losers who can't hack medical school.[5]

In fact, a large body of research shows that the care of NPs and other advanced practice registered nurses (APRNs) is at least as effective as that of physicians.[6] In the 1960s nurses began training as advanced practitioners in primary care and other fields that included work traditionally done by physicians.[7] Advanced practice nursing evolved mainly to provide care to disadvantaged persons who were not receiving physician care. APRNs, most with at least a master's degree, now provide care in many specialties.[8] They practice mainly in the United States but increasingly also in other nations.[9] APRNs are especially likely to provide care to underserved urban and rural populations.[10] Like other nurses, APRNs use a holistic care model that emphasizes prevention, health maintenance, and overall quality of life.[11] APRNs are adept at identifying subtle problems and managing serious chronic conditions. Thus, expanding APRN care is a key part of the reforms of the 2010 Affordable Care Act (ACA), which increased funding for APRN education and APRN-run health clinics as part of its overall effort to improve health in a cost-effective way.[12] A massive 2010 report from the National Academy of Sciences' highly regarded Institute of Medicine (IOM) called for the expansion of APRN practice for the same reasons. The report was called *The Future of Nursing: Leading Change, Advancing Health*.[13]

In the United States there were more than 200,000 advanced practice nurses employed in 2012. More than 105,000 are practicing NPs, specializing in many fields. There are more than 34,000 certified registered nurse anesthetists (CRNAs), and they make up 53 percent of the anesthesia providers in the United States. More than 5,700 certified nurse midwives (CNMs) provide obstetrics and gynecology (OB/GYN) care and deliver babies using a natural care model, one many other developed nations use to achieve better patient outcomes at lower cost. More than 70,000 graduate-prepared clinical nurse specialists (CNSs) provide clinical leadership to direct care nurses.[14]

In the new millennium, direct care nurses suffered the effects of the global shortage. Nurse midwives struggled to cope with increasing practice costs. CNSs had grown in number and improved care greatly through the early 1990s, but hospitals eliminated many CNS positions in the managed care era, undermining clinical leadership in nursing.[15] Still, the practice of NPs and CRNAs continued to expand. NP-staffed health clinics based in retail stores—like those selling the Nurse Quacktitioner—have grown quickly.[16] Nursing leaders now plan to establish the existing four-year doctorate of nursing practice (DNP) degree as the standard for all new APRNs by 2015.[17] These last two developments sparked fierce resistance from some physician groups. However, cost-effective NP-directed care offers not only a way to enhance access to care for underserved populations, but also an advanced hybrid practice model that could change the future of health care for everyone.

Media portrayals of APRNs have been mixed. Hollywood has offered a few well-meaning television portrayals suggesting that NPs are moderately skilled assistants to physicians. But at their worst, television depictions have expressed overt contempt for APRNs, and many recent shows have suggested that able RNs want to become physicians. Some news stories have provided helpful information about APRN practice. There has been reporting on the cost-effectiveness of APRN care in the ACA era, on physician efforts to limit APRN practice, and on the growth of the DNP degree. But APRNs are largely ignored as general health experts, and the media's relentless suggestions that practitioner care is provided only by "doctors" continue unabated in news pieces and advertising. Doubt it? Just "ask your doctor"! Some press accounts have wrongly suggested that APRNs are capable only of treating minor problems. Deference to physicians remains so strong that often, the media allows physicians to express uninformed criticism of APRN care without even consulting APRNs or the relevant research.

However, some physicians are receptive to the idea that APRNs make valuable contributions to modern health care. In 2002 the US Department of Health and Human Services (HHS) launched an annual campaign to increase visits to primary care providers. It was called "Take a Loved One to the Doctor Day." We led nurses in trying to persuade HHS to change the name to one that would not exclude the APRNs who provide vital primary care to the very minority populations the campaign targets. In July 2005 HHS—with the leadership of Assistant Secretary for Minority Health Garth Graham, MD, MPH—actually changed the name to "Take a Loved One for a Checkup Day." HHS used that name in ensuing years, although HHS has recently played a less active role in the campaign. HHS did give its campaign partners discretion to use the old name, and popular ABC Radio host Tom Joyner and some others still insist on using the "Doctor Day" label.[18] (We find that a bit confusing, since "every day is a doctor day," as Jackie Peyton drily noted in a June 2011 episode of *Nurse Jackie*.) But some do use "Checkup Day" for the minority health campaign.[19] Some similar events have long been on the right track, like "National Women's Checkup Day," also sponsored by HHS and so named since 2002.[20] Next up: "Improve a Loved One's Understanding of APRNs Day!"

Who Are APRNs and How Good Is Their Care?

APRNs are skilled health professionals who provide advanced care, including diagnosis and treatment traditionally done by physicians, in a great variety of settings. These range from major teaching hospitals to small clinics, and from the military to public health services.

Because APRNs take a holistic approach, they are especially skilled at cost-effective preventive care, the management of chronic disease, coordinating care among different providers, and long-term health maintenance. Many APRNs focus on underserved poor communities where physicians choose not to practice, so APRNs are a vital health resource for millions who would otherwise receive little or no health care. APRNs' work has become even more critical in light of dramatically rising healthcare costs and as fewer physicians choose to pursue less lucrative primary care practices. On the other hand, some nursing advocates have argued that the growth in APRN practice has drawn nurses away from the bedside and from teaching positions, exacerbating the nursing shortage. In an era in which severe short-staffing has made bedside practice difficult, these are understandable concerns.

The first NP program (in pediatrics) was developed by public health nurse Loretta Ford, EdD, and pediatrician Henry Silver, MD, at the University of Colorado in 1965.[21] Today NP specialties include family practice, intensive care, emergency care, oncology, cardiology, mental health, and surgery, among many others. As described by the American Association of Nurse Practitioners,

> Nurse Practitioners (NPs) have been providing primary, acute and specialty healthcare to patients of all ages and walks of life for nearly half a century. NPs assess patients, order and interpret diagnostic tests, make diagnoses, and initiate and manage treatment plans—including prescribing medications. They are the healthcare providers of choice for millions of patients. An NP is truly Your Partner in Health.[22]

Nurse anesthetists provide high-quality, cost-effective anesthesia services. Nurse midwives give advanced OB/GYN and prenatal care, and they deliver babies under a care model that treats the birth process as a natural one, rather than an illness. CNSs provide vital clinical leadership to direct care nurses and direct care in some community settings. They practice in a variety of specialties, including pediatrics, geriatrics, emergency care, critical care, and psychiatric care. The US National Association of Clinical Nurse Specialists explains:

> In addition to providing direct patient care, Clinical Nurse Specialists influence care outcomes by providing expert consultation for nursing staffs and by implementing improvements in health care delivery systems. Clinical Nurse Specialist practice integrates nursing practice, which focuses on assisting patients in the prevention or resolution of illness, with medical diagnosis and treatment of disease, injury and disability.[23]

In the United States APRNs are licensed by each state, bound by legal and ethical duties, and subject to malpractice actions. Their legal rights to practice without collaborating with physicians vary by state. APRNs are eligible for Medicare and Medicaid reimbursement, and they can prescribe most medications. In some states, APRNs run successful independent health practices, although the extent of their rights to prescribe medication and to receive insurance reimbursement has been hotly disputed.[24]

Some people regard physician training as superior to that of APRNs. Physician training in the United States includes a four-year undergraduate degree with some rigorous science courses and a demanding four-year graduate medical degree, in addition to several years of training in residency programs. On the other hand, APRNs have a four-year bachelor's degree in nursing science and two or more years of intense graduate education in nursing science.[25] Many now undertake one-year residencies[26] and all receive the informal training in the first years of practice that any serious professional receives. In most cases, they also have years of highly relevant experience practicing as RNs before their graduate education. Many APRNs have doctorates. APRNs follow an effective care model that emphasizes health maintenance and addresses all facets of human well-being, not simply a specific condition or symptom.

Nevertheless, some physician groups have questioned the safety of APRN care and fought to restrict the scope of APRN practice, claiming that APRNs require physician "supervision," as some state laws still provide.[27] Many physicians, and even some APRNs, refer to APRNs as "physician extenders"[28] or "mid-level providers."[29] These contemptuous terms suggest that APRNs are the extremities of physicians, perhaps helping them reach things on a high shelf, and also that only physicians are "high-level." Presumably RNs are "low-level." Of course, the term "advanced practice" nurse itself may suggest that RNs are not advanced, and so that term could probably be improved.

We are aware of no scientific basis for physicians' safety claims about APRNs. In fact, a vast body of research indicates that APRN care is *at least as good* as that of physicians.[30] Some studies have found differences, but overall these suggest that if anyone's care is better, it is that of APRNs.

A review of 107 studies conducted between 1990 and 2008, published in a 2011 issue of the journal *Nursing Economic$*, determined that for a wide variety of patient care, outcomes for APRN-led teams that included physicians were *at least as good on all measures* as physician-led teams with no APRNs.[31] Nurses outperformed physicians on such measures as controlling blood pressure, controlling blood glucose and lipid levels, reducing length of hospital stay, enabling patients to function better in activities of daily living, and giving patients a higher perceived level of health, as well as on many important measures related to childbirth, including achieving lower rates of cesarean sections and episiotomy and higher rates of breastfeeding. Physicians did not outperform advanced practice nurses on *any* of the eighteen health indicators measured.

A study by the Research Triangle Institute, published in *Health Affairs* in 2010, looked specifically at the care of nurse anesthetists.[32] The study analyzed inpatient mortality and complication rates from nearly half a million hospitalizations covered by Medicare between 1999 and 2005. The researchers found no evidence that nurse anesthetists working without physician "supervision" posed any greater risk to patients than did physician anesthesiologists. Indeed, as the American Association of Nurse Anesthetists has noted, "Numerous outcomes studies have demonstrated that there is no difference in the quality of care provided by CRNAs and their physician counterparts."[33]

In 2003 the *American Journal of Public Health* published a study of low-risk obstetric patients funded by the US Agency for Health Care Research and Quality. The study compared two groups of patients, one of which received 95 percent of their care from CNMs and 5 percent of care from OB physicians, whereas the other received care only from physicians. The two groups had comparable rates of morbidity, preterm birth, and low birth weight, but in other respects the nurse midwife team had better outcomes at a lower cost, because patients spent less time as inpatients and had fewer cesarean sections, episiotomies, inductions, and vacuum- or forceps-assisted vaginal births.[34]

In 2002, Horrocks, Anderson, and Salisbury published a meta-analysis of thirty-four clinical studies in the *British Medical Journal* indicating that patients were more satisfied with their care if it was delivered by an NP than if by a physician. NPs read X-rays equally well, identified more physical abnormalities, communicated better, and taught patients how to provide self-care better. NPs also spent more time with patients than did physicians (14.9 versus 11.2 minutes).[35]

Nursing leaders are on schedule to make the DNP degree the standard APRN degree by 2015, as noted previously.[36] The DNP degree includes four years of graduate education, plus a one-year residency, after the bachelor's degree. In addition to providing fodder for hilarious "Dr. Nurse" wordplay in media reports,[37] the idea appears to be to expand the knowledge base of APRNs and to promote greater parity with primary care physicians in formal education. Of course, as we have explained, research shows APRN care is at least as good as physician care even though most APRNs do not yet have doctoral-level education. Some nurses have expressed concerns that the move to the DNP standard could effectively require current APRNs to obtain more graduate education, that it implies current APRN abilities are inadequate, and that it could lead to the "medicalization" of APRN practice.

Predictably, the plan has also encountered strong resistance from some physician groups.[38] They argue that further "blurring the lines" between the professions will endanger patient health. In June 2008 the American Medical Association (AMA) House of Delegates passed resolution 214, which stated that DNPs should be supervised by physicians and that the National Board of Medical Examiners should not offer a certifying examination for DNPs.[39] (The National Board of Medical Examiners went ahead with the examination and posted a long list of FAQs explaining why on its website.)[40] But the AMA delegates rejected a proposed resolution (232) seeking to limit the use of the terms "doctor" and "residency" in clinical settings to physicians, dentists, and podiatrists. The American Nurses Association objected to that resolution and gave this account of the AMA meeting about it:[41]

> Unfortunately, the use of the term "doctor" by doctorally-prepared health care providers really struck a raw nerve with many physicians. A parade of impassioned AMA members cited a "barrage of surrogates" and "assault by wannabes" . . . the purported inadequacy of 500 hours of clinical training for a DNP; the capacity for "grievous harm," bordering on homicide. . . . One delegate stated that AMA needs to take a hard stance against "dabblers" and "encroachers."[42]

The rejected proposal would have prevented not just nurses but also psychologists, social workers, and others from describing their own qualifications. Maybe the problem was that the proposal did not go far enough. To really protect the physician brand, we suggest barring the very issuance of doctorates in any field but medicine. Nurses aren't the only ones who need to learn their place!

"Doctor" jokes aside, we believe that APRNs have developed a hybrid care model with the potential to revolutionize advanced practitioner care. Are they the ones to help liberate the public from the current healthcare morass?

"Midwifs" and Minor Ailments: APRNs in Hollywood

Entertainment television has taken some notice of APRNs. In fact, some shows have presented ostensibly positive visions of APRNs, but they have also suggested that APRNs treat only simple conditions in an environment rightly controlled by physicians. No major television product has really conveyed the nature or value of the APRN practice model. Probably the most notable recent portrayals have been the nurse-midwife characters on *Strong Medicine* and *Private Practice*, a show that repeatedly mocked nurse midwifery. Many shows, including *ER*[43] and *Private Practice*,[44] and even *Mercy*[45] and *HawthoRNe*,[46] have suggested that ambitious nurses want to become physicians, even though in reality nurses are one hundred times more likely to attend graduate nursing school.[47] In its last season *ER* did indicate that nurse anesthetist student Sam Taggart would have considerable skill and autonomy as a CRNA.[48] Recent films have generally ignored APRNs, although there have been helpful minor depictions in Mike Nichols's *Angels in America*[49] and Abby Epstein's *Business of Being Born* documentaries.[50] In addition, episodes in the first season of the documentary series *24 Hours in A&E* showed NPs providing skilled emergency care, although without really explaining who NPs are or how they differ from physicians.[51]

Strong Medicine's nurse-midwife character Peter Riggs has probably been serial US television's best portrayal of an APRN.[52] He did not figure heavily in most episodes, and he did not spend much time actually delivering babies or seeing outpatients, as a real nurse midwife would. But he did seem to operate with some autonomy, treating patients in a clinic run by primary care physician Luisa Delgado. One September 2005 episode had Riggs establishing and skillfully running a "baby boot camp" for gangbanging boyfriends of his patients who were not meeting their fathering responsibilities.[53] Riggs clearly took a holistic approach to care, which the show both honored and mocked. Riggs reported to Delgado and the show's other physicians, and he generally deferred to them in clinical matters, with minor exceptions. In one episode, Riggs did confront a powerful OB-GYN physician who had performed an unnecessary cesarean section, resulting in a hysterectomy. But as a result of Riggs's advocacy, Delgado had to save his job, as discussed in Chapter 6. In the September 2005 episode mentioned previously, Riggs briefly argued with a major surgeon character about which of them had delivered more babies and so would be more qualified to deliver the baby of their friend Delgado. In the February 2006 series finale, Riggs resisted pressure from his girlfriend, a physician resident, to go to medical school.[54] Riggs said he preferred to be a nurse, although he gave only the vague reason that medicine would not make him "happier." Viewers got no sense that he regarded advanced practice nursing to be as valuable as medicine generally.

Peter Riggs had his moments, but as we've seen, the Dell Parker character on *Private Practice* was mostly an APRN disaster.[55] At first Dell was a receptionist with a "nursing degree" who was studying midwifery; even after he become a midwife, he still seemed to have office administrative duties. Early episodes mocked midwifery, as superstar OB/GYN Addison Montgomery uttered the word "midwif" as if she had never heard of such an outlandish pursuit. In the September 2007 series premiere, Dell asked her if he could help with a delivery for "field experience for my midwife training"—as if his clinical training consisted of whatever ad hoc assistance he could offer clinic physicians, rather than the midwife-directed graduate degree training he would get in real life.[56] Addison repeatedly rejected his help. Dell eventually lost it:

DELL: You don't take me seriously. . . . You think I'm some dumb surfer boy, you think I'm eye candy. You have no respect for me or my midwifery skills.

ADDISON (STRUGGLING NOT TO LAUGH): I have total respect for you and your . . . mid*wif*ery skills? Is that even a word—mid*wif*ery?

DELL (PETULANTLY): It's a word. (*Pause.*) It's definitely a word!

Of course the show was poking fun at the elite surgeon surrounded by Southland nuts, but it was also laughing at Dell's midwifery. Even accounting for Addison's arrogance, which the show celebrated by pretending to condemn, it's unlikely that an OB/GYN physician would really be unfamiliar with the word *midwifery*. But Addison didn't know about it, we were meant to assume, because it's largely irrelevant to serious maternal-child health care. And receptionist Dell was not likely to cite the studies showing that nurse midwives' care is at least as effective as that provided by OB/GYNS such as Addison.

In later seasons, the portrayal of Dell improved somewhat. He occasionally showed some tentative clinical aptitude, usually under Addison's supervision, as when he performed a vacuum-assisted delivery in a February 2009 episode.[57] In a January 2010 episode, he managed to perform a solo delivery and showed psychosocial skill, although the show made fun of the natural birth model the mother insisted on following. Even Dell seemed to find it odd.[58] In March 2010, Dell got to deliver a baby by himself in the field. Because he successfully executed a risky maneuver to free the baby, who was stuck in the birth canal, physician Cooper later credited Dell with saving two lives.[59]

But Dell remained essentially a subordinate, and the show did not provide helpful information on advanced practice nursing, to say the least. On the contrary, a March 2009 episode showed a distraught Dell hooking up with young women by pretending to be a physician. That earned amused derision from the elite physician characters—and from us, because the plotline reinforced the harmful wannabe-physician stereotype that real APRNs confront.[60] Of course, Dell's elation at having been admitted to medical school just before his May 2010 death had the same effect. In a May-June 2010 issue of *TV Guide*, show creator Shonda Rhimes explained that Dell was "a midwife in a world of doctors. Babies can only be delivered in so many episodes. Dell got lots of coffee, answered lots of phones."[61] Rhimes lauded Chris Lowell, who played Dell, by noting that "an actor of his caliber should be doing Shakespeare, not handing people charts." In other words, nurses and midwives don't do much of interest, which is why Dell spent so much time doing receptionist work and why he eventually had to go. But at least he went to that great medical school in the sky!

One of the few other notable APRN characters appeared in late 2004 on CBS's *Dr. Vegas*, a flashy, short-lived drama about a Las Vegas casino physician named Billy Grant. Grant's casino clinic sidekick was NP Alice Doherty, who did show some health knowledge and a willingness to push for more holistic care.[62] At one point she argued successfully for alcoholic rehabilitation for an abusive patient when Grant wanted to treat the man's minor wounds and cut him loose. However, Doherty was basically just a skilled assistant to Grant. The show's final episode delivered a remarkably direct attack on NP practice. Doherty, struggling to handle her unrequited love for Grant, got drunk with the son of the casino manager's old friend. Then, when this son injured himself, Doherty brought him back to the clinic and forged Grant's signature on an OxyContin prescription. Meanwhile, her date stole the prescription pad, and a hotel guest later OD'd and almost died. Grant saved the day by telling the police that he had authorized Doherty to write the prescription. But the plotline suggested that NPs are flighty females who can't be trusted with the power of the prescription pad.

Even the most realistic of other hospital shows, *ER*, never quite had a major APRN character. Nurse character Sam Taggart did start a nurse anesthetist program in the show's final season. A few plotlines sent helpful messages about her career path, although we did not learn that it was a graduate program or where she was studying. In an October 2008 episode Taggart explained to a condescending physician intern that Taggart would indeed be handling her own anesthesia cases when she finished the program.[63] The episode also indicated that her knowledge of anesthesia had already surpassed that of her boyfriend, physician resident Tony Gates. In December 2008 episodes, Taggart impressed senior physicians by using her growing knowledge to improve critical care, at one point persuading the chief of surgery to let her use an innovative combination of drugs and interpersonal methods to extubate a patient early.[64] The NP character Lynette Evans appeared in nine *ER* episodes from 1998 to 1999.[65] But as discussed in Chapters 3 and 6, *ER* often suggested that nurses achieve by going to medical school.

In recent years popular Hollywood shows have continued that theme. On *The Glades*, the lead detective character's fiancée Callie Cargill was always a bright, skilled nurse—and an off-and-on medical student.[66] Summer 2013 episodes found Callie "dying" to get back to medical school while doing a fellowship with a crusty senior surgeon. Once he warmed to Callie, the surgeon became fond of saying that she would make "a hell of a doctor"—and he left her a great deal of money when he died so she could finish medical school. Even nurse-focused shows have relied on the wannabe-physician stereotype. On *HawthoRNe*, nurse Ray Stein was pining for medical school right up until his final episodes on the show in July 2010, although he had failed his MCAT examination the first time.[67] In a May 2010 episode of *Mercy*, the bright young nurse Chloe Payne got praise from one physician for "thinking like a doctor" after she diagnosed a case of airport malaria. In the series finale, Chloe vowed that she would attend medical school, apparently to show another physician that she was worthy of his affections—a truly pathetic final note for an otherwise impressive nurse character.[68]

In any case, on most recent hospital shows, APRNs are conspicuously absent. No advanced practice nurse has appeared on the 2009 US nurse shows. Perhaps this reflected the nurse shows' overall sense of the nurse characters as being smart and pragmatic, but not necessarily having a lot of formal education, as the physician characters did. *HawthoRNe* said nothing about its chief nursing officer character's educational background. Although a September 2009 episode of *Mercy* revealed that Chloe Payne had a masters degree, she practiced as an inexperienced RN, not an APRN.[69]

However, in a June 2014 episode of *Nurse Jackie*, the excellent Zoey Barkow announced that she wanted to get a masters degree and become an NP. Jackie was very supportive and—being Jackie—soon told a patient that Zoey already was an NP, giving the younger nurse the chance to try to evaluate him as an NP might. Zoey seemed to do well in diagnosing and counseling the patient about his dangerous high blood pressure.[70]

To our knowledge no APRNs have ever appeared on *Grey's Anatomy*, but the show did eventually get around to expressing contempt for them. In a January 2010 episode, surgeon Derek Shepherd confronted fellow surgeon Miranda Bailey about a postoperative patient who was getting weekly follow-up visits with Bailey herself. In fact, she was covering up an error made by the chief of surgery.[71] Shepherd noted that the patient was "getting some high-class care. Six visits with a surgeon? A nurse practitioner can do this." Shepherd's premise, of course, was that surgeon care is much better. In noting that NPs "can" do the follow-up care, he meant that even they are capable of it. In fact, he had previously called that care "easy." The idea was clearly that this is simple care requiring little expertise, not that it is a job for NPs because they are so good at monitoring patients and explaining how to cope with a difficult recovery.

Both *House* and *Scrubs* actually had nurse characters confront the idea of becoming NPs, although both shows sent damaging messages about NP education. A February 2007 *House* episode included nurse Wendy, then-girlfriend of House's underling physician Foreman.[72] Foreman cleverly broke up with Wendy by telling her that he'd make "a few calls" and get her into an elite hospital-based NP program in a distant city. This plotline would likely suggest to viewers that the most prestigious NP preparation is nondegree training to which entry can be had at the whim of physicians, rather than NP-directed graduate degree programs at major universities with rigorous admissions requirements.

The treatment of NP education on *Scrubs* was oddly similar. In a November 2002 episode, surgeon Turk signed up his future wife, nurse Carla Espinosa, for an NP program as a surprise gift.[73] Unlike Foreman, Turk was trying to do something nice, and the episode made clear that Carla was well qualified for the program: attending physician Perry Cox said so! But Carla chose not to pursue it so she could spend more time with Turk. Like Foreman in the *House* episode, Turk apparently had the power to simply enroll Carla in NP training. In both episodes, the nurses' boyfriends seemed to assume that any nurse would leap at the chance to pursue NP training. The nurse characters did not leap, for their own reasons, but neither defended the value of bedside nursing either.

One revealing portrayal of an NP on a nonhealthcare show was that of Jorge on ABC Family's *Switched at Birth*. Jorge supervised main character Daphne during her community service at an urban clinic. He occasionally displayed autonomy and health expertise, for instance in caring for a pediatric asthma patient in a March 2014 episode.[74] He also vied with the medical student Campbell for Daphne's romantic attention. But Daphne began to explore premed programs, with no mention of nursing, even though virtually all of her clinical interactions were with Jorge, not Campbell. Everyone was impressed by Daphne's new interest in becoming a physician, and the clinic's head physician encouraged her to pursue it despite potential obstacles (she is deaf). It did not seem to occur to anyone, including Jorge, that the bright, promising Daphne might consider a nursing career. On the romantic side, Campbell also seemed to come out on top, although Daphne at least struggled more with that decision than she had about the medical school choice. Jorge did maintain his dignity, both as a serious health professional at the clinic and as an apparently unsuccessful suitor.

In September 2004, the syndicated television quiz show *Jeopardy!* included a clue about NPs. On the show, contestants receive the answer to a question, and they must provide the correct question to win points. In this episode, there was an "answer" stating, "Minor ailments can be treated by NPs (nurse practitioners) & PAs (these)." The contestant responded "correctly" by saying, "What are physician's assistants?"[75] This answer wrongly suggested that major ailments, such as cardiac disease, cancer, and diabetes, are beyond NPs. Nurses contacted the show with their concerns, and in June 2005 an episode featured this clue: "The Golden Lamp Awards are bestowed for the best portrayals of these health professionals in the media."[76] These were the awards the Center for Nursing Advocacy was giving annually at that time to recognize good and bad portrayals of nursing (we now call them the Truth About Nursing awards). Although we might have preferred a clue that communicated more of the substance of nursing, the way the clue played out illustrated the very attitudes that lead to poor understanding of the profession. Upon the reading of the clue, one contestant—a medical student—quickly, almost gleefully, responded, "What are doctors?"

Hollywood films have generally taken little notice of APRNs. However, Mike Nichols's HBO adaptation of Tony Kushner's *Angels in America*, discussed in previous chapters, did include the NP Emily, a minor character who directed the major character Prior's AIDS care. No physician was shown treating Prior. Emily expertly assessed his condition, monitored his treatment, and helped him confront his fears. Emily did not share Prior's cultural knowledge—she had not heard of the Bayeux Tapestry—but her steadfast positivity made Prior's friend Louis look painfully inadequate.[77]

Abby Epstein's documentaries *The Business of Being Born* (2008) and *More Business of Being Born* (2011), produced by and featuring former talk show host Ricki Lake, offered compelling arguments that the United States return to an empowering midwifery-driven home birth model. The first film presented US obstetric care as a dysfunctional business that has consigned midwives to the periphery so that physicians who don't understand natural birth can perform dangerous, unnecessary interventions, while the rest of the developed world achieves better outcomes for less money using midwives for most births.[78] The four follow-up films released in 2011 featured conversations with pioneering lay midwife Ina May Gaskin; celebrities discussing their birth experiences; and explorations of such topics as birth centers, doulas, cesarean sections, and vaginal birth after cesarean.[79]

The films were not the portrayals of *nursing* that they might have been. The first film did include a powerful portrait of New York City nurse midwife Cara Muhlhahn, who came off as a birth expert as she visited patients and delivered babies at home. Muhlhahn was articulate and passionate in explaining her role as "guardian of safety" and "witness to [the mother's] process." But the films largely ignored the work of nurse midwives in hospitals and never explained how nurse midwives differ from lay midwives. The 2011 films did briefly include a few knowledgeable nurse midwives, but mainly to explain policies at the hospital birth centers of which the films were critical. The nurses were identified only by name and "CNM," so viewers may not have known who they were. Overall the later films presented the birthing world as a divide between generally interventionist physicians and enlightened lay midwives who embrace natural birth. So the films failed to convey that nurse midwives have long combined advanced health skills and a holistic approach to birthing. Maybe the general disregard of nurses was conscious: Is nursing too closely associated with female subjugation for some progressives to embrace it?

One recent bright spot for APRNs on television has been the UK documentary series *24 Hours in A&E*, which has included some helpful portrayals of NPs treating patients in the emergency setting. For example, episodes broadcast in the United States in November 2011 featured NPs Nancy and Kim providing authoritative physical and psychosocial care to an older woman with an ear infection as well as patients who had had nasty encounters with panes of glass.[80]

The Doctorate of Splinter Diagnosis: APRNs in the News and Advertising Media

The news media's treatment of APRNs has been mixed. They have received some good recent coverage as a new wave in health care, and even as an alternative to the physician care model, particularly in light of the reforms associated with the ACA and the perceived shortage of primary care physicians. Positive articles have focused on the work of NPs and nurse midwives, marveling at APRN autonomy, patient satisfaction, and even skill. Nurse anesthetists do not appear to have received as much fair coverage, and CNSs seem to receive little coverage of any kind.

But most media items about the work of advanced health practitioners simply ignore APRNs, discussing the work of "doctors" even when APRNs play a critical role in the care at issue. Prominent marketing for drugs still typically advises the audience to "ask your doctor" about the advertised product. Even many news items about APRN care show contempt for it, often relying solely on uninformed criticism from physicians rather than the relevant scientific research. Physician objections seem to have intensified as APRNs work increasingly in middle-class care settings in which physicians themselves have an economic interest. The objections may grow stronger to the extent that health-financing reforms increase the number of patients seeking primary care.

Fair Reporting on APRNs

Recent reports have described in positive terms the growing role of NPs in primary care. Some even discuss the research demonstrating the high quality of APRN care.

In October 2012 *The New York Times* posted Tina Rosenberg's excellent "The Family Doctor, Minus the M.D.," an articulate and well-reasoned plea for the United States to expand the authority and scope of practice of APRNs, as part of the paper's "Fixes" series.[81] Rosenberg argued forcefully that expanding APRN practice would improve access to care and likely reduce healthcare costs. She suggested that physician groups' opposition appears to be driven more by concerns about lost income and authority than by any well-founded concern for patients. Her main focus was the hundreds of NP-run health clinics, like a couple of clinics in Indiana that are part of Purdue University's School of Nursing. These clinics serve mostly uninsured patients who come for "family care, pediatrics, mental health and pregnancy care," including "chronic problems: obesity, diabetes, hypertension, depression, alcoholism." Rosenberg explained NPs' educational credentials and noted that they "do everything primary care doctors do, including prescribing, although some states require that a physician provide review." She also observed that "like doctors, of course, nurse practitioners refer patients to specialists or a hospital when needed." Rosenberg discussed the apparent shortage of primary care physicians and noted that those physicians are not well-distributed, with very few working in rural areas or the poor parts of major cities, treating the underinsured.

Rosenberg addressed head-on the concern that a nurse-run clinic is "second-class primary care," stating flatly that "it is not." First, she noted, the actual alternative for many is no primary care at all, because there are so few physicians in some areas. So patients might eventually end up in the emergency department, but often much sicker than necessary. Rosenberg continued:

> Just as important, while nurses take a different approach to patient care than doctors, it has proven just as effective. It might be particularly useful for treating chronic diseases, where so much depends on the patients' behavioral choices. Doctors are trained to focus on a disease—what is it? How do we make it go away? Nurses are trained to think more holistically. The medical profession is trying to get doctors to ask about their patients' lives, listen more, coach more and lecture less—being "patient-centered" is the term—in order to better understand what ails them.

In other words, the medical profession is trying to get physicians to act more like nurses. Jennifer Coddington, a pediatric NP who was "co-clinical director" at the Indiana clinics, explained to Rosenberg that she spent a lot of time teaching patients and families about how to manage diseases, mindful of their educational and economic levels. Rosenberg also described the research on APRN care, citing the 2011 *Nursing Economic$* review comparing physician-led and NP-led clinics; she noted pointedly that there were "no measures on which the nurses did worse."

In October 2004 the *Wall Street Journal* published another extraordinarily good article of this type by Andrew Blackman: "Is There a Doctor in the House? Perhaps Not, as Nurse Practitioners Take on Many of the Roles

Long Played by Physicians."[82] Long before the IOM report and the current ACA debates, Blackman reported that nurse-run primary care practices "may be critical to the future of health care in the U.S." The story suggested that NPs' holistic, thorough, preventive approach may be uniquely suited to an aging population with long-term illnesses. In particular, the piece explained how the nurses' focus on patients' environments, psychological factors, and practical issues leads to solutions to long-term problems. Blackman discussed hurdles that NPs have yet to overcome, including legislative limits on their autonomy. Noting concerns that NPs might miss a diagnosis, the article concluded that "studies have shown that when it comes to patient outcomes, nurse practitioners are just as good as doctors."

At the core of Blackman's piece was its description of the Columbia Advanced Practice Nurse Associates (Capna), a pioneering NP-run practice founded in 1994 by the Columbia University School of Nursing. Capna was the first nurse-run US clinic to win full privileges to admit patients to hospitals and the first to gain insurance compensation at the same rate as physicians.[83] One Capna patient praised the comprehensive, unhurried approach of the NPs. She faulted the physicians she had seen before for being rushed and having "no bedside manner." Another patient compared NP-physician collaboration to his own experience as a business school graduate in partnership with a lawyer. The patient suggested that perhaps "the future of health care is to find a way to combine the different skills of each one." However, Blackman's piece made clear that the NPs were not just filling gaps but winning over patients who could easily be seeing physicians instead. Columbia nursing dean and Capna founder Mary Mundinger emphasized that she chose an exclusive Madison Avenue address for one Capna office precisely so the NPs could compete directly with physicians.

Indeed, any piece with Mundinger in it is likely to include some strong pro-APRN advocacy. In December 2009 the *New York Observer* published an extensive profile of the "controversial" leader, who was then retiring as dean after a quarter century of fighting to strengthen advanced practice nursing. Dana Rubinstein's article had flaws, but it was a thoughtful examination of how far nurses have come and what the future might hold.[84] The piece noted that Mundinger "argues that, if anything, primary care physicians are overeducated." It included an anecdote about the time she had spoken to the Federation of State Medical Boards and a primary care physician asked if he had "wasted" his time going to medical school. Mundinger: "I wanted to say, yeah."

Other reports have emphasized APRNs' focus on underserved populations. In April 2004, the *Atlanta Journal-Constitution* ran a very good article by Patricia Guthrie about local NP Dorothy Gallaway.[85] Gallaway's clinic provided low-income families with primary care and preventive health services, such as vaccinations, family planning, sexually transmitted disease diagnosis, and treatment of high blood pressure and asthma. Gallaway said the clinic was also "seeing more insured patients because they like nurse practitioners." In November 2003, in an enthusiastic piece about the growing role of NP-run primary care centers, *Philadelphia Daily News* columnist Ronnie Polaneczky described a clinic in a public housing development where NPs "do everything primary-care physicians do."[86] Polaneczky cited research showing that the nursing center patients saw their practitioners more often than patients in traditional care settings, but they used emergency departments 15 percent less and had shorter hospital maternity stays, lower prescription costs, and better preventive child health programs.

Some pieces have presented APRNs as innovative leaders in developing new care models. In January 2013 Minnesota Public Radio aired an excellent report by Laura Yuen about sexual abuse of runaway girls that featured NP Laurel Edinburgh.[87] Broadcast on National Public Radio's *All Things Considered* program, the report noted that Edinburgh had "helped create the beginnings" of the Ramsey County Runaway Intervention Program a decade earlier. Her research had shown that the program improved outcomes. The piece reported that Edinburgh had devised a set of questions that St. Paul police used to screen runaways for signs of physical and sexual abuse. Several recent items, including one by Joseph Shapiro that ran on NPR in July 2009, have explained the work of transitional care nurses, many of whom are NPs.[88] These nurses help patients navigate the healthcare system after hospital stays, preventing needless readmissions and saving money. Shapiro's very helpful piece focused on professor Mary Naylor's Transitional Care Model program at the University of Pennsylvania, showcasing NPs' psychosocial and health management skills.

Nurse midwives have received some attention, perhaps because of recent interest in different approaches to birthing. In July 2008, the *Post and Courier* (Charleston, South Carolina) ran Jill Coley's report on the Charleston Birth Place as a new alternative for mothers who want a natural birth but also access to emergency care if needed.[89] The Birth Place's owner, nurse midwife and family NP Lesley Rathbun, noted that a "culture of fear" has developed around birth in the United States, with women in labor "screaming" in the popular media. In January 2006 Rhode Island's *Providence Journal* ran a profile of nurse midwife Mary Breckinridge by Stanley M. Aronson, dean of medicine emeritus at Brown University. "Kentucky's Intrepid Nurses on

Horseback" discussed Breckinridge's globally influential work in founding and leading the Frontier Nursing Service, which has provided care to poor mothers and children since 1925.[90] The piece said that today, Brown medical students "may spend up to three months in rural service supervised by these indomitable nurse midwives."

There has also been some good coverage of threats to APRN practice. In a powerful May 2007 cover story in the *Washington Post Magazine*, Phuong Ly described the struggle of midwifery pioneer Ruth Lubic to keep birth centers for low-income urban women open, despite rising malpractice rates.[91] The piece explained that over the previous several decades, Lubic had established nurse midwife-staffed birthing centers in New York City and Washington, DC and "defied doctors to transform the way American women give birth." In July 2005, the *Savannah Morning News* posted Don Lowery's story about a local primary care physician serving an eight-month sentence in federal prison, apparently in part for signing blank Schedule II substance prescription refills for NP colleagues to use.[92] Such NP prescription was then unlawful in Georgia. The physician reportedly wrote the prescriptions so that the rural clinic where he practiced could handle its huge patient load. The following year Georgia NPs finally gained statutory prescription authority.[93]

Some news outlets have reported on the plan to make the DNP the standard APRN degree by 2015. In April 2008 the *Wall Street Journal* ran Laura Landro's "Making Room for 'Dr. Nurse.'"[94] The piece presented the DNP, pioneered at Columbia University, as a "possible solution" to the perceived shortage of primary care physicians. Patient Judith Gleason praised the preventive care and keen diagnostic skills of the DNPs at Capna. But the piece fell short in suggesting that NPs "fear the doctoral programs might be raising the bar too high for their profession," which implied either that nurses think they can't handle doctoral training or that nursing is not important enough to warrant it.

Although it's still rare, the media has even consulted APRNs as health-care experts. In January 2013 the Richmond, Virginia CBS television affiliate WTVR (Channel 6) ran a short segment in which CVS Minute Clinic NP Anne Pohnert debunked common myths about the flu. Pohnert explained simply and clearly that you can't get the flu from the flu shot and that it's important to get the vaccine every year.[95] Pohnert's segment was remarkable not just because it represented an appearance by a nurse as a health expert but because the station made a point of mentioning that Pohnert practiced at CVS. In the early days of quick clinics, the major corporate players almost seemed to apologize for staffing their clinics with NPs. But the references to

CVS here suggested that the company was actually promoting its clinics with the expertise of NPs, at least in this case.

In June 2010, the *Houston Chronicle* ran a "Sunday Q&A" feature by Cindy George in which University of Texas NP and nursing professor Elda Ramirez gave advice on coping with the very hot days her region experiences.[96] Like Pohnert, Ramirez displayed an ability to convey practical health information in a direct, engaging way. Her advice ranged from hydration strategies to how to avoid leaving children in vehicles: "In the summertime, a lot of grandparents or other people have the children who don't normally have that responsibility. Have a backup system. . . . Have a picture of the baby right by the speedometer or on the rearview mirror. Always have something that reminds you: I have the baby. And if you're going in the store, always take the kid out. Don't be lazy."

The News and Advertising Media Often Ignores or Disrespects APRNs

APRNs are rarely mentioned or consulted in health items that are not specifically about them. A constant assumption in the advertising and news media's treatment of health issues is that only "doctors" provide advanced practitioner care and that only "doctors" need be consulted in discussion of that care. That is the case even in areas in which APRNs in fact play a critical role, such as primary care, obstetric care, and public health.

A striking example of the absent APRN is Deirdre Kennedy's April 2008 National Public Radio report about the expanding use of online "doctor-patient" communication.[97] As is typical, the five-minute piece referred relentlessly to "doctors," as if the 200,000 US APRNs did not exist. But nursing did get one disdainful mention: At one point, Kennedy noted that some "doctors" were using a physician-designed Web portal that asked patients preliminary questions about their conditions, using "branching logic." Kennedy referred to this computer system as an "electronic advice nurse."

Advertising is not traditionally the place to look for progressive ideas, and the subject of APRN care is no exception. With the growth of APRN practice, some may see profit-making potential in reinforcing the false idea that only physicians have real health care expertise. In early 2013 a television commercial aired in the southern United States for American Family Care, an aggressively expanding chain of urgent care clinics that planned to have more than 110 locations in twenty-eight states by the end of 2013.[98] The advertisement featured two people texting back and forth about where to seek health care. At the end, one texter recommended that the other go to American

Family Care because there patients get to see "a doctor, not a nurse." Despite those reassuring words about the company's high-quality care, in March 2014 its website's "staff openings" section listed five open Family Nurse Practitioner positions in Alabama—in the "Physician Services" Department.[99]

When news items do discuss APRN care, they too may indicate that APRNs are poor substitutes for physicians. Many pieces have relied for expert comment solely on physicians, who seem to assume that APRNs can't handle serious conditions simply because they have not been educated as physicians. Often, reports do not even give APRNs the chance to respond to uninformed attacks on the care they give. A November 2002 *Redbook* article entitled "Advice Docs Give Their Own Families" included a physician warning: "Don't let yourself be brushed off onto a Nurse Practitioner."[100] The piece presented no NP response. Here again, it must be enough to just "ask your doctor"!

Even more substantial news reports may fall into this trap. In an October 2010 *Kaiser Health News* article posted on the MSNBC website, Andrew Villegas and Mary Agnes Carey gave a fairly detailed account of the 2010 IOM report's significance for APRNs.[101] The piece included physician leaders' claims that APRNs are unqualified to practice independently, with specific quotes from representatives of the AMA and the American Society of Anesthesiologists. Yet the piece quoted *no nurses on that subject*—in an article about a report urging nursing empowerment. The piece did include general quotes from IOM panel member Donna Shalala on the need to use all resources to meet healthcare needs, but that did not counter the physician attacks.

Sometimes physicians themselves create such media. An August 2008 *Washington Post* piece by physician Benjamin Natelson bemoaned the decline in physicians' ability and willingness to make difficult diagnoses, which the author attributed mainly to modern healthcare economics. Natelson wrote that a "partial solution to the growing gap in primary care providers" is "physician extenders," who are "trained to deal with commonly occurring, easy-to-diagnose problems: a flu, hay fever, a splinter, even severe chest pain."[102] However, he claimed, those "extenders" usually have not "had enough training to give them the know-how to sort through a complex medical history to arrive at a diagnosis that isn't immediately evident. When they're stuck, they have to call the physician, and by then, the 30-minute visit is very often over." Natelson wrongly conflated years of formal education with the ability to diagnose, and diagnosis with all of health care, as in *House*. In fact, NPs have used their advanced listening skills to diagnose many life-threatening conditions that physicians did not. But more generally, NPs achieve good patient outcomes because they are adept at the full range of what practitioners should do, including preventive health and patient education. Ironically, another NP asset is just what Natelson seems to disdain: NPs' willingness to consult with others when they do not know something. Plus, with those graduate science degrees, NPs are super at splinters!

Nurse anesthetists have received critical reviews from high-end plastic surgeons in the media. In June 2004 *Vogue* ran a piece by Ariel Levy about cosmetic surgery that quoted Santa Monica surgeon R. Patrick Abergel, whose patients included Hollywood stars, as follows: "It's not illegal for surgeons to administer anesthesia themselves, and a lot do—or they work with nurse anesthetists. Both are unsafe."[103] Of course, the actual research proves otherwise. As with the American Family Care advertisement discussed previously, we have to wonder if elite plastic surgeons may be doing a bit of medical upselling, justifying high fees in part through their association with anesthesiologists.

Coverage of the proliferation of clinics in supermarkets and drugstores has rarely conveyed much respect for NPs. For example, in a March 2014 segment about the ACA (Obamacare) on the Fox News show *The O'Reilly Factor*, host Bill O'Reilly denigrated the clinics because they were not staffed by physicians: "If I want a strep throat diagnosis, I don't want Lenny who just came out of the community college."[104] Guest Ezekiel Emanuel, a physician who helped design Obamacare, responded: "Excuse me, those are nurse practitioners, it's not Lenny out of a community college." Emanuel did not explain NP education, and rather than defending NP diagnostic skill, he went on to emphasize that such diagnosis is straightforward. Still, with luck viewers would at least understand that NPs have more education than an associate's degree. Emanuel did stress that physicians are not required for every aspect of health care. In any case, the exchange showed that uninformed disdain for APRNs remains widespread in influential media.

A July 2006 *Houston Chronicle* report, Brett Brune's "In-Store Clinics Not a Cure-All, Doctors Warn," described the AMA's efforts to limit the rapid expansion of retail clinics.[105] Physician Michael Speer of the Texas Medical Association allowed that the idea of the clinics had "some degree of merit" for things like flu shots, simple abrasions, colds, and other "minor illnesses." But he suggested that (in the reporter's words) "if stitches are needed or a cough gets deeper, it's time to go to a doctor." The *Chronicle*'s main source on NP skill was AMA board member Dr. Rebecca Patchin, who at the time was using her status as a "former nurse" to bolster misleading press attacks on NPs in retail clinics. In the *Chronicle*, Patchin said the AMA wanted

> to make sure the public understands when it's appropriate to use a store-based clinic and when they should utilize an emergency room or a doctor's office. . . . When I was a nurse, I didn't know as much as I know now. . . . The extra years of training as a physician provide added experience, exposure and depth of knowledge regarding patients, illness, disease process and treatment.

But that is not a fair comparison of NPs and MDs because Patchin was never an NP. Patchin also asserted that physicians (in Brune's words) "have at least five more years of education than nurse practitioners." This formulation wrongly equates NPs' undergraduate education, which includes two years of healthcare education, with physicians' undergraduate education, which does not include healthcare education. It also wrongly counts physician residencies as education but not NP residencies, the early years of NP practice, or the many years of prior RN practice that most NPs have. Like all who claim that NPs are unsafe, Patchin ignored the wealth of research showing the contrary.

In an apparent stab at balance, the *Chronicle* piece included reaction from a retail clinic company CEO. He said that most customers have no primary care provider but that they are discouraged from making the clinics their "medical home" for anything other than "routine episodic care." Of course quick clinics should be clear about their scope of care. But like most comments by retail clinic executives in similar articles, this one did not convey that NPs are skilled professionals who can themselves provide comprehensive primary care in a setting that allows for it. There was no recognition that the type of vaccinations and basic screenings the retail clinics provide have saved millions of lives around the world. No NP was consulted for the piece, suggesting that physicians are the only health experts with anything useful to say about NP care. And there was no hint that retail-based clinics can be viewed not just as a clever business initiative, but as a promising new basic care model.

An August 2009 article by Julian Drape on the Western Australia news website *WAtoday* was headlined "Nurse Clinics are 'Supermarket Medicine.'"[106] That was the view of the only expert quoted, Australian Medical Association president Andrew Pesce, who objected to one company's plan to open 180 pharmacy-based clinics staffed by NPs. Pesce also offered this analysis: "Nurse practitioners tend to be highly trained in a narrow area of health care and are not skilled or experienced in providing holistic care." Really? Perhaps the

NPs also tend to be greedy and arrogant! The only response to Pesce in the report came from Health Minister Nicola Roxon, who did not defend NP skill, but emphasized that the NPs would have to make "collaborative agreements" with physicians.

Similarly, in November 2005 NBC's *Today* show included a short, troubling segment about retail clinics by reporter Janice Lieberman.[107] While stressing that the clinics offer convenience and affordability for basic care, the report also degraded the NP care available "on the cheap" at what it called "quickie" clinics. It ignored NPs' vital role in more comprehensive primary care and suggested that autonomous NP care presents safety risks, relying on a quote about the supposed need for "supervision" of the "non-physician providers" from AMA president Edward Hill. The only audible NP response the NBC News product offered its audience consisted of an NP, identified as "Kathy," saying "ready?" to indicate that she was set to give Lieberman a flu shot.

In September 2009 *Today* returned to the APRN beat with a report by Peter Alexander that aired with the title "The Perils of Midwifery," though NBC later changed the online title to "The Perils of Home Births."[108] The biased report focused on the death of a baby under the care of Cara Muhlhahn, the prominent nurse midwife who appeared in *The Business of Being Born*. Relying on interviews with the grieving parents, the report used this one tragic death to question the safety of home births and (as the initial title showed) midwifery. The piece did show another couple who had a good home birth experience, and it stated the basic argument Abby Epstein's film makes against hospital births, including comment from one of the film's home birth advocates. But the report ignored the research demonstrating the high quality of nurse-midwife care, and it included no expert comment from midwives or their associations. It presented physicians as the only source of true healthcare expertise.

Even press items that support APRN practice may convey subtle disdain. In a May 2012 piece on *The Atlantic* website, "Why Nurses Need More Authority," physician John Rowe argued with some force that allowing APRNs to do more would improve primary care and probably reduce healthcare costs.[109] He also suggested that the objections from physician groups were unfounded. Noting that the physician groups "argue that physicians with more years of training under their belts must necessarily know more than an APRN ever could," Rowe responded that "of course they know more, but it is well established that they do not know more about providing the core elements of basic primary care." However, as we have seen, APRNs typically have six to eight years of university-level education, four to six of it in nursing, and most have spent years in clinical practice. It is absurd to suggest that medical training means that a physician knows more than an APRN "ever could." Rowe also asserted that letting APRNs "handle routine care frees up physicians to focus on diagnostic dilemmas and more complex management issues while dramatically reducing waiting times for care," expanding on an earlier reference to APRNs treating "uncomplicated" acute illness. In fact, APRNs—who have an advanced holistic practice model and excellent interpersonal skills—are quite capable of going beyond "basic" and "routine" care to handle complex diagnoses and care management.

Indeed, consider a 2010 article that KJ Lewis posted on the University of Central Florida's *Today* site about Arden Monroe-Obermeit, who appeared as a morgue technician on the Discovery Channel reality show *Dr. G: Medical Examiner*. Monroe-Obermeit was about to enter the university's DNP program.[110] The article reported that her new career path was inspired partly by an NP who had diagnosed her Cushing disease when many physicians could not.

Some news items praise APRNs in a way that denigrates other RNs. The April 2008 *Wall Street Journal* piece about the development of the DNP degree included a chart comparing the education and practice of DNPs, master's-prepared APRNs, and RNs.[111] Under the heading of "Professional Authority," the chart listed the APRNs' prescription authority; for the RNs, it stated "None." Nonsense. RNs cannot prescribe drugs, but that does not mean they have no professional authority, as the nurse practice acts discussed in Chapter 4 make clear.

In February 2005 the *Australian* ran a generally good piece by Adam Cresswell about the growing role of Australian NPs in managing chronic heart failure. "The rise of the super nurse" emphasized the positive effect of the holistic nursing model on patient outcomes.[112] But the term "super nurse," even more than "advanced practice nurse," may suggest that RNs are nothing special.

Similarly, a January-February 2005 issue of *U.S. News & World Report* featured a massive special health report entitled "Who Needs Doctors?"[113] Describing how other professionals are increasingly providing care that used to be the exclusive province of physicians, the report took an unusually positive look at the work of APRNs. But parts of the report suggested that APRNs are worthy of attention because they're doing things physicians do, whereas other nurses remain engaged in their subservient, limited traditional work. One NP was quoted as saying that when she started out (in about 1980) "nurses were not told we could think for ourselves" and "just did what a doctor planned out for us," which is incorrect. Some nurses may have internalized the idea that they have not been thinking for themselves, but autonomous thinking has been a critical part of nursing practice since at least Nightingale's time, as we discuss in Chapter 4. The feature stated that "through the 1980's, the idea of nurses doing more than just assisting doctors gained acceptance" as patients began seeking out nurses as their primary care providers. That statement obviously implies that RNs simply assist physicians, which is false. For centuries, nursing has been an autonomous science profession with its own distinct sphere of practice. That is true even though nursing has traditionally had less power than medicine, as we discuss in Chapter 4, and not enough nurses have yet embraced their autonomous decision-making, as we discuss in Chapter 11.

Thus, even in some pro-APRN media pieces, a troubling theme remains: Now that APRNs can do work that physicians have been doing, who needs RNs?

Notes

1. CFNA, "Duck Soup," TAN (December 2005), http://tinyurl.com/l2fj2ej.
2. William T. Jarvis, "Some Notes on Quackery," National Council Against Health Fraud (1996), http://tinyurl.com/kuyw2of.
3. CFNA, "Mattel on the 'Nurse Quacktitioner': Problem? What Problem? Oh—and Did We Mention the New Nurse Barbie?," TAN (January 11, 2006), http://tinyurl.com/lde6v7w.
4. CFNA, "Some U.K. Physicians to Mattel: Keep That Anti-Nurse Hatred Coming!," TAN (January 9, 2006), http://tinyurl.com/ohjwq8u.
5. Bryan Moore and Chris Peterson, writers, Victor Gonzalez, director, "Bionic Showdown," *Lab Rats*, Disney XD (August 5, 2013), TAN, "Nurse Practitioner Evil!" (August 5, 2013), http://tinyurl.com/mzuzud9; TAN, "Lab Rats Experiment a Success!" (February 2014), http://tinyurl.com/njtnk46.
6. Robin P. Newhouse, Julie Stanik-Hutt, Kathleen M. White, Meg Johantgen, Eric B. Bass, George Zangaro, Lily Fountain, et al., "Advanced Practice Nurse Outcomes, 1990–2008: A Systematic Review," *Nursing Economic$* 29, no. 5 (September-October 2011): 230–250, http://tinyurl.com/l58y243; TAN, "Do Physicians Deliver Better Care than Advanced Practice Registered Nurses?," http://tinyurl.com/yd7r3yv.
7. American Association of Nurse Practitioners, "Historical Timeline," accessed February 17, 2014, http://tinyurl.com/myzmvty.

8. University of California, San Francisco School of Nursing, "Areas of Specialty, M.S. Program," accessed February 17, 2014, http://tinyurl.com/le2xdqw.
9. Victorian Government Health Information, "Nursing in Victoria" (February 5, 2014), http://tinyurl.com/pz4bpdc; Nursing Council of New Zealand, "Nurse Practitioner," accessed February 17, 2014, http://tinyurl.com/lsopbkb; Galadriel Bonnel, "Evolvement of French Advanced Practice Nurses," *Journal of the American Association of Nurse Practitioners* 26, no. 4 (April 2014): 207–219, http://tinyurl.com/m7wt4pl.
10. American Association of Colleges of Nursing, "Nurse Practitioners: The Growing Solution in Health Care Delivery," accessed February 17, 2014, http://tinyurl.com/lyd793m.
11. Carla Mariano, "Holistic Nursing," *Imprint* (February/March 2005): 48–51, http://tinyurl.com/m5f82cc.
12. US Senate, "Expanding the Primary Care Workforce," accessed February 17, 2014, http://tinyurl.com/olkjk4g.
13. Institute of Medicine of the National Academies, "The Future of Nursing: Leading Change, Advancing Health" (October 5, 2010), http://tinyurl.com/2brrusk.
14. US Department of Labor, Bureau of Labor Statistics, "Query System: Occupational Employment Statistics: Registered Nurses, Nursing Instructors and Teachers, Postsecondary (251072); Registered Nurses (291141); Nurse Anesthetists (291151); Nurse Midwives (291161); Nurse Practitioners (291171); Licensed Practical and Licensed Vocational Nurses (292061)" (May 2012), http://data.bls.gov/oes/; National Association of Clinical Nurse Specialists, "Clinical Nurse Specialist" (2012), http://tinyurl.com/lcn9eaj; American Association of Nurse Practitioners, "NP Fact Sheet," accessed February 20, 2014, http://tinyurl.com/o28aq3j.
15. Susan Trossman, "A Calculated Approach," *American Nurse Today* 4, no. 4 (April 2009), http://tinyurl.com/m7s4t3f.
16. Phil Galewitz, "Urgent Care Centers Are Booming, which Worries Some Doctors," *Washington Post* (September 17, 2012), http://tinyurl.com/blqybt2.
17. American Association of Colleges of Nursing, "The Impact of Education on Nursing Practice" (January 21, 2014), http://tinyurl.com/6uvr58r.
18. Black America Web, "A Note from Tom Joyner," accessed March 26, 2014, http://tinyurl.com/ldkpyzq; Greenville Health System, "Take a Loved One to the Doctor Day," accessed March 26, 2014, http://tinyurl.com/lhtpvt4.
19. National Institutes of Health, "The National Diabetes Education Program Supports Take a Loved One for a Checkup Day" (September 20, 2005), http://tinyurl.com/kr55qoh.
20. US Department of Health and Human Services, Office on Women's Health, National Women's Health Week (May 12–18, 2013), http://tinyurl.com/mw3cvrt.
21. Eileen M. Sullivan-Marx, Diane O. McGivern, Julie A. Fairman, and Sherry A. Greenberg, eds., *Nurse Practitioners: The Evolution and Future of Advanced*

Practice, 5th ed. (New York: Springer Publishing Company, 2010), http://tinyurl.com/.ofd9y59.
22. American Association of Nurse Practitioners, "All About NPs," accessed February 22, 2014, http://www.aanp.org/all-about-nps.
23. National Association of Clinical Nurse Specialists, "CNS FAQ's: What is a Clinical Nurse Specialist?," accessed February 22, 2014, http://tinyurl.com/blokbrk and http://tinyurl.com/lqhjwgp.
24. American Association of Nurse Practitioners, "Legislation/Regulation," accessed February 22, 2014, http://tinyurl.com/kc3canc; Reimbursement Task Force and APRN Work Group of the WOCN Society National Public Policy Committee, "Reimbursement of Advanced Practice Registered Nurse Services: A Fact Sheet," *Journal of Wound, Ostomy & Continence Nursing* 39, no. 2S (March/April 2012): S7–S16, http://tinyurl.com/m9cj8eo.
25. American Association of Nurse Practitioners, "All About NPs: Education and Training," accessed February 22, 2014, http://tinyurl.com/l9mm6tf.
26. Kate Darby Rauch, "Are Residencies the Future of Nurse Practitioner Training?," *Science of Caring* (January 2013), http://tinyurl.com/kwmjuhw.
27. Rebecca Patchin, "AMA Responds to IOM Report on Future of Nursing," American Medical Association (October 5, 2010), http://tinyurl.com/mvku7xu.
28. Carolyn Rogers, "Physician Extenders: PAs, NPs, and. . .Athletic Trainers?," American Academy of Orthopaedic Surgeons (October 2008), http://tinyurl.com/qj26cbw.
29. American College of Cardiology, "Mid-Level Providers," accessed February 23, 2014, http://tinyurl.com/p56wyfo.
30. TAN, "Do Physicians Deliver Better Care than Advanced Practice Registered Nurses?," accessed March 28, 2014, http://tinyurl.com/yd7r3yv.
31. Robin P. Newhouse, Julie Stanik-Hutt, Kathleen M. White, et al., "Advanced Practice Nurse Outcomes 1990–2008: A Systematic Review," *Nursing Economic$* 29, no. 5 (September-October 2011): 230–250, http://tinyurl.com/l58y243.
32. Brian Dulisse and Jerry Cromwell, "No Harm Found When Nurse Anesthetists Work without Supervision by Physicians," *Health Affairs* 29, no. 8 (August 2010): 1469–1475, http://tinyurl.com/kbxmqja.
33. American Association of Nurse Anesthetists, "Certified Registered Nurse Anesthetists at a Glance," accessed March 28, 2014, http://tinyurl.com/75ykpqd.
34. Debra J. Jackson, Janet M. Lang, William H. Swartz, Theodore G. Ganiats, Judith Fullerton, Jeffrey Ecker, and Uyensa Nguyen, "Outcomes, Safety, and Resource Utilization in a Collaborative Care Birth Center Program Compared with Traditional Physician-Based Perinatal Care," *American Journal of Public Health* 93, no. 6 (June 2003): 999–1006, http://tinyurl.com/mtm9xrv.
35. Sue Horrocks, Elizabeth Anderson, and Chris Salisbury, "Systematic Review of Whether Nurse Practitioners Working in Primary Care Can Provide Equivalent Care to Doctors," *British Medical Journal* 324 (April 6, 2002): 819–823, http://tinyurl.com/lkhmyqy.

36. American Association of Colleges of Nursing, "DNP Fact Sheet" (January 2014), http://tinyurl.com/puq85ex.
37. Joe Mantone, "Say Hello to 'Dr. Nurse,'" *Wall Street Journal* (April 2, 2008), http://tinyurl.com/mojg28h.
38. Melissa Waterbury, "American Medical Association Opposition to the DNP," Non-Thesis Masters Paper, Washington State University (December 2008), http://tinyurl.com/mcnf6ff.
39. Eileen Shannon Carlson, "ANA Advocates for Nurses at American Medical Association Meeting: Resolution 214 and Resolution 232," *Capitol Update*, American Nurses Association (August 4, 2008), http://tinyurl.com/ll4guyf; Amy Lynn Sorrel, "AMA Meeting: Physicians Demand Greater Oversight of Doctors of Nursing," *American Medical News* (July 7, 2008), http://tinyurl.com/l375wcs.
40. National Board of Medical Examiners, "DNP Certifying Exam—Q&A," accessed February 24, 2014, http://tinyurl.com/pb5arff.
41. Rebecca Patton and Linda Stierle, "Letter to David Lichtman, President of the American Medical Association" (June 11, 2008), http://tinyurl.com/pmjwlna.
42. Eileen Shannon Carlson, "ANA Advocates for Nurses at American Medical Association Meeting: Resolution 214 and Resolution 232," *Capitol Update*, American Nurses Association (August 4, 2008), http://tinyurl.com/ll4guyf.
43. Lydia Woodward and Lisa Zwerling, writers, Paul McCrane, director, "Ruby Redux," *ER*, NBC (April 28, 2005); CFNA, "Judas in a Lab Coat," TAN (April 28, 2005), http://tinyurl.com/ksyumg7.
44. Fred Einesman, writer, Mark Tinker, director, "In the Name of Love," *Private Practice*, ABC (May 6, 2010); Debora Cahn, writer, Jeannot Szwarc, director, "The End of a Beautiful Friendship," *Private Practice*, ABC (May 13, 2010); TAN, "A Midwife in a World of Doctors" (August 2010), http://tinyurl.com/qh9mzjd.
45. Liz Heldens and Colleen McGuinness, writers, Andrew Bernstein, director, "That Crazy Bitch Was Right," *Mercy*, NBC (May 12, 2010); TAN, "It Droppeth as the Gentle Rain from Heaven" (May 2010), http://tinyurl.com/psomrge.
46. John Masius, writer, Mikael Salomon, director, "Pilot," *HawthoRNe*, TNT (June 16, 2009); TAN, "Chief Nursing Officer" (June 16, 2009), http://tinyurl.com/o5ce4yw.
47. CFNA, "Nurses Are About 100 Times More Likely to Attend Graduate Nursing School than Medical School," TAN (2002), http://tinyurl.com/p7orchc.
48. Shannon Goss, writer, Lesli Linka Glatter, director, "The High Holiday," *ER*, NBC (December 11, 2008); Karen Maser, writer, Christopher Chulack, director, "Haunted," *ER*, NBC (October 30, 2008); TAN, "The Extubating Babysitter" (March 29, 2009), http://tinyurl.com/mavyu3b; TAN, "Helping You Remember Complicated Facts" (October 30, 2008), http://tinyurl.com/lpvlnf4.
49. Tony Kushner, writer, Mike Nichols, director, *Angels in America*, HBO Films (2003); CFNA, "Angels in America," TAN (2003), http://tinyurl.com/mqcbd3l.

50. Abby Epstein, director, *The Business of Being Born*, Ample Films, Barranca Productions (2008); CFNA, "The Business of Being Born," TAN (January 14, 2008), http://tinyurl.com/pk9kay7.
51. Nick Curwin, Hamo Forsyth, Jonathan Smith, executive producers, *24 Hours in A&E*, Channel 4/BBC America (2011-), http://tinyurl.com/3onwxsw.
52. CFNA, "Peter Riggs, CNM (2000–2006)," TAN (February 4, 2006), http://tinyurl.com/n5y7nb6.
53. Darin Goldberg and Shelley Meals, writers, Catherine Jelski, director, "It Takes a Clinic," *Strong Medicine*, Lifetime (September 18, 2005); CFNA, "The Baby Man," TAN (September 18, 2005), http://tinyurl.com/kgqwf5q.
54. Dianne Messina Stanley and James Stanley, writers, John Perrin Flynn, director, "Special Delivery," *Strong Medicine*, Lifetime (February 5, 2006); CFNA, "The Way Out of Strong Medicine," TAN (February 5, 2006), http://tinyurl.com/kwtypzf.
55. TAN, "*Private Practice* Episode Analyses" (2013), http://tinyurl.com/lecehka.
56. Shonda Rhimes, writer, Mark Tinker, director, "In Which We Meet Addison, a Nice Girl from Somewhere Else," *Private Practice*, ABC (September 26, 2007), http://tinyurl.com/lh29vxs; CFNA, "Private Practice: Is That Even a Word?," TAN (September 26, 2007), http://tinyurl.com/kwahd79.
57. Michael Ostrowski, writer, Steve Gomer, director, "Acceptance," *Private Practice*, ABC (February 5, 2009); TAN, "Not a Doctor, But. . ." (April 29, 2009), http://tinyurl.com/mr7232d.
58. Patti Carr and Lara Olsen, writers, Bethany Rooney, director, "Best Laid Plans," *Private Practice*, ABC (January 21, 2010), http://tinyurl.com/lqor6me; TAN, "It Hurts" (January 21, 2010), http://tinyurl.com/k7ydej2.
59. Kathy McCormick, writer, Ann Kindberg, director, "Pulling the Plug," *Private Practice*, ABC (March 25, 2010), http://tinyurl.com/lqltz4l; TAN, "Saving Two Lives, in the Field, with No Equipment" (August 2010), http://tinyurl.com/kjv2tw7.
60. Craig Turk, writer, Eric Stoltz, director, "Do the Right Thing," *Private Practice*, ABC (March 26, 2009); TAN, "Not a Doctor, But. . ." (April 29, 2009), http://tinyurl.com/l8v7fus.
61. Shonda Rhimes, "Shonda Rhimes on Dell's Death," *TV Guide* (May 24–June 6, 2010); TAN, "Postmortem: Shonda Rhimes on Dell's Death" (May 24–June 6, 2010), http://tinyurl.com/msqfqpu.
62. John Herzfeld and Jack Orman, creators, *Dr. Vegas*, CBS (2004–2005); CFNA, "Dr. Vegas," TAN (March 4, 2005), http://tinyurl.com/pk8yo7n.
63. Karen Maser, writer, Christopher Chulack, director, "Haunted," *ER*, NBC (October 30, 2008); TAN, "Helping You Remember Complicated Facts" (October 30, 2008), http://tinyurl.com/lpvlnf4.
64. Joe Sachs, writer, Charles Haid, director, "Let it Snow," *ER*, NBC (December 4, 2008), http://tinyurl.com/l5l3nzh; Shannon Goss, writer, Lesli Linka Glatter,

director, "The High Holiday," *ER*, NBC (December 11, 2008), http://tinyurl.com/m3u43nn; TAN, "The Extubating Babysitter" (March 29, 2009), http://tinyurl.com/mavyu3b.

65. IMDb, "*ER* (1994–2009): Full Cast & Crew," accessed February 25, 2014, http://www.imdb.com/title/tt0108757/fullcredits.
66. Clifton Campbell, creator, *The Glades*, A&E (2010–2013), http://tinyurl.com/ks9p3qt; Matthew J. Lieberman, writer, Donna Deitch, director, "Magic Longworth," *The Glades*, A&E (June 17, 2013); TAN, "Hell of a Doctor" (August 2013), http://tinyurl.com/l2gfpxd.
67. TAN, "*HawthoRNe* Episode Analyses" (2011), http://tinyurl.com/jwd7neg.
68. Peter Elkoff and Joe Sachs, writers, Timoth Busfield, director, "Too Much Attitude and Not Enough Underwear," *Mercy*, NBC (May 5, 2010); Liz Heldens and Colleen McGuinness, writers, Andrew Bernstein, director, "That Crazy Bitch Was Right," *Mercy*, NBC (May 12, 2010); TAN, "It Droppeth as the Gentle Rain from Heaven" (May 2010), http://tinyurl.com/psomrge.
69. Liz Heldens, writer, Adam Bernstein, director, "Can We Get That Drink Now?," *Mercy*, NBC (September 23, 2009); TAN, "Traffic Is Backed Up in the Tunnel Heading into Respect" (September 23, 2009), http://tinyurl.com/m76xbzs.
70. Carly Mensch and Heidi Schreck, writers, Seith Mann, director, "Sidecars and Spermicide," *Nurse Jackie*, Showtime (June 15, 2014).
71. Debora Cahn, writer, Randall Zisk, director, "Blink," *Grey's Anatomy*, ABC (January 14, 2010), http://tinyurl.com/kjr8sy5; TAN, "*Grey's Anatomy*: Have Fun Playing Nurse: High Class Care" (August 2010), http://tinyurl.com/kk7w3m4.
72. Matthew V. Lewis, writer, Deran Sarafian, director, "Insensitive," *House*, Fox (February 13, 2007), http://tinyurl.com/k7q56mm; CFNA, "They Dare to Be Do-Able," TAN (February 13, 2007), http://tinyurl.com/l96xcq2.
73. Mike Schwartz, writer, Lawrence Trilling, director, "My First Step," *Scrubs*, NBC (November 7, 2002), http://tinyurl.com/lpf7npo; TAN, "*Scrubs* TV Series Review" (2010), http://tinyurl.com/lq9hjmq.
74. Lizzy Weiss and Michael V. Ross, writers, Millicent Shelton, director, "Dance Me to the End of Love," *Switched at Birth*, ABC Family (March 3, 2014).
75. CFNA, "What Are Nurse Practitioners?," TAN (September 7, 2004), http://tinyurl.com/otoxgzt.
76. CFNA, "What Are Doctors?!," TAN (June 23, 2005), http://tinyurl.com/kz45y2q.
77. Tony Kushner, writer, Mike Nichols, director, *Angels in America*, HBO Films (2003); CFNA, "Angels in America," TAN (2003), http://tinyurl.com/mqcbd3l.
78. Abby Epstein, director, *The Business of Being Born*, Ample Films, Barranca Productions (2008); CFNA, "The Business of Being Born," TAN (January 14, 2008), http://tinyurl.com/pk9kay7.
79. Abby Epstein, director, *More Business of Being Born*, independent release, Ricki Lake, executive producer (2011), http://tinyurl.com/lxsvky7.

80. Nick Curwin, Hamo Forsyth, Jonathan Smith, executive producers, *24 Hours in A&E*, Channel 4/BBC America (2011-), http://tinyurl.com/3onwxsw.
81. Tina Rosenberg, "The Family Doctor, Minus the M.D.," *New York Times* (October 24, 2012), http://tinyurl.com/9cjwrvj; TAN, "Fixes" (October 24, 2012), http://tinyurl.com/ke7dmo8.
82. Andrew Blackman, "Is There a Doctor in the House? Perhaps Not, As Nurse Practitioners Take on Many of the Roles Long Played by Physicians," *Wall Street Journal* (October 11, 2004), http://tinyurl.com/42mqk; CFNA, "Excellent Wall Street Journal Article Highlights Potential Importance of Nurse Practitioners to Future of Health Care," TAN (October 11, 2004), http://tinyurl.com/mfbtwjs.
83. Robert Wood Johnson Foundation, "Is There a Nurse in the House? Evaluating a Nurse-Run Primary Care Practice" (September 2001), http://tinyurl.com/m6v2j2q.
84. Dana Rubinstein, "The Nurse-Crusader Goes to Washington," *The New York Observer* (December 8, 2009), http://tinyurl.com/q7hshzr; TAN, "The Nurse-Crusader" (December 8, 2009), http://tinyurl.com/m5ymmt7.
85. Patricia Guthrie, "Nonprofit Clinic Reaches Out to Underserved Community," *Atlanta Journal-Constitution* (April 28, 2004); CFNA, "*Atlanta Journal-Constitution*: Nurse Practitioner Clinic Provides Vital Care to Low-Income Patients," TAN (April 28, 2004), http://tinyurl.com/lz3cngv.
86. Ronnie Polaneczky, "Nurses Make a Difference: Practitioners Could Ease Doctor Shortage," *Philadelphia Daily News* (November 13, 2003), http://tinyurl.com/m7herra; CFNA, "Polaneczky: Nurse Practitioners Provide Excellent Primary Care to the Poor; Why Not to Everyone?," TAN (November 13, 2003), http://tinyurl.com/mo2svgy.
87. Laura Yuen, "Runaway Girls Focus of Minn. Fight to Curb Sex Trafficking," Minnesota Public Radio (January 11, 2013), http://tinyurl.com/mnsbvx9; TAN, "Living Antisocial" (January 11, 2013), http://tinyurl.com/mcr2hzq.
88. Joseph Shapiro, "Transitional Care Cuts Hospital Re-Entry Rates, Costs," National Public Radio (July 28, 2009), http://tinyurl.com/pw58vw; TAN, "I Like Getting to Prevent Things" (August 9, 2009), http://tinyurl.com/n4ngyqv.
89. Jill Coley, "Birthing Center Delivers Options," *Post and Courier* (July 21, 2008), http://tinyurl.com/mzwr38e.
90. Stanley M. Aronson, "Kentucky's Intrepid Nurses on Horseback," *Providence Journal* (January 23, 2006), http://tinyurl.com/klfmv96; CFNA, "Brown Physician Salutes Mary Breckinridge and Her 'Indomitable Nurse Midwives,'" TAN (January 23, 2006), http://tinyurl.com/l5g52te.
91. Phuong Ly, "A Labor without End," *Washington Post Magazine* (May 27, 2007), http://tinyurl.com/ypevt9.
92. Don Lowery, "A Doctor's 'Conviction' Violates the Law," *Savannah Morning News* (July 30, 2005), http://tinyurl.com/ld5bqlr; CFNA, "Power, Justice, and Little White Pieces of Paper," TAN (July 30, 2005), http://tinyurl.com/kn3kqvy.

93. California Healthcare Foundation, "Scope of Practice Laws in Health Care: Rethinking the Role of Nurse Practitioners" (January 2008): 4, http://tinyurl.com/aoxw2fx.
94. Laura Landro, "Making Room for 'Dr. Nurse,'" *Wall Street Journal* (April 2, 2008), http://tinyurl.com/md9zlkl.
95. Anne Pohnert, "Nurse Busts Top 5 Flu Myths," WTVR (January 6, 2013), http://tinyurl.com/lrr884t; TAN, "The Mythbuster" (January 6, 2013), http://tinyurl.com/kx7pzj3.
96. Cindy George, "Don't Sweat It: Here Are Tips to Survive the Heat," *Houston Chronicle* (June 13, 2010), http://tinyurl.com/lf8snzb; TAN, "Don't Be Lazy" (August 2, 2010), http://tinyurl.com/kt2bvm9.
97. Deirdre Kennedy, "Doctor-Patient 'Web Visits' Spur Privacy Concerns," National Public Radio (April 3, 2008), http://tinyurl.com/63wcrg.
98. TAN, "American Family Care Clinics: You Get to See a Physician, Not a Nurse!" (May 31, 2013), http://tinyurl.com/pkfg5pz.
99. American Family Care, "Staff Openings," accessed March 1, 2014, http://tinyurl.com/nbm6rh8.
100. CFNA, "Redbook Magazine: 'Don't Let Yourself Be Brushed Off onto a Nurse Practitioner,'" TAN (November 2002), http://tinyurl.com/m86lv5v; Jolynn Tumolo, "NP Spotlight: *Redbook* Article Raises the Ire of Nurse Practitioners," *Advance for Nurses* (October 21, 2002), http://tinyurl.com/kxz4o2o.
101. Andrew Villegas and Mary Agnes Carey, "Nurses Need a More Independent Role, Report Argues," *Kaiser Health News*, NBC News (October 5, 2010), http://tinyurl.com/mcmvkxh; TAN, "A Terrible Thing to Waste" (November 18, 2010), http://tinyurl.com/kzxnkud.
102. Benjamin Natelson, "Lost in a System Where Doctors Don't Want to Listen," *The Washington Post* (August 3, 2008), http://tinyurl.com/5zf4gx; CFNA, "'Physician-Extenders' Lack 'Know-How' to Diagnose Complex Stuff, but Are Really Good at Taking Out Splinters," TAN (August 3, 2008), http://tinyurl.com/m7l36na.
103. CFNA, "Prominent Hollywood Plastic Surgeon Tells Vogue Readers That Use of Nurse Anesthetists Is 'Unsafe,'" TAN (June 2004), http://tinyurl.com/mg8qzw2.
104. Bill O'Reilly, "American Doctors and Obamacare," *The O'Reilly Factor*, Fox News (March 4, 2014), http://tinyurl.com/mlyjn42.
105. Brett Brune, "In-Store Clinics Not a Cure-All, Doctors Warn," *Houston Chronicle* (July 9, 2006), http://tinyurl.com/mcpwesn; CFNA, "But When I Became a Physician, I Put Away Nursing Things," TAN (July 9, 2006), http://tinyurl.com/lsdfc3w.
106. Julian Drape, "Nurse Clinics Are 'Supermarket Medicine,'" Australian Associated Press (August 13, 2009), http://tinyurl.com/k4n5tcv; TAN, "Nurse Clinics Are 'Supermarket Medicine'" (August 13, 2009), http://tinyurl.com/k8rxtw8.

107. CFNA, "Fast, Cheap, and Out of Control," TAN (November 14, 2005), http://tinyurl.com/kmqzu62.
108. Peter Alexander, "The Perils of Midwifery," renamed "The Perils of Home Births," *Today Show*, NBC (September 11, 2009), http://tinyurl.com/lycjspz; TAN, "Love and Commerce" (September 11, 2009), http://tinyurl.com/lyy76ny.
109. John W. Rowe, "Why Nurses Need More Authority," *The Atlantic* (May 7, 2012), http://tinyurl.com/lb6zxr9; TAN, "Fixes" (October 24, 2012), http://tinyurl.com/m9tp37t.
110. Kimberly Lewis, "Former 'Dr. G' Cast Member Becomes Nurse," *UCF Today* (August 2, 2010), http://tinyurl.com/2e6ao4e; TAN, "Don't Be Lazy: Dr. M-O" (August 2, 2010), http://tinyurl.com/l44zjxq.
111. Laura Landro, "Making Room for 'Dr. Nurse,'" *Wall Street Journal* (April 2, 2008), http://tinyurl.com/md9zlkl (chart not included in current online article).
112. Adam Cresswell, "Rise of the Super Nurse," *The Australian* (February 12, 2005), http://tinyurl.com/m89hlgv; CFNA, "The Australian: 'Rise of the Super Nurse,'" TAN (February 12, 2005), http://tinyurl.com/krdo9p6.
113. *U.S. News & World Report*, "Who Needs Doctors?" (January 31, 2005—February 7, 2005), http://tinyurl.com/kxbnb8j; CFNA, "*U.S. News & World Report*: 'Who Needs Doctors?,'" TAN (January 31, 2005–February 7, 2005), http://tinyurl.com/lv45u9o.

III SEEKING BETTER UNDERSTANDING OF NURSING—AND BETTER HEALTH CARE

10 HOW WE CAN ALL IMPROVE UNDERSTANDING OF NURSING

One afternoon we drove in the rain along the winding Rock Creek Parkway in Washington, DC. Suddenly we saw a commotion ahead. A car had just slid off the road and flipped upside down. A small crowd had gathered, but paramedics had not yet arrived. We stopped, and Sandy got out to help, having practiced emergency nursing at major trauma centers for many years.

Sandy approached the overturned car. The driver was suspended upside down by her seat belt. She was conscious but understandably anxious. A group of about ten people, mostly men, was frantically trying to figure out how to remove the driver from her car. Sandy spoke loudly: "I'm a nurse. Do you need help?" The crowd ignored Sandy and continued preparing to move the woman. If the woman had had a serious neck injury, moving her without immobilization precautions could have caused paralysis or even death. Sandy said loudly, "Is anyone else here a health professional?" Again no one replied. So Sandy said, "OK then, I'm an ER nurse, I'm in charge here."

Very reluctantly, the crowd gave Sandy enough room—barely—to push through to examine the upside-down patient in the car. A few men in the crowd demanded that Sandy let them get the woman out. Sandy had to back them off several times as she assessed the woman's neck and general condition. She had no apparent serious injury, so Sandy let the crowd take her down.

Every day, people in situations like this depend on nurses to advocate for them. But in this case, as in many others, the nurse was barely able to protect the patient. It's hard to escape the conclusion that this danger arises from the public's misunderstanding of nursing. The crowd at Rock Creek conveyed confusion, even anger, that a nurse would purport to direct them on a life-threatening health condition, even though no one else present had health expertise.

Perhaps the crowd, like surgeon character Cristina Yang on *Grey's Anatomy*, would have been happy to let Sandy know if a bedpan needed emptying! But if Sandy had announced that she was a physician, it is hard to imagine the crowd having the same reaction.

We have shown how the media reinforces the undervaluation of nursing. In 2006 a Brazilian nursing professor wrote us to say that she shared our concerns about the show *House*, which was popular in Brazil and around the world. The professor said nursing was very different in Brazil, where, she said, nurses do not report to physicians but to a nurse manager.[1] Of course, US nurses also report to senior nurses, not to physicians. But *House* and other Hollywood shows offer a persuasive enough vision of US health roles that even the nursing professor believed the inaccuracy.

We have also seen that public disrespect for nursing has grave consequences for nurses and patients. Disrespect underlies many of the more immediate causes of the deadly nursing shortage. It leads governments and foundations to allot meager funding for nursing education and research. That in turn undermines the nursing profession, leaving too few qualified nurses and nursing educators, and people die. We rightly spend billions on alleviating deadly diseases, but we spend relatively little on the poor nursing infrastructure that allows the diseases to spread in the first place. Disrespect leads hospital administrators to replace registered nurses (RNs) with technicians, who can't tell when a patient is deteriorating, so patients suffer, even die. Disrespect leads patients to ignore nurses' health advice, and the patients suffer, even die. Disrespect undermines nurses' sense of their own autonomy and worth, deterring them from advocating for themselves and their patients.

We can change this situation. Poor public understanding of nursing, and the resulting harm to public health, is not inevitable. Of course changing the way the world thinks is a challenge, but even the most ingrained social biases can change over time. Nurses have already managed to improve understanding, in ways large and small.[2] Nurses have persuaded or helped some media creators to produce more accurate news articles and even entertainment media. Nurses have convinced advertisers to reconsider degrading naughty nurse depictions. We've seen how in 2005 nurses persuaded the US government to change the name of the Take a Loved One to the Doctor Day campaign to Take a Loved One for a Checkup Day, a name that does not exclude the advanced practice RNs who provide primary care to the minority populations the campaign targets.

But understanding does not improve only when we change media products that reach millions. All of us can have a powerful effect simply through the way we think and act every day. Sandy was raised in a family with a strong focus on mechanical and computer science, but she considered nursing to be undesirable handmaiden work until, as a teenager, she worked at a nursing home. She was awed by the skill and autonomy she saw in the nurses there. She began nursing school. Not all nurses would have inspired that choice. That those nurses did is a testament to their professional strength and vision.

Everyone should play a role in increasing understanding of nursing. Of course nurses must take the lead, as we'll discuss in detail in Chapter 11. Nurses must believe in themselves and project that belief to others. Nurses should work to persuade the media to provide a more accurate picture of the profession and they should consider creating new media themselves.

But nurses cannot improve understanding by themselves because they are underpowered, even in their own spheres of expertise. The Institute of Medicine's landmark 2010 report, *The Future of Nursing: Leading Change, Advancing Health*, correctly argued that nurses should play a far greater role in healthcare decision-making.[3] Few nurses serve as hospital CEOs or as directors on hospital boards, even though hospitals exist mainly to provide nursing care. A March 2012 analysis by the Truth About Nursing suggested that of the directors of the top seventeen US hospitals as selected by *U.S. News & World Report*, only a handful were nurses.[4] We know of no major hospital board on which nurses are even 5 percent of the members; often there are no nurses at all. In 2012 the Center to Champion Nursing in America, a project of the AARP and the Robert Wood Johnson Foundation, launched an initiative to put more nurses on hospital boards of directors, and they have been making some progress![5] MinuteClinic, the CVS retail clinic group with more than 750 US locations in early 2014, did at that time include two nurses (and two physicians) on its eight-member management team.[6] But overall, few nurses hold powerful positions in government or the private sector. In addition, few nurses have significant input on influential media.

Many other segments of society can help nurses by influencing both media portrayals of nursing and people's understanding of nursing generally. We can all listen to nurses and watch what actually happens when we interact with the healthcare system: What are the nurses doing? Do the media we see reflect that? Tell a friend! What are our assumptions and actions when it comes to nursing, including our language; do we credit physicians for things nurses really do? How can we apply our new understanding to push for more resources and respect for the skilled nurses almost all of us will one day need?

Some parts of society have special influence. In particular, those who create media should try harder to provide a fair picture of nursing. Creators of news and entertainment media can learn from nurses about what they really do. Nurses make great expert sources, because a key part of nursing education is learning how to convey complex health information to lay people. In addition, advertisers should consider the effects of nursing stereotypes and try to find alternative ways to sell their products.

Private sector health executives should ensure that their public speech reflects an understanding of nursing. Managers of hospitals and other clinical facilities should promote nursing as they do medicine, and publicize their efforts to strengthen the profession. Insurers and drug companies can advertise without suggesting that health care revolves solely around "doctors."

Government leaders and other health policy makers should also work to communicate an understanding of what nurses really do. They should publicize their efforts to invest in nurses' clinical practice, education, and research, and place qualified nurses in visible positions of authority. Foundations should consider creating prizes and museums to build public appreciation for nursing.

Nurses' healthcare colleagues can also play a key role. Physicians must learn about what nurses really do for patients, and they should do what they can to stop the crediting of physicians for work that nurses really do, from Hollywood to your bedside. Other health workers should ensure that they are not mistaken for nurses.

What will the future look like when the global public truly values the nursing profession? *Understanding that nurses save lives will itself save lives*—by enabling nurses to get the resources and respect they need to do their work. Adequate resources for clinical settings are only the beginning. Through their holistic, preventative focus, nurses can intervene before conditions become severe, so that patients don't end up dead or in expensive hospitals. Teams consisting of community health nurses and advanced practice nurses, working in local settings, can prevent or manage a great deal of the illness the world now suffers. With such programs, malaria might kill millions fewer children, because the nurse teams could work to eliminate standing pools of water and increase use of mosquito nets. Obesity-related problems like heart disease and diabetes might no longer cripple health systems if nurses were educating and advocating in the community for better diet and exercise. Millions of critically ill infants might be home with their families because nurses would have the resources to teach mothers how and why to breastfeed. Emergency departments might no longer burst with patients waiting twenty hours for care, because nurses would be keeping many patients out of the hospital system.

Here is a prospectus for a global investment in nursing:

Value of nurses saving thousands of additional lives every day:
Trillions of dollars.
Value of nurses teaching millions more people how to live healthier lives:
Trillions of dollars.
Value of nurses keeping families, workplaces, communities, and nations strong:
Priceless.

Everyone can do *something* to increase knowledge of what nurses really do and thereby improve health. Below are some ideas, conveniently organized for specific categories of people. Clip 'n' save!

I'm a Citizen of the World. What Can I Do?

We can all learn more about nursing—what it is and is not. When you are in the healthcare system, or meet a nurse, try to learn what nurses really do. We can all look critically at what the media tells us about nursing. Does that news story or show treat nursing fairly? If not, is that acceptable in the midst of a nursing crisis? We can all consider the messages that we ourselves send, through things as basic as our clothes and our language. What each of us does matters particularly now, because with the Internet, virtually anyone can create media accessible to the rest of the world, all day, every day.

"What Do You Do All Day, Anyway?"

When you meet a nurse, try asking what was exciting or worthwhile about the care he or she provided to patients in recent days. Try to focus on what the nurse actually did for the patient: How did he improve the patient's outcome? Did she save (or lose) a life? The nurse will get a chance to practice explaining what nursing involves and perhaps gain reassurance that it matters. You'll probably learn something new about nursing and health care generally.

"You Could Be a Doctor!"

Let's say you are a patient or family member who is impressed by a nurse's competence. Or perhaps a nurse tells you a fascinating story and you are floored by his skilled, autonomous interventions. (Stay with us, this often happens when people really listen.) Try to resist the urge to tell him, "You could be a doctor!" We know that people mean that as a compliment, but it suggests that any nurse who displays knowledge or skill is exceptional and ought to be a physician, because nurses do not need such qualities. In fact, knowledgeable, skilled nurses are not the exception but the rule. Nurses must have those qualities to detect and overcome subtle threats to patient health and thereby save lives. So a better way to compliment that excellent nurse might be, "Please stay in nursing!"

Don't Believe the Hype

We can all look more critically at what the media presents to us. The next time the news media consults only physicians for a story about something in which nurses are expert, like hospital conditions or community health, consider why nurses were ignored—and what the story is not telling you as a result. Research shows that even the entertainment media affects our thinking, as we explained in Chapter 2. So when a hospital drama shows physicians providing all skilled hospital care, ask yourself how likely is that to occur. Would nurses be providing much of that care? Ask media creators why they do not give a fair account of nursing. It's fun!

Try to Resist That Naughty Nurse's Charms

Naughty nurse pornography, lingerie, and costumes remain popular, although they reinforce a tired, damaging stereotype. Sexual fantasies cannot be simply wished away, of course, but we can consider new ways to think about nurses. We urge those who profit from naughty nurse products to seek other ways to prosper.

Say you're invited to a Halloween party. You could wear some naughty nurse costume. But the naughty nurse really is a corpse bride, because she scares away the resources nurses need to save lives. So consider telling some other tale from the crypt.

What's My Name?

Language is powerful. Unfortunately, too many common words and phrases, with deep roots in our culture, reinforce damaging assumptions and stereotypes about nursing. Many of these usages degrade nurses' professional identity or credit others for their work. Of course, purposely changing language is difficult, but you can start with yourself. You may expand your mind—and improve your health. Table 10.1 outlines some troubling usages and suggests alternatives.

Table 10.1 How Word Choice Can Help Nursing

Common word or phrase	Better words or phrases	Why consider the change?
Angel	Nurse	When we refer to nurses as "angels," we imply that they are unskilled spiritual beings who don't need salaries, rest, or resources. "Angels" can take care of ten patients on sixteen-hour shifts and never make a deadly mistake. Humans can't.
Baby nurse	Newborn nanny or caregiver	Many people refer to infant caregivers as "baby nurses," but these workers do not have a nursing education, and most have little or no health education.
Doctor	Physician	Using "doctor" to describe only physicians elevates them above other health workers and gives the false impression that physicians are the only health workers who can earn a doctoral degree.
Doctor or physician (to refer to those who provide primary or other practitioner care)	Health provider	Most of us have spent a lifetime being told to "ask your doctor" about healthcare products and confronting forms that ask us to name our "doctor" or "physician." These usages should change so as not to exclude advanced practice nurses.
Former nurse	Nurse	Like physicians, nurses do not stop being nurses when they stop providing direct care. Nursing involves thinking, not just physical tasks at the bedside. Thus, when a nurse is managing other nurses, teaching nursing, doing research, creating policy, or advocating for change, he or she is still a "nurse."
Medical center	Hospital	Many vital health professionals besides physicians work in hospitals. Yet because only physicians practice "medicine," the term "medical center" suggests hospitals are all about physicians.

(*continued*)

Table 10.1 (Continued)

Common word or phrase	Better words or phrases	Why consider the change?
Medicine (to mean all health care)	Health care	Medicine, which physicians practice, is one type of health care, but many others are also important. Health professions like nursing are not subsets of medicine but distinct, autonomous fields.
Nurse (to mean anyone who provides nonphysician care)	Nurse's aide, nursing assistant, patient care technician, or whatever they really are	Only nurses should be called "nurse." When nonnurses are called "nurse," people interacting with them may reasonably conclude that nurses know far less about health care than they really do. Many family members admirably provide care for their loved ones, but that does not make them "nurses."
Nursing or wet nursing (to mean breastfeeding)	Breastfeeding	Using "nursing" or "wet nursing" to mean breastfeeding subtly suggests that nursing is something we can do without health education, and of course that only women can be nurses, which is not the case.
Order	Prescription or care plan	Nurses don't take "orders" from physicians. If nurses do not agree with a physician plan, they are legally and ethically obligated to work for a better plan.
She (to refer to a nurse of indefinite gender)	He, or he or she	Some nurses prefer female pronouns, because most nurses are women, and women predominate in few professions. But one way to undermine the prevailing social bias that nurses are all female is to use "he" when discussing nurses of indefinite gender.
Student nurse	Nursing student	Nursing students are awesome, but they are not yet nurses, and describing them as such lessens the value of the term "nurse." So just as we do not refer to medical students as "student physicians," we should not refer to nursing students as "student nurses."
Work as a nurse	Practice nursing	Nurses are health professionals who "practice" nursing, just as physicians practice medicine.

(*continued*)

Table 10.1 (Continued)

Common word or phrase	Better words or phrases	Why consider the change?
Advanced practice nurse	?	We ourselves use "advanced practice nurse," for lack of a better way to describe the group that encompasses nurse practitioners, nurse midwives, nurse anesthetists, and clinical nurse specialists. But the term wrongly suggests that other nurses are less than "advanced." Can you help find a better term?
Nurse	?	The term "nurse" has been linked so closely and for so long to unskilled tending, especially by females—from "nursing a baby" to "nursing a drink"—that we wonder if it can ever properly name a modern, nongendered profession. Can you help find a better term?

I'm a Member of the Media. What Can I Do?

As the global population ages, it becomes even more interested in health. If you create media about health care, we urge you to learn all you can about what nurses really do. Whether you write or edit for a newspaper, a magazine or book publisher, a website, an advertising agency, or Hollywood, please listen to nurses when they point out inaccuracies, distortions, and other damaging messages about their profession. The input will improve your work.

No media creator is immune from sending unhelpful messages about nursing, because our social assumptions are so deeply embedded and awareness of nursing's media issues remains so limited. Consider the Wolters Klower company Lippincott Williams & Wilkins (LWW), which publishes many excellent materials in nursing and other health fields. But LWW also has a publication and series of texts it markets under the name *Nursing made Incredibly Easy*.[7] We understand the appeal to overwhelmed nursing students, but would a major company publish a series of texts called *Medicine made Incredibly Easy*? *Brain Surgery made Incredibly Easy*?

Because of the media's influence on how people think, media creators should pay special attention to the language issues discussed previously. For example, it remains common for the entertainment media to refer to minimally trained nurse's aides as "nurses," which is a problem even when the characters are positive, because such references still undervalue nursing knowledge and skill. One example is "Nurse John," a character in the 2009 film *Precious*.[8] An unusual twist on this problem appeared in the recent HBO series *Getting On*, which follows the staff at an extended care facility. One major character is Didi, who is sometimes called a "nurse"[9] and who appears to be a licensed vocational nurse (with about one year of nursing education). But in the November 2013 series premiere, Didi seemed to refer to herself as an "orderly,"[10] which is a term sometimes used to describe nursing assistants with perhaps six to eight weeks of training.[11] The show went to the trouble of having the character wear an "L.V.N." I.D. badge—why would it also suggest that the term "nurse" could be applied to someone with six to eight weeks of training?

Report on the Nurse at the Bedside

The bedside nurse saves lives and sees it all, and some reports have given readers a sense of that. But the news media has barely skimmed the surface. Nurses save lives in countless ways, managing high-tech interventions, catching subtle but deadly errors, and spearheading public health programs. Don't forget nursing errors: the media generally assumes that only physician errors matter, but in fact nurses affect patient outcomes just as much, and so their care deserves the same scrutiny. Nurses spend far more time with patients than anyone else, and they see people at their best and their worst. Nursing is vital and exciting. News consumers would be interested in what nurses do and what they know, if only the consumers heard more about it. Be receptive to what nurses tell you, and ask them questions. Too many reporters and editors rely on inaccurate assumptions about nursing, or on physicians, who, sadly, often don't know much about nursing either. Physicians dominate media like the *New York Times* and CNN, creating many stories themselves. But when nurses get the chance—as the *Times* has given oncology nurse Theresa Brown, who began contributing in 2008 to Tara Parker-Pope's "Well" blog and later to Brown's Opinionator series "Bedside"—they too can create compelling and informative pieces.

Discover 2.5 Million Women in Science

There are scientific breakthroughs all the time—and they're published in peer-reviewed nursing journals like LWW's *American Journal of Nursing*. The news media's audience would be interested in many of these, such as the studies about how hospital conditions affect patients, the latest advances in pain control, and innovative health initiatives addressing problems like HIV and diabetes. Nursing should be presented as the cutting-edge health science it is, and the profession's leaders, like those discussed in Chapter 1, should be considered among the world's health leaders. The media sometimes runs stories about women in science, but these reports typically overlook the 2.5 million female RNs in the United States, including the 340,000 with master's or doctoral degrees.[12] In fact, nurses have long done fascinating, groundbreaking work. The work of nursing pioneers like nurse midwife Mary Breckinridge and public health nurse Lillian Wald remains influential even today. Informing your audience about these nursing pioneers may pique interest in the profession's current leaders.

Consider Nurses as Expert Sources in All Health Stories

Nurses make great media health experts. They combine advanced health knowledge with the ability to communicate important health ideas to lay people, as part of their focus on patient education.

Unfortunately, nurse experts often struggle to be heard. Some news outlets consult nurses when the topic is some aspect of nursing, such as the nursing shortage. But nurses rarely appear as experts when the topic is health in general. The website Help A Reporter Out (www.helpareporter.com) posts queries from reporters looking for sources, and those seeking health expertise often seem to assume that only a physician can help them. Nurse Wendie Howland has long monitored the site and she recommends nurses when the topic is one in which nurses are at least as expert as physicians.

Virtually no hospitals have public relations officials devoted to promoting their nurses in the media, as almost all do for physicians. But Georgia Peirce of Massachusetts General Hospital is one such publicist. When reporters call Peirce looking for an expert, she often suggests a stellar nurse who has expertise in the area of interest. Nevertheless, the reporters usually insist on a physician despite her recommendation.

Similarly, physicians remain the overwhelming favorite choice for health-care speaking engagements—even when the audience is a large group of nurses. In 2013, one nursing school representative in Texas told us that she had repeatedly asked a speaker's bureau for a nursing leader to speak at a conference, only to be repeatedly offered physician speakers. Indeed, many nurses themselves plan nursing conferences featuring physicians as the most prominent speakers. It is as if the nurse planners do not know that engaging nurse experts could fill their speaking slots, or they do know but believe physicians have the real health expertise or would be more appealing even to an audience of nurses.

When the media doesn't see nurses as experts, and so does not present them that way, the public shares that view. The public does not understand why nursing requires many resources, and it takes nurses' health advice less seriously, in clinical settings and otherwise. The public also comes to see health through a physician-centered lens, as something that involves the diagnosis and treatment of illness. If the media used more nurses as expert sources, the public might develop a stronger sense of health as attaining and maintaining wellness. Consulting nurse experts would create richer media, help reshape debates on health, and offer new ideas to repair the broken healthcare system.

The few media programs that do routinely use nurse experts show how effective the practice can be. One that may use nurse experts more than any other is *HealthStyles*, the weekly radio show on New York's WBAI, hosted since 1986 by nurses Diana Mason, former editor-in-chief of the *American Journal of Nursing*, and Barbara Glickstein. On that show, nurse experts discuss health topics we don't often hear elsewhere, such as the movement in care of the dying from a "do not resuscitate" focus toward plans to "allow a natural death."[13] Vancouver nurse Maureen McGrath hosts the *Sunday Night Sex Show* on local station CKNW, relying on nurses and other experts to address a range of topics related to sexual health. In 2008 nurses Casey Hobbs and Shayne Mason started *Nurse Talk*, a radio show sponsored by the union National Nurses United that is irreverent but also addresses health policy and issues direct care nurses face.[14] Nurse Donna Cardillo has appeared on television to explain health issues to the public;[15] Cardillo has also served as an expert blogger at DrOz.com.[16] And nurses Barbara Dehn[17] and Nancy Reame[18] have appeared on iVillage to discuss maternal-child issues.

Make Clear That Nurse Experts Are Nurses

When nurse experts do appear in media items, their status as nurses is often hidden. When the media identifies an expert only as "Dr. Pugh" most people assume the expert is a physician. This actually works against nursing by reinforcing the sense of physicians as the only health experts and suggesting that yet another health expert is not a nurse. Even when a nurse expert's PhD is noted, few realize he or she is a nurse unless the piece says so. The media should identify experts as nurses so that the profession receives credit for the knowledge they provide. When one nurse expert we know appeared on a major national talk show, producers told her she had to choose only one identifier—her RN or her PhD. We understand that anyone who has earned a PhD would want to be identified with it. But we believe it is more important for the nursing profession that the RN appears than the "Dr." or the PhD. People will know the nurse is expert and well-educated by the way she or he speaks. But they won't know she or he is a nurse unless that is specified.

Create Television Shows about Nurses

Although real nursing is dramatic and exciting, relatively few television shows have featured nurses as main characters. Instead, they have presented nurses as peripheral to serious care and have focused almost solely on physician characters—who are shown spending much of their time doing what *nurses* do in real life. *Grey's Anatomy* is the most obvious recent example, but there have been dozens of such shows, from short-lived flops to long-running hits, such as *House, ER, St. Elsewhere*, and *M*A*S*H.*

There have been a few recent exceptions. As we explained, in 2009 three new nurse shows appeared on US television, and *Nurse Jackie* has survived at least six seasons. But *Mercy* was canceled after one season, and *HawthoRNe* survived only three seasons as a summer cable show with a limited audience. *Call the Midwife* has aired at least three seasons, although each has had fewer than ten episodes. MTV's recent *Scrubbing In* has given nursing the kind of attention it doesn't need.[19] In any case, the rarity, limited reach, and inconsistent value of these exceptions prove the rule.

But Aren't Hollywood's Current Nurse Advisers Enough?

Nurses have served as advisors to many popular Hollywood shows, such as *Grey's Anatomy* and *House*, but their main role seems to have been teaching the actors playing physicians how to behave credibly on set. Obviously, "nursing advice" that has no evident impact on how the show actually depicts nursing does not help the profession. As with the news media, physicians dominate in providing the advice that drives the story lines. Even the recent nurse-focused shows, apart from *Call the Midwife*, have at times reinforced the handmaiden and other stereotypes. Only meaningful advice on scripts by nurses who understand nursing's media issues can help, and producers must be more open to it.

In Chapter 2 we described how a nurse who is an international expert in her specialty got a telephone call from producers of a popular television hospital show. After she gave the producers the information they wanted, she tried to educate them about why they should include more nursing in their show. That was a great effort, but not surprisingly that one interaction wasn't enough to change the show. In fact, although the producers were stunned to learn that our friend was a nurse—an expert and a nurse!—they still told her that they and their audience were interested only in physicians.

But How Can I Sell Things Without Using Nursing Stereotypes?

With imagination, you can advertise your product without resorting to tired and demeaning stereotypes. It's true that the naughty nurse has been an advertising mainstay, and other advertisements have presented nurses as handmaidens or relatively unskilled. But that need not be so. If advertisers wonder if they are using nursing imagery in a responsible way, they should consult with those familiar with nursing's image issues.

One recent example of an advertisement that conveyed respect for nursing was a full-page magazine advertisement the University of Phoenix ran in *The New Yorker* in April 2011. The advertisement featured a woman in a business suit looking upward and the headline: "Offering a faculty of industry professionals to inspire tomorrow's health care leaders." The woman was identified as "Diane Wilson, MSN/MHA, College of Nursing, Chief Operating Officer, Community Tissue Services."[20] The advertisement explained the University's "cutting-edge" healthcare management curriculum, noting that because

> many of our students are experts in their fields, they can share industry insights gained through years of experience. It's an approach to education where accomplished students like Diane Wilson, already a CEO before enrolling, can debate new ideas on how to build a more reliable, efficient and sustainable health care system for all of us.

"Community Tissue Services" is a major Ohio-based nonprofit tissue bank. Ironically, the tissue bank—Wilson's own employer—apparently failed to identify her as a nurse in its online leadership profiles until early 2014, when it did finally include a helpful biographical sketch of her.[21]

Some advertisers have been commendably flexible when nurses bring issues to their attention. Advertisers do not wish to alienate consumers, and some, like Skechers, have curtailed advertisements that relied so heavily on nursing stereotypes that they could not be salvaged.[22] Others, including Walmart[23] and CVS,[24] have modified advertisements to eliminate nursing stereotypes, with no apparent loss of effectiveness. For example, in 2007 Heineken brand Dos Equis launched an amusing set of beer advertisements in a mock-serious tribute to a character presented as "the most interesting man in the world."[25] The advertisements showed him bench-pressing two chairs in which sat attractive, giggly women in short white dresses with nurses' caps. In response to our concerns, Heineken digitally altered the spots to change the color of the dresses and eliminate the nursing caps. We encourage other advertisers to show similar flexibility and imagination.

"I Wouldn't Stereotype Nurses—My Mom's a Nurse!"

Please don't be one of those media creators who claim that they could not possibly create media that harms nursing because they're related to nurses or really love nurses. Just as it makes no difference that a nurse was involved in creating a television show if that show harms nursing, it makes no difference that a media creator is close to nurses if his show, advertisement, or other product stereotypes them. For instance, even though *House* regularly degraded nursing, a show representative once suggested to us that the show couldn't harm nursing, in part, because the mother of show creator David Shore was a nurse, and she just loved the show! We have heard from other media creators that their shows couldn't harm nursing because close relatives of the show creators are nurses (as with Dr. Phil[26] and Sean Hannity,[27] both of whom have sisters who are nurses) or the creators previously expressed appreciation for nurses (as with David Letterman).[28] But there's no reason to think the *effects* of these shows change because of the relatives or intentions of the creators. We urge media creators to consider whether the images they *actually present* to the public conform to their positive sentiments about nursing.

I'm a Private Sector Healthcare Executive. What Can I Do?

If you are an executive at a hospital or other organization that provides health care (like the Red Cross or Doctors Without Borders), or at a health insurance company or pharmaceutical company, there is much you can do to help nurses improve understanding of their profession. Whether you realize it or not, you play a key role in shaping how the media treats nursing and how the public sees it.

Hospitals and Other Health Facilities Should Promote Nursing

Hospital and other clinical care executives should take steps to learn what nurses *really* do. Then they should promote the hospitals' nursing to the media, on their websites, and in other ways. Hospital nurses play a central role in patient outcomes and cost control. Long-term care institutions are essentially nursing facilities; thus the name "nursing homes." Of course, many urgent care and retail "quick" clinics rely primarily or exclusively on advanced practice nurses. Because your facility's nursing is at least as important as its medicine, nursing deserves to get at least as much attention. In January 2014, Valley Health Services of Herkimer, NY, actually issued a press release to let the community know about the clinical background and plans of the facility's new cardiac rehabilitation nurse, a recent BSN graduate! As a result a local newspaper, *The Telegram*, ran a short but helpful story on the nurse's arrival.

Sadly, that kind of effort to promote nursing is rare. The Truth's 2012 analysis of the top seventeen US hospitals as ranked by *U.S. News & World Report* also examined the hospitals' websites, and it revealed an almost complete failure to publicize the expertise of nurses.[29] In stark contrast to the attention lavished on physicians and medical care, the sites typically offered little about nursing care or the hospitals' nursing leaders, beyond some basic information directed at recruiting nurses themselves. We searched the websites for information or links to information about nursing from the main, "about us," "patient information," "patient services," and health specialties pages. We found those pages to be devoid of any mention of nursing, except that the bottom of Duke's "about us" page included the header "Nursing," and beneath it the link, "Get information about nursing at Duke." That was almost certainly aimed at prospective nurses, and we doubt many patients would click on it, but at least it did lead to a page with short biographies of the hospital's nursing leaders. A couple of hospitals mentioned their membership in the Magnet Recognition Program of the American Nurses Credentialing Center, but those pages were also aimed at prospective nurses, not the patients who might be interested if they knew that research showed that nurses are more likely to save their lives at a Magnet hospital.[30] Typical hospital web pages that were directed at patients were like the extensive "Why Choose Mayo Clinic" page, which had 521 words about the expertise of the Clinic's physicians but not a single word about nursing.[31] The site's discussions about a long list of medical "departments" did not include anything on nursing.[32] Likewise, urgent care and retail clinics did not initially seem eager to acknowledge that their care was mainly provided by nurses,[33] although that seems to have started to change somewhat recently.[34]

Executives should also promote nursing within hospital and clinic walls, to physicians, to patients, and to the nurses themselves: many need reminding of their own importance! Encourage physicians to follow nurses for a few days, just as physicians accompany paramedics in periodic "ride-alongs" in ambulances. Give patients information about what your nurses do and why, the qualifications of your nurses, and the hospital's efforts to strengthen nursing. Download, print, and hang our "I Am Your Registered Nurse" poster, which explains a nurse's role in simple terms, so patients and visitors can see it.[35] Adjust forms, records, and software so that staff and patients are not compelled to provide the names of physicians when the relevant provider may actually be an advanced practice nurse. Similarly, change the word "orders" to "prescriptions" to help disabuse physicians of the notion that they are in charge of nurses.

Help your nurses tell everyone who they are. In today's clinical settings, many different staff wear similar uniforms, and in some cases this trend has obscured the practice of replacing nurses with cheaper unlicensed personnel. Instead, facilities should encourage nurses to wear distinctive uniforms and use other identifiers, like RN patches.[36] Some have argued persuasively that a true professional does not need a patch with big letters on it. But we think that at this point in the development of public understanding of nursing, nurses need some way to ensure that they receive the credit (and blame) they deserve, so that awareness of their true role in heath care grows.

Of course, there is one widespread exception to the general rule of nursing invisibility at hospitals: the annual Nurses Day or Nurses Week in May. However, as we suggested in Chapter 7, we are ambivalent about those celebrations. Their heavy reliance on angel imagery undercuts the sense of nurses as skilled professionals, and the events arguably reflect the once-a-year "pat on the head" often given to underpowered jobs as a substitute for real respect and resources. In a June 2011 episode of *Nurse Jackie*, the main character dismissed the celebrations as "patronizing."[37] If hospitals do observe Nurses Day or Week, they should focus on nursing skill, not hearts and flowers.

Invest in Public Relations for Nursing

Every hospital should have a public relations professional to promote the facility's nurses—their stories, research, and community activities—and to direct media inquiries to nurses when their expertise is called for. Yet we know of only one hospital that has a public relations officer who works solely on promoting the nursing profession. If you know of others, please tell us!

Georgia Peirce is the public relations person for nursing at Massachusetts General Hospital.[38] She is not a nurse, but she persuaded the *Boston Globe* to follow nurses in the hospital and to create one of the best newspaper accounts of nursing practice that we have seen in the last decade.[39] The result was the excellent four-part October 2005 series about the hospital's intensive care unit (ICU) nurses, especially a formidable veteran who was training a new nurse, as described in Chapters 3 and 4. Reporter Scott Allen and photographer Michele McDonald followed the nurses intermittently for nine months. Their series, which remains available online, educates society about the vital, skilled, and difficult work that nurses do.

To make the *Globe* series happen, Peirce spent time picking the right medium and the right writer. She geared her pitch around a high-autonomy area for nursing, the ICU. She focused on nurses in a mentor/apprentice role, so that it would be easier for the reporter to learn what was going on inside their heads. That might otherwise have been difficult, because nurses are still socialized to defer and mask their skills. It took Peirce many weeks to overcome the *Globe*'s skepticism, but after she persuaded the reporter to come observe, he found plenty of interest and he agreed to pursue the story.

Publicize Efforts to Improve Nurses' Working Conditions

If you're an executive at a healthcare institution during today's nursing crisis, you probably want to improve the morale of your nursing staff and reduce turnover. The best way to do that is to strengthen nursing. Reversing the denursification of health care can save hospitals money and save patients' lives.[40] But if you publicize what you're doing—as some hospitals have publicized their Magnet status—through advertising and other media, you can also improve understanding of nursing. You will not only present your institution in a positive light but also explain nursing to society and encourage others to take similar steps. That was the effect when Philadelphia's Hahnemann Hospital decided to end the use of nursing assistants and adopt an all-RN staffing model, as the February 2012 coverage of that move in *The*

Philadelphia Inquirer showed.[41] *Inquirer* reporter Stacey Burling described how the all-RN staffing in a pilot program improved care by enabling better front-line surveillance, thereby reducing the number of bedside emergencies, patient falls, bedsores, and trouble with blood thinners, while at the same time improving patient satisfaction, especially with pain control. That kind of specific information is valuable to nursing because it improves public understanding—and ultimately valuable to patients, who deserve to be monitored and evaluated by *nurses*.

Specific ideas to publicize include:

- increasing RN-to-patient ratios and eliminating the use of assistants and "techs" for nursing tasks;
- helping nurses improve their education levels, including through tuition reimbursement, and providing rigorous continuing education and professional development programs;
- empowering nurses by including them in authoritative positions and roles, including on your governing board and ethics committees, as well as in morbidity and mortality conferences, patient-family meetings, and nurse-driven daily rounds;
- creating multiyear nursing residencies;
- ensuring that each unit has 24/7 coverage by clinical nurse specialists; and
- instituting zero tolerance for abuse policies.

There are many more suggestions on the Truth About Nursing's website page about Magnet status.[42] If you implement changes like these, tell the world: you're helping to resolve the nursing crisis.

Public Health Organizations Can Help Promote Nursing

Nurses play central roles in some of the most respected and well-known nongovernmental health institutions, and it is vital that these institutions convey respect for nursing as well. But some groups could do far more. For instance, in mid-2008 the American Red Cross—127 years after nurse Clara Barton founded the organization—eliminated its chief nursing officer position as part of budget cutbacks.[43] Fortunately, the Red Cross reinstated the position in April 2009,[44] although it does not appear to be in the organization's top leadership group.[45] The Red Cross website's history page notes that Clara Barton founded the organization, but not that she was a nurse![46] The site's 969-word biography of Barton does mention, near the very end, that "she nursed, comforted, and cooked for the wounded"—using "nurse" in the layperson sense.[47]

Consider the Nobel Prize–winning Médecins Sans Frontières (MSF) or Doctors Without Borders. This international aid group was founded by a small group of physicians and journalists, but today more nurses than physicians work for MSF, and nurses have played leadership roles in the organization. Yet its name sends the public the message that the physicians provide most or all of its health care. That message is especially influential because the group receives tremendous media attention for its work on disasters worldwide; not surprisingly, news and entertainment media that refer to MSF regularly suggest that it is essentially a group of physicians. We and other nursing advocates have asked MSF to consider a more inclusive name, such as Soins Sans Frontières (Health Care Without Borders). So far, MSF has refused.[48]

Healthcare Billing

Typically, skilled nursing care provided in US hospitals is not billed and reimbursed as a distinct item but is instead included in "room and board" charges. However, health insurance companies and the health institutions they reimburse should keep the nursing out of the mashed potatoes. Nursing care should be billed and reimbursed as a professional service, just like the work of physicians and others. When nursing is lumped in with the bed sheets and hospital food, people are encouraged to see nurses as interchangeable widgets, not professionals who provide a distinct health service. Early nurses provided the full range of care that patients needed, including physical therapy, occupational therapy, speech-language therapy, and social work.[49] Although nurses are still responsible for basic care in those fields, over time the fields evolved and became distinct professions, most of which now bill independently for their specialized work. Nursing is no less skilled. Allowing nurses to bill separately would open up a dialogue that would encourage decision makers, the media, and the public to learn about and articulate the nature of nursing work.

Drug Companies Should Ask Their Nurses

As we all know, advertising for medications and other healthcare products typically advises consumers to "ask your doctor" whether the product is right for them. That phrase reflects the assumption that only physicians have expertise in such products and prescription authority, but neither of those ideas is correct. Nurses, especially advanced practice nurses, are the primary care providers for millions of health consumers, and these tremendously influential advertising campaigns should recognize that. In 2008 the American Academy of Nurse Practitioners launched a campaign to persuade pharmaceutical companies to change the language in their commercials to "ask your provider."[50]

As health products makers, drug companies also have a special responsibility to advertise in a way that recognizes the contributions of the nurses who actually administer most of their products in hospital settings. In 2006 a Bristol Myers-Squibb television commercial featured Sharon Blynn reciting a poem on fighting cancer that included the line "Doctors who tell jokes in the chemo room are beautiful."[51] However, virtually all chemo room work is done by nurses. Although Johnson & Johnson deserves credit for putting tens of millions of dollars into its campaign to help resolve the nursing shortage, as we have explained in previous chapters, it should also work to reduce its heavy reliance on damaging angel and handmaiden imagery. Like hospitals, influential drug companies can enhance their own images by promoting nursing, but in doing so they should communicate that nurses are highly skilled professionals who save lives and improve patient outcomes. We have also asked the company to refrain from advertising on shows that degrade nursing, such as *Grey's Anatomy*, but as of early 2014, it has refused.[52]

I'm a Government or Health Policy Maker. What Can I Do?

We urge government and health policy makers to learn the value of nursing and convey their knowledge wherever they can. They should publicize the urgency of the nursing shortage and their efforts to address it, which will tell the public that nursing has value. Major foundations should consider funding various initiatives to improve understanding of nursing, including prizes, museums, and popular media programming.

Governments Should Communicate the Value of Nursing

The government has great power to direct the flow of information to the media and the public. Government leaders should use that power to convey the true nature and importance of nursing. In 2009, President Barack Obama repeatedly used nurses in his efforts to promote the health reforms that eventually became the Affordable Care Act of 2010.[53] Much of Obama's praise for nurses reflected an unusual understanding of the profession, including nurses' work to advocate for patients and help underserved communities, although some comments did focus on nurses' caring and virtue, rather than their life-saving skills. Public health campaigns are also useful in getting the word out.

Occasionally national policy can affect the nursing image directly. In 2010, Wales launched a new program under which all 36,000 Welsh nurses and midwives were to wear a national uniform, in solid colors determined by their specialties and levels of authority.[54] The idea was to make it easier for confused patients to see who was who, a chronic problem because of the proliferation of different workers with similar uniforms in modern hospitals.

Another notable recent idea is nurse Teri Mills's proposal to establish a National Nurse position within the US Public Health Service. The main purposes of the National Nurse would be to promote public health through media-driven preventative health education and the deployment of community health nurses, as well as to highlight the key role that nurses play in health care and the threat posed by the nursing shortage. Mills has pursued this initiative for many years and it has been introduced in Congress, most recently in 2013. The National Nurse would appear to offer a promising way to increase public understanding of the profession.[55]

Governments Should Give Nurses a Seat at the Table

Leaders should also appoint qualified nurses to visible positions of authority, as President Bill Clinton did in choosing nurse Kristine Gebbie as the first "AIDS czar" in 1993[56] and Obama did in appointing nurse Mary Wakefield to head the Health Resources and Services Administration in 2009.[57] As the American Nurses Association's then-president Rebecca Patton said in 2009, if nurses don't have a seat at the policy-making table, they will be part of the menu.[58] Increasing the role of nurses in decision-making was also an important recommendation of the Institute of Medicine's 2010 report *The Future of Nursing*.[59] Taking such steps makes for better health policy, but it also shows the public that nurses have valuable knowledge and skills.

Governments Should Publicize Efforts to Address the Shortage

Government and other health policy leaders at all levels should communicate their efforts to support nursing and address the nursing shortage. That would not only attract support for the initiatives of these leaders but also highlight the importance of nursing and inspire the private sector to follow suit.

Specific improvements that public sector health leaders should consider include:

- investing far more in nursing education, clinical practice, residencies, and research, because nursing currently gets only a tiny fraction of the government resources that medicine does;[60]
- passing *minimum* nurse staffing legislation to address the denursification of clinical settings, as well as measures to limit mandatory overtime and provide whistle-blower protection;
- vastly increasing funding for community health nursing projects, such as school nursing and nurse-family partnerships, which would enhance health, reduce costs, and educate the public about nursing; and
- making it a major public priority to resolve the nursing shortage, including the formation of working groups and policy discussion at the highest levels.

Leaders should regularly address these issues in their interactions with the media, and discussions about the Affordable Care Act provide a good vehicle to do so.

Foundations and Other Health Policy Makers Should Honor Nursing and Include the Profession in Policy Initiatives

Health policy makers, including major foundations, should consider bold measures that could radically change the way the media and the public sees nursing. In a 2006 *Baltimore Sun* op-ed, Sandy and Kristine Gebbie argued that nurses deserve a Nobel Prize or comparable annual award.[61] We noted that nursing leaders have long been at the forefront of health research and clinical practice, reinventing health systems, pioneering new therapies, and improving community health, from AIDS treatment to neonatal care. The Nobel Prize in Nursing would shine a light on the profession's achievements and help show how important it is that nursing get the resources it needs to overcome the global shortage.

Foundations should also consider creating an International Museum of Modern Nursing to educate the public about nursing. We envision an interactive science museum that would show that nursing is an exciting profession whose members use the latest technologies to help people regain and maintain health. Visitors would be invited to put themselves in the place of nurses on the front lines, in settings ranging from the extreme high-tech of teaching hospital ICUs to humanitarian relief projects around the world. The museum would also demonstrate that nurse scholars work on the cutting edge of global health research.[62]

Foundations can fund television shows and educational materials about nursing, including documentaries and scripted dramas. Foundations might also consider creating videos to educate the media, physicians, career seekers, and students about nursing. A November 2013 report by the Foundation Center indicated that US foundations had given $1.86 billion in media-related grants from 2009 to 2011, with marked growth in giving to new media and large grants to public radio and television—on which *Call the Midwife* airs.[63]

Foundations and health policy makers should include nurses in advisory groups and in joint efforts to shape health policy. In 2007 Google created a Health Advisory Council with twenty-five members, and although many were physicians, not a single one appeared to be a nurse.[64] The powerful media company refused requests to place nurses on the panel despite our letter and many follow-up telephone calls.[65] Health initiatives like this cannot succeed without the input of nurses. Of course, including nurses in such high-profile positions would tell the public that nurses are health experts whose work has value.

Nurses are often missing from joint health policy efforts that directly implicate nursing concerns, even though the physician and public health communities are included. For example, in September 2011 the Pew Charitable Trusts organized a joint letter to Members of Congress warning of the link between the overuse of antibiotics in food animal production and drug-resistant infections in humans. Original signatories included the American Medical Association, the American Academy of Pediatrics, the American College of Preventive Medicine, and the American Public Health Association.[66] Not a single nursing group signed at that time, although nurses are deeply involved in these preventive public health issues. As of early 2014 the number of organizations signing had reached 453, and there were 37 national and state nursing organizations among them. That was still only about 25 percent of the health organizations that signed (not all organizations were health-related), even though nursing is the largest health profession. Of course, it may be that some nursing organizations were asked and declined—nurses have long had an unfortunate habit of keeping their heads down—but the underrepresentation of nurses in efforts like this is so common that it is critical for all who advocate for better health to ensure that nurses are part of the picture.

I'm a Health Worker but Not a Nurse. What Can I Do?

Nurses' healthcare colleagues, particularly physicians, can help nurses improve public understanding.

Physicians

Physicians wield unmatched authority over how the media presents health care and how the public sees it. Unfortunately, much of the worst media about nurses, such as Hollywood dramas, is created in collaboration with physicians. Physicians write for and advise television shows, and they consult on many media programs and news articles. It's no shock that these media generally show little interest in nursing. But the collaborating physicians often cause or allow the media to give physicians credit for the work that nurses really do and to present nurses as low-skilled physician subordinates.

We need physicians to try to understand nursing better. It appears that few physicians learn much about what nurses really do in medical school or afterward. With only common social and professional stereotypes to go on, many physicians wrongly assume they are "in charge" of nurses and that nursing care is rudimentary. The media they create reflects that.

There are exceptions, almost all in the print media. Physician Pauline Chen has written some pieces for the *New York Times* that reflect an unusual awareness of the value of nursing.[67] Physician Richard Gunderman and Michigan nurse practitioner Peg Nelson have teamed up to write end-of-life care articles in *The Atlantic* since at least 2009. In December 2013 the magazine published "Midwives for the Dying," a piece that consisted mainly of Gunderman interviewing Nelson, as a palliative care expert, on how to give excellent end-of-life care.[68] Later that month, the *New York Times* posted physician Barron Lerner's generally helpful blog review of a book about nurse "Sister" Elizabeth Kenny, a pioneer in polio care.[69] And in March 2014, physician Victoria Sweet published a very thoughtful piece in the *Times* about Florence Nightingale's work. Sweet admitted that she once thought of Nightingale in handmaiden and angel terms, but she later learned that the "Lady with the Lamp" actually transformed health care through research and advocacy in areas like hospital design, health statistics, and of course nursing. Sweet observed that Nightingale was "a fighter" whose study of hospitals led her to conclude that "patients get the best care when no single power is ascendant, rather when there is the 'perpetual rub' between doctor, nurse and administrator."[70]

One promising way to improve physicians' understanding is through structured interactions during their training, such as joint classes in which nursing and medical students learn together. Even a video explaining the basics of nursing would help medical students understand the profession better. Consider the joint program of Dartmouth's medical school and hospital in which medical students shadow nurses for six lengthy sessions. The students ask nurses questions and meet later to discuss what they have learned. As Ellen Ceppetelli, the nursing codirector of the program, said, "You cannot collaborate with people unless you see them as competent."[71] In 2012, nurse Megan LeClair conducted research at the University of Wisconsin showing that even a four-hour shadowing program of that type was effective in improving physician views on collaborating with nurses.[72]

Medical Technicians and Nursing Assistants

Some healthcare personnel who are not nurses allow patients and physicians to call them nurses, and some even call themselves nurses. The result is that nurses lose control of their image. Only those whose title includes "nurse" should call themselves nurses.

Receptionists and Appointment Clerks

Personnel who provide support to health professionals play a role in shaping how nurses are perceived. Some ask patients things like, "Would you like an appointment with Dr. Kumwenda or with Eve, our nurse practitioner?" Please refer to advanced practice nurses with honorifics if you do the same for physicians. In this example, you might call Eve "Dr. Peyton" if she has a doctoral degree, or "Nurse Practitioner Peyton" if she does not.

Using the ideas in this chapter, nurses' colleagues and supporters can help increase understanding of the profession. That will help nurses get the resources they need to resolve the nursing crisis and meet the health challenges of the twenty-first century.

Notes

1. Renata Flavia, Personal email exchange (September 10, 2006).
2. TAN, "Our Success Stories," accessed March 2, 2014, http://tinyurl.com/mxjfpnk.
3. Institute of Medicine of the National Academies, "The Future of Nursing: Leading Change, Advancing Health" (October 5, 2010), http://tinyurl.com/2brrusk.

4. TAN, "Nursing Representation on the Websites and Boards of Directors at the Top 17 Hospitals Ranked by *U.S. News and World Report* in 2012" (March 2012), http://tinyurl.com/n8hp4kr.
5. Susan Reinhard and Susan Hassmiller, "The Future of Nursing: Transforming Health Care," *AARP International: The Journal* (February 2012), http://tinyurl.com/lnavaja.
6. CVS MinuteClinic, "Management Team" (March 2, 2014), http://tinyurl.com/k7qo834.
7. Lippincott Williams & Wilkins, "Nursing made Incredibly Easy," accessed March 2, 2014, http://tinyurl.com/ycuntu7.
8. Geoffrey Fletcher, screenplay based on the novel *Push* by Sapphire, Lee Daniels, director, *Precious*, Lionsgate (2009); TAN, "*Precious*" (May 30, 2010), http://tinyurl.com/l67gxmk.
9. Jo Brand, Vicki Pepperdine, Joanna Scanlan, Mark V. Olsen and Will Scheffer, creators, *Getting On*, HBO (2013-), http://www.hbo.com/getting-on.
10. Mark V. Olsen and Will Scheffer, writers, Miguel Arteta, director, "Born on the Fourth of July," *Getting On*, HBO (November 24, 2013), http://tinyurl.com/n79t62g.
11. US Department of Labor, Bureau of Labor Statistics, *Occupational Outlook Handbook, 2014–15 Edition*, "Nursing Assistants and Orderlies" (January 8, 2014), http://tinyurl.com/pj2f44n.
12. US Department of Labor, Bureau of Labor Statistics, "Query System: Occupational Employment Statistics: Registered Nurses, Nursing Instructors and Teachers, Postsecondary (251072); Registered Nurses (291141); Nurse Anesthetists (291151); Nurse Midwives (291161); Nurse Practitioners (291171)" (May 2012), http://data.bls.gov/oes/; National Association of Clinical Nurse Specialists, "Clinical Nurse Specialist" (2012), http://tinyurl.com/lcn9eaj.
13. CFNA, "Allowing a Natural Death," TAN (March 16, 2007), http://tinyurl.com/nybnaae.
14. NurseTalk, accessed March 2, 2014, http://nursetalksite.com.
15. CFNA, "How to Survive the Plague of Short-Staffing: *Weekend Today* Features Nurse as Health Expert," TAN (October 4, 2003), http://tinyurl.com/lp7sspm.
16. Donna Cardillo, "Donna Cardillo, RN, MA, Blog Posts," *The Dr. Oz Show* website, accessed March 27, 2014, http://tinyurl.com/kamd7g4.
17. iVillage, "iVillage Live: Episode Info" (February 16, 2007), http://tinyurl.com/kkydwv7; Barbara Dehn, "Entries by Barbara Dehn," *Huffington Post*, accessed March 27, 2014, http://tinyurl.com/jww5zyh; Barbara Dehn, "Nurse Barb's Daily Dose," accessed March 27, 2014, http://www.nursebarb.com.
18. NBC Universal Archives, "iVillage Contributor Professor Nancy King Reame Discusses Getting Pregnant in the New Year" (January 5, 2007), http://tinyurl.com/pjmdg9k.
19. TAN, "Scrubbing Less" (November 16, 2013), http://tinyurl.com/k6otvht.

20. TAN, "The Talk of the Town" (December 2011), http://tinyurl.com/mu88h9u.
21. Community Tissue Services, "Executive Officers and Boards," accessed March 2, 2014 http://tinyurl.com/mab2rvl.
22. CFNA, "Skechers Pulls Christina Aguilera 'Nurse' Ad After Receiving More Than 3,000 Letters from Nursing Supporters," TAN (August 17, 2004), http://tinyurl.com/lfz2ebb.
23. CFNA, "Wal-Mart Changes Brain Surgeon Ad," TAN (April 2, 2005), http://tinyurl.com/m553h35.
24. CFNA, "CVS Pharmacist Returns from Matrix; Can Now Download Entire Nursing Curriculum Into Your Brain in Four Hours!," TAN (January 24, 2006), http://tinyurl.com/mwvx9bj.
25. CFNA, "The Most Interesting Nurse Ad in the World," TAN (October 25, 2007), http://tinyurl.com/lf2ch7z.
26. CFNA, "Dr. Phil Responds to Nurses," TAN (November 30, 2004), http://tinyurl.com/leml5oh.
27. CFNA, "Are There Any Hot Nurses at Walter Reed? Sean Hannity Is on the Case!," TAN (January 18, 2006), http://tinyurl.com/kanxna6.
28. Caryn James, "Here's David: Letterman Returns, True to Form" (February 22, 2000), http://tinyurl.com/mb55494; CFNA, "The Gash Cam," TAN (December 19, 2005), http://tinyurl.com/ly74f66.
29. TAN, "Nursing Representation on the Websites and Boards of Directors at the Top 17 Hospitals Ranked by *U.S. News and World Report* in 2012" (March 2012), http://tinyurl.com/n8hp4kr.
30. Matthew McHugh, Lesly A. Kelly, Herbert L. Smith, Evan S. Wu, Jill M. Vanak, and Linda H. Aiken, "Lower Mortality in Magnet Hospitals," *Medical Care* 51, no. 5 (May 2013): 382–388, http://tinyurl.com/n2a4cer.
31. Mayo Clinic, "Why Choose Mayo Clinic," accessed March 3, 2014, http://tinyurl.com/ltbz7eo.
32. Mayo Clinic, "Medical Departments & Centers," accessed March 3, 2014, http://tinyurl.com/mlk7jle.
33. CFNA, "Quick Clinic NPs: Neos in the Health Care Matrix?," TAN (July 18, 2004), http://tinyurl.com/lcsygyd.
34. Anne Pohnert, "Nurse Busts Top 5 Flu Myths," WTVR (January 6, 2013), http://tinyurl.com/lrr884t; TAN, "The Mythbuster" (January 6, 2013), http://tinyurl.com/kx7pzj3.
35. TAN, "I Am Your Registered Nurse" (April 2011), http://tinyurl.com/lhjaoyx.
36. TAN, "Wear the RN Patch! Join Us in Creating a Professional Nursing Uniform," accessed March 3, 2014, http://tinyurl.com/l2ycoez.
37. Liz Flahive, writer, Linda Wallem, director, "Batting Practice," *Nurse Jackie*, Showtime (June 13, 2011); TAN, "Thank You, Nurses!" (May 2012), http://tinyurl.com/kp5kder.
38. Massachusetts General Hospital, "Georgia Peirce," accessed March 3, 2014, http://tinyurl.com/jwebpg7.

39. Scott Allen, "The Making of an ICU Nurse," *Boston Globe* (October 23–26, 2005), http://tinyurl.com/yje5d62; CFNA, "As I Lay Dying," TAN (October 23–26, 2005), http://tinyurl.com/mnm2zkh.
40. Jack Needleman, Peter I. Buerhaus, Maureen Stewart, Katya Zelevinsky, and Soeren Mattke, "Nurse Staffing in Hospitals: Is There a Business Case for Quality?," *Health Affairs* 25, no. 1 (2006): 204–211, http://tinyurl.com/m7kdm3l.
41. Stacey Burling, "Hahnemann Boosts Use of Registered Nurses in Bid to Improve Care," *Philadelphia Inquirer* (February 7, 2012), http://tinyurl.com/6sdfvsj; TAN, "America's Top RN Model?" (February 7, 2012), http://tinyurl.com/pk7kjlc.
42. TAN, "Magnet Status: What It Is, What It Is Not, and What It Could Be," accessed May 9, 2014, http://tinyurl.com/79mxv8y.
43. Maureen "Shawn" Kennedy, "*AJN* Report: American Red Cross Drops Chief Nurse Position," *American Journal of Nursing* 108, no. 7 (July 2008): 22–23, http://tinyurl.com/q8naqr4.
44. Maureen "Shawn" Kennedy, "Red Cross Reinstates Chief Nurse Position and Appoints Sharon Stanley," *AJN Off the Charts* (April 10, 2009), http://tinyurl.com/ky628mh.
45. American Red Cross, "Leadership," accessed March 6, 2014, http://tinyurl.com/plzajal.
46. American Red Cross, "A Brief History of the American Red Cross," accessed March 3, 2014, http://tinyurl.com/pq3lrk2.
47. American Red Cross, "Founder Clara Barton," accessed March 3, 2014, http://tinyurl.com/cow9h3s.
48. CFNA, "Infirmieres Sans Frontières," TAN (December 8, 2006), http://tinyurl.com/k6tlodb.
49. US Department of Health and Human Services, Centers for Medicare & Medicaid Services, Medicare.gov, "Your Medicare Coverage," accessed March 7, 2014, http://tinyurl.com/jwdw39g.
50. CFNA, "Nurse Practitioners Urge Drug Companies to End Media Bias," TAN (April 9, 2008), http://tinyurl.com/oercebm.
51. Bristol-Myers Squibb and Sharon Blynn, "Beautiful People," YouTube (November 2006), http://tinyurl.com/kwuzf9x.
52. TAN, "J&J Stops Advertising on *Scrubbing In*, But Keeps on Advertising on *Grey's Anatomy*" (November 25, 2013), http://tinyurl.com/oqbkl9d.
53. TAN, "It's Time for Us to Buck Up" (July 15, 2009), http://tinyurl.com/ldwmyap.
54. BBC, "Nurses Start Wearing National Uniform in Wales" (April 8, 2010), http://tinyurl.com/nfyf24w; TAN, "Who Are You?" (April 8, 2010), http://tinyurl.com/mfgnr3z.
55. The National Nurse for Public Health, accessed March 3, 2014, http://nationalnurse.org.
56. Richard L. Vernaci, "Clinton Names Nurse, Health Administrator As First AIDS Czar," Associated Press (June 25, 1993), http://tinyurl.com/mc5cupz.

57. Philip Rucker, "Mary Wakefield Picked as HRSA Chief," *Washington Post* (February 20, 2009), http://tinyurl.com/at7j7k.
58. Rebecca Patton, Presentation to the Vermont Nurses Association Annual Conference, November 12, 2009.
59. Institute of Medicine of the National Academies, "The Future of Nursing: Leading Change, Advancing Health" (October 5, 2010), http://tinyurl.com/2brrusk.
60. TAN, "Just How Undervalued and Underfunded is Nursing?" (November 15, 2009), http://tinyurl.com/k7m4wep.
61. Kristine Gebbie and Sandy Summers, "Nurses' Achievements Merit International Recognition," *Baltimore Sun* (December 8, 2006), http://tinyurl.com/metcefz; CFNA, "The Nobel Prize in Nursing," TAN (December 8, 2006), http://tinyurl.com/mnuq2c9.
62. CFNA, "Q: Should We Create an International Museum of Modern Nursing to Show the World How Vital, Exciting, and Technologically Advanced Nursing Really Is?," TAN (February 29, 2008), http://tinyurl.com/l8dsbay.
63. Denise Lu, "Foundation Support Booms for Web, Mobile Media Projects," Public Broadcasting Service Idea Lab (November 22, 2013), http://tinyurl.com/lw2274g; Knight Foundation, "Growth in Foundation Support for Media in the United States" (November 12, 2013), http://tinyurl.com/kskbkxh.
64. Google, "New Advisory Group on Health" (June 27, 2007), http://tinyurl.com/29ptre.
65. Sandy Summers, Letter to Missy Krasner, Google (July 5, 2007), http://tinyurl.com/o7ukv84.
66. Pew Foundation, Letter to Congress: "Sound Science: Antibiotic Use in Food Animals Leads to Drug Resistant Infections in People" (September 6, 2011), http://tinyurl.com/lfylfc7.
67. Pauline W. Chen, "Doctor and Patient: When It's the Nurse Who Needs Looking After," *New York Times* (July 5, 2012), http://tinyurl.com/7w2dd2p; Pauline W. Chen, "Doctor and Patient: Nurses' Role in the Future of Health Care," *New York Times* (November 18, 2010), http://tinyurl.com/26jtfsq; TAN, "Oh, Inverted World" (July 5, 2012), http://tinyurl.com/lm3q8nl; TAN, "A Terrible Thing to Waste" (November 18, 2010), http://tinyurl.com/lrhudxg.
68. Richard Gunderman, "Midwives for the Dying," *The Atlantic* (December 16, 2013), http://tinyurl.com/msj3x75.
69. Barron Lerner, "A Nurse Gains Fame in the Days of Polio," *New York Times* (December 26, 2013), http://tinyurl.com/kdpj2jq.
70. Victoria Sweet, "Florence Nightingale's Wisdom," *New York Times* (March 3, 2014), http://tinyurl.com/ks97vzb.
71. Sion E. Rogers, "'Me and My Shadow' Is Mantra for a New Medical Student Elective," *Dartmouth Medicine Magazine* (Summer 2005), http://tinyurl.com/ybt5d29.
72. Megan LeClair, "Advancing Interdisciplinary Collaboration: Medical Students Partnering with Nurses" (July 2012), http://tinyurl.com/jwjcpop.

11 HOW NURSES CAN IMPROVE THEIR OWN IMAGE

For understanding of nursing to improve, nurses and nursing students must exert more influence on their own image. They must educate society and the media about what nurses really do and why it matters, so that the profession can attract the resources and respect it needs to resolve the global nursing crisis. No one else can do this—nurses are the key.

Everyone in nursing can help. Consider the work of nursing scholar Diana Mason, who has spent decades advancing public understanding of nursing in ways that range from cohosting the *HealthStyles* radio show to pushing the mainstream media to cover nursing research when she was editor of the *American Journal of Nursing*; nurse life care planner Wendie Howland, who has tirelessly monitored the Help a Reporter Out website to suggest nursing experts for reporters who might otherwise consider only physician sources; nurses Milka Stojanovic (at the time a nursing student) and Tyler Kuhk, who used a variety of social media to generate massive support for the petition in protest of the damaging MTV reality show *Scrubbing In* in 2013.

The first hurdle in this advocacy is self-image. Some nurses will need to focus first on believing in their own profession and in their power to effect meaningful change for it. Then nurses should consider ways they can project a professional image in their everyday interactions, from the way they act to the way they dress. Nurses will then be ready to analyze and change the media. Nurses should learn ways to improve how the media portrays nursing. And nurses should consider how to create their own media, to tell the public directly why nursing deserves more respect and support.

There is often more than one way to see a given issue or media product. But nurses must find common ground and work together, because it's the only way they'll effect change. Consider what Benjamin Franklin said at the signing of the US Declaration of Independence: "We must, indeed, all hang together, or most assuredly, we shall all hang separately."[1]

Nurses Have the Power

After many decades of damaging media and social disrespect, improving nursing's image will not be easy. But it must be done. The first thing is to believe that it *can* be done, and more basically, to believe in nursing. Nurses have the power to change the way society sees their profession.

Take Credit for Nursing's Life-Saving Work

Nurses must take credit for the value of their work. We're not saying nurses should become braggarts, but too many nurses seem to think they must avoid any credit or attention, whether from a lack of confidence or a belief that professional modesty is the greatest virtue. However, to borrow former US Vice President Dick Cheney's famous 2001 remark about energy conservation,[2] nursing modesty "may be a sign of personal virtue, but it is not a sufficient basis for a sound, comprehensive [public] policy." Some nurses don't even seem to respect their own profession. Perhaps they have internalized society's undervaluation of nursing and are expressing frustration at their position in the one acceptable direction: at each other. In fact, some nurses tell reverential stories about physician colleagues, but not about nurse colleagues. Nurses save lives every day too. Until it's clear that people understand that, nurses should make sure they do. If nurses would rather not tell people about the value of their own work, they should consider letting others know about the heroic work that their nurse colleagues are doing.

To encourage more credit for nurses, we created a bumper sticker that says "Save Lives. Be a Nurse." It is a recruitment message, but we designed it primarily to tell people the most important thing they need to learn about nurses—*nurses save lives*. Is it boasting? Perhaps, but not unjustifiably. The Truth About Nursing will send a bumper sticker to anyone who asks for one.[3]

Take Responsibility

The media generally suggests that physicians are responsible for all of health care, including errors. Some articles blame physicians for the errors nurses make. Many nurses seem happy to let this go—happy to have dodged the bullet. But these pieces effectively tell people that nurses are marginal players who report to physicians; they undermine the sense of nursing as an autonomous profession with its own legal and ethical duties. To be seen as true professionals, nurses must accept credit when things go well and responsibility when things do not.

Take the Lead

Some nurses believe that they can rely on others to fix problems within nursing. Some have actually suggested to us that physicians or their professional groups will or should lead the way. But the troubling role many physicians and their groups have played so far in nursing practice and in media about nursing suggests that is extremely unlikely. Of course, physicians and others can help nurses improve their image, as discussed in Chapter 10, but *nurses* must lead the way.

Your Voice—Yes, Just Yours—Can Make a Critical Difference

One nurse can change the world. When operating room nurse Francine Brock of Placentia, California, visited Las Vegas in 2006, she saw IGT's *Nurse Follies* slot machine, which features naughty nurse and battle-axe imagery. She wrote to Wynn Las Vegas. The casino quickly began converting its eight to ten *Nurse Follies* slot machines to another theme, at a cost of $2,000 per machine. Of course, not every change can be made this way. But if nurses believe in the power of their voices, so might others.

Projecting a Professional Image Every Day

Everything nurses do reflects on the nursing profession. Of course no nurse can be expected to carry that burden 24/7, but we urge nurses to consider how their everyday actions affect how nurses are viewed.

Accentuate the Positive: Promoting Nursing in Hard Times

The first rule of novelist Chuck Palahniuk's Fight Club may have been to not talk about Fight Club, but the first rule of Nurse Club is you *do* talk about it. We know that working conditions for nurses across the globe are difficult now. But however understaffed and overworked nurses may be, building up the profession requires nurses to talk about it and emphasize what is good about it. Nurses have to set aside feelings about difficult workplace conditions and instead focus on how they've made a tangible difference in someone's life—interactions with patients and the life-saving actions they have taken, the things that make nursing so incredibly fulfilling. Workplace conditions can and will change when nurses work together to strengthen nursing. A big part of that collective action is attracting a new generation of nurses who are enthusiastic about their profession and eager to join in saving lives. The Truth About Nursing's recruitment page offers career seekers information about the many ways in which nursing is a great choice.[4]

Recall the story in Chapter 6 about the Chicago artist who told two nurses that she was sad about the downward trajectory of her daughter's career aspirations, from medicine to nursing. Sandy was one of the nurses. Sandy's nurse friend was speechless. But when there was an opportunity, Sandy said, "You know, there's this perception in society that being a nurse is less valuable than being a physician, but that's actually not true." Sandy and her nurse friend went on to describe some of the things nurses do to help patients live better lives. The artist began to learn about nursing. Increasing understanding of nursing begins with you teaching the person in front of you.

Identify as a Nurse

Many nurses introduce themselves to patients and colleagues by their first name, or they don't introduce themselves at all. This sure is down-to-earth, but sadly, it can also undermine respect for nurses. Nurses don't need to be formal and cold to convey that they are serious professionals. Consider this: "Hi, Ms. Jones. My name is Rich Kimball. I'll be your registered nurse until seven a.m. If you have any problems or questions about your illness or your care, just ask for me, and I will help you, OK?"

Who Put Cartoon Characters All over My Uniform?

Nurses should consider whether their uniforms convey that they are professionals. We love Hello Kitty and SpongeBob Squarepants, but not on nursing uniforms. In 2006 host Matt Lauer of *The Today Show* remarked that nurses "look like they're going on vacation" in their scrubs.[5] Physician Patricia Raymond published a 2004 piece in the *Sacramento Bee* respectfully chastising nurses: "You're the only thing between [your] patients and death, and you're covered in cartoons."[6]

Nurses' uniforms should also make clear that nurses are nurses. When nurses wore caps, patients could identify them. But caps were annoying and carried deadly infections, so most nurses ditched them in the 1980s. Now many bedside positions are filled by far less educated personnel, and everyone dresses in scrubs. Patients don't know who is who—or who can address their questions and concerns. In 2004 both the *Pittsburgh Post-Gazette*[7] and the *Kansas City Star*[8] ran articles focusing on patients' right to know who is providing their care, and it has become common for lists of hospital patients' rights to include the right to know the roles of different caregivers.[9]

To address this problem, we have embraced the registered nurse (RN) patch created by J. Morgan Puett and Mark Dion as part of a 2004 exhibit on nursing uniforms at the Fabric Workshop and Museum in Philadelphia.[10] In 2005, with permission from the artists, we created additional nurse patches, all in bold red and white, to help identify who's who. (You can get them by visiting truthaboutnursing.org/patch.) We have also seen some hospital identification badges with a big, bold "RN," which has the same effect. As noted in Chapter 10, not everyone favors this kind of RN identifier, but it is one way for nurses to make sure others know who they are.

Another way to identify nurses is by uniform color. In recent years some institutions have gone back to all-white nurse uniforms. While we applaud the effort to reclaim a professional image, nurses work with a lot of body fluids and substances like charcoal. White uniforms do show stains and may evoke the unhelpful angel image discussed in Chapter 7. Also, people often use chlorine bleach on whites, which degrades the environment that nurses should protect for their patients. In addition, some men do not favor all-white outfits, and it is vital that nursing not create additional barriers to increasing the number of men in the profession. A January 2013 report by the New York City NBC television affiliate Channel 4 described the displeasure of nurses at one local hospital group at being required to wear just white scrub *tops*. Distinct solid colored scrubs might be a better option. Consider the system of nursing uniforms that Wales introduced in 2010, with different shades indicating different specialties and levels of authority, as discussed in Chapter 10. In 2012, nursing student Ani Burr wrote an opinion piece for *Scrubs Magazine* describing how she felt "like the Michelin Tire man" in her all white uniform. In a later rotation in pediatrics, where all-white was considered too scary for kids, Burr changed to teal-colored scrubs. She reported that kids, parents, and healthcare colleagues suddenly treated her like part of the team and less like an outsider.[11]

Acceptance by others in the workplace is critical for anyone, but nurses must balance that general need with their profession's unique ones. A lack of clear RN identifiers might lessen awareness of the need to have RNs make nursing assessments—and make it easier for decision-makers to replace nurses with unlicensed caregivers, which has been happening since the early 1990s. Some nurses have told us that their employers actually *forbade* nurses to wear RN identifiers because that would signal to patients just how few RNs were on the floor.

When Texas nurse practitioner Margaret Helminiak accepted a new job, the business manager of the practice offered to buy her scrubs "like we do for the medical assistants." Helminiak thanked him, but declined: "No, I don't wear scrubs. I didn't go to school for eight years to be mistaken for one of the medical assistants."[12] She wears a laboratory coat with "Nurse Practitioner" embroidered on it.

Nursing Out Loud

Nursing is more about thinking than it is about busy hands. But society doesn't realize it when nurses keep all their thinking to themselves. Unlike physicians, nurses cannot count on the assumption that they *are* thinking.

Accordingly, nurses should consider nursing out loud. Patients, families, and colleagues would learn far more about nursing if nurses would say more of what they are thinking, consistent with patient confidentiality and sensitivity. For example: "Ms. Keating, when I listen to your lungs, they sound like they are half-filled with fluid. You probably know this is related to your congestive heart failure, but I'm concerned that the fluid is decreasing your oxygen level. Are you having trouble breathing? It seems that you are, so I'm going to look into your fluid balance and see if you might need some more diuretics to get rid of the fluid around your lungs. Let me also check your blood oxygen level to see if some nasal oxygen would help you breathe more easily. Do you feel up to taking a walk? That would help you get oxygen to all the tiny distant pockets in your lungs, prevent pneumonia, and strengthen your heart and lungs."

When nurses think out loud, others get a sense of nurses' education and skill. Nursing professor Rhea Sanford suggests that if nursing students and new nurses practice out loud, they can "transfer classroom knowledge into quality clinical practice" and assess their own performance, while "providing needed education to their patients."[13] She incorporates "nursing out loud" into her curriculum on the Planetree patient-centered model of care.[14] In fact, some hospitals' hourly rounding programs require nurses to introduce themselves and explain what they are doing.

Walk the Walk

Nurses live stressful lives, and understandably, some cope in unhealthy ways. Unfortunately, unhealthy behavior may undermine the public's sense of nurses as health professionals. Some nurses have a difficult relationship with food.[15] When nurses become overweight, they may not seem like people who embrace healthy living. So patients and the public may doubt their credibility on any health issue, not just nutrition. If you need help attaining a healthy weight, consider an easy plan we put together to help you at www.truthaboutnursing.org/healthy. It is also important to get enough exercise and try to stop smoking. If you exercise, you can teach exercise principles and motivating techniques to your patients. In addition, patients may not regard nurses who smoke as serious health professionals.[16]

Act for Change

When nurses are off duty, their actions still say something about nursing. We urge nurses to consider acting as a health resource for their families, friends, and communities. Nurses can offer friendly advice on a wide range of health issues. They can also advocate for public health issues at their kids' school and in other settings. Doing so educates those who nurses help and those who nearby that nurses have health expertise.

Nurses can also advocate for public health. Consider working for health financing reform; more school nurses; or better dietary policies in schools, restaurants, and grocery stores. Sometimes nurses' professional organizations lead the way, and nurses might look to them for ideas. For example, consider the US National Association of Pediatric Nurse Practitioners' public opposition to corporal punishment, which got good coverage on the Examiner.com website in August 2011,[17] or the New Zealand Nurses Organisation's endorsement of World Smokefree Day, which got helpful coverage from Dunedin's Channel 39 in May 2010.[18] Nurses might try helping to improve the environment, reduce greenhouse gases, or find alternative sources of energy. Nurses might even signal their personal virtue by conserving energy. Or work to address preventable global diseases. Nurses who fight for global health send the message that they believe in their profession and that they fight for their patients' needs whether they are at the bedside or elsewhere. We're not saying nurses have to run for Congress or Parliament or something—although that might not be a bad idea, because we do need more nurses in power.

Educate Physicians and Medical Students

Nurses already teach physicians a great deal about health care in clinical settings, but they could do more to tell them about nursing. In addition to nursing out loud, nurses might reach out to local medical schools to promote the interprofessional training and shadowing programs discussed in Chapter 10. Nurses also might consider what nurse practitioner Margaret Helminiak does: "When my physician colleague calls for a nurse but really means a medical assistant, I go into the room and tell her, 'You called for a nurse. I am the only nurse here. Everyone else is a medical assistant.' "[19]

Equal Rights for Equal Work

Nurses should address physicians as physicians address them. If a physician calls a nurse by his or her given name, the nurse should call the physician by the same. If a physician asks to be called "Dr. Jones," the nurse should be called "Nurse Smith." If only senior physicians receive an honorific, senior nurses should be treated the same way. This makes it clear to all—including the media—that physicians are not nurses' masters or betters. Really. Nurses and doctors are colleagues, each worthy of respect.

Explaining Nursing's Role to Patients

Nurses often have difficulty acting as the patient advocates they have been trained to be, especially when that role brings them into conflict with physicians. We propose a basic statement that nurses might consider making available to their patients and colleagues. The statement could go something like this:

I Am Your Registered Nurse

During your stay here, it is my duty to protect you from all harm. That means any harm from your illness and its symptoms, from external forces including the care environment, and from other people. As an autonomous health professional who reports only to senior nurses, it is my job to protect you from poor or misguided health care from any source. I am your advocate. I vow to do my best to protect you as if you were a member of my family.

The Truth About Nursing has developed a downloadable poster of this statement, which we encourage nurses to hang in every patient's room![20]

Educating the Media about Nursing

Once nurses have embraced their power to create change and considered what they can do every day to improve the image of nursing, they should take a look at what the media is saying about their profession. Does it reflect the stereotypes we have discussed in this book? Next we discuss some ideas we have found useful in helping the media improve.

Develop Media Expertise and Get Coverage for Nursing

Nurses must stand up and be someone when the media is interested in health care in which nurses play a role—not simply defer to physicians, or slink into corners, as some nurses do. Here are some basic suggestions for nurses, prospective nurses, or anyone interested in the topic.

1) **Read *From Silence to Voice*.** The excellent book by Bernice Buresh and Suzanne Gordon is *the* how-to manual for nurses seeking to relate to the media.[21] Every nurse should read it.
2) **Observe experts on major media outlets.** Every day, experts in various fields present their views on television and radio networks, and in print media articles. Consider how these experts relate to journalists, how they present their basic positions and respond to questions. Consider how well prepared they are. Then practice presenting your points. Have a friend pose possible questions and practice responding to them.
3) **Study examples of good coverage of nursing wherever they appear.** Many press items worldwide have effectively highlighted nursing practice or research. A short December 2013 item in the *Southern Reporter* (Scotland) reported that a "pioneering" care model in the early recognition of patient decline developed by nurses at Borders General Hospital had attracted the attention of Danish specialists.[22] An August 2012 article in the *Peterborough Examiner* (Ontario) reported that

nurses at the local Kawartha Sexual Assault Centre had launched the "Don't Be That Guy" awareness campaign, primarily to convey to men that having sex with a woman who is too drunk to consent is rape.[23] In October 2008, the *New York Times* published a report about the research of Kristine Williams and colleagues at the University of Kansas, who found that use of "elderspeak" ("dear," "sweetie," "honey") causes patients to become aggressive and sends a message of incompetence, which starts them on a downward health trajectory.[24] In March 2006 the *Mainichi Daily News* published a piece about research by Japanese nurses who showed that when patients listened to relaxing enka music during cardiac catheterizations, it lowered their blood pressure by forty-four points—thereby decreasing the risk of potentially lethal punctures to their blood vessels.[25] Consider the information nurses gave the media to get this coverage.

4) **Make it a priority to help media creators understand nursing when they ask.** When the media contacts us, we put everything else aside and talk for as long as they wish. We treat every reporter as if he or she writes for the *New York Times* or *The Economist*. We follow up immediately by sending documents or other resources to supplement the information we provided and answer any additional questions the media may have. In addition to providing input on stories about nursing in the media, we have been quoted in pieces discussing the nursing shortage, nursing uniforms, Magnet status, men in nursing, sexual abuse in nursing, how military medics might become nurses, and other topics. We also refer the media to other nurses with expertise.
5) **Step up and respond, promptly.** The media moves quickly and media opportunities are usually fleeting. We once had a great television opportunity lined up for the director of a state nursing association, but she "had a meeting" that afternoon and couldn't do it. The issue was controversial, but this director could have used the chance to present her perspective and let viewers know that nursing leaders are responsive health professionals with opinions about public policy issues. In 2009 and 2010, after the small wave of new Hollywood nurse shows hit, NYU physician Marc Siegel consulted Sandy several times for expert comment on the shows as part of his occasional *Los Angeles Times* column "The Unreal World," which analyzed the realism of health-related entertainment television. These consultations entailed very quick turnarounds, but Sandy made it a priority to provide prompt and professional responses, parts of which did appear in the columns.[26]

6) **Establish relationships with local media and persuade them to cover nursing.** Invite your local media people to lunch or coffee, and tell them about the diverse work of nurses. Set up a luncheon or roundtable at which local nursing leaders talk to the media about their innovative practices or research. Invite the media to nursing meetings and seminars. Establish a Be a Nurse for a Day program so the media can follow nurses at work. Nurse researchers should consider the last step in their publication process to be coverage in the lay media. Send the media your research and tell them why their readers would find it compelling. Nursing journal editors should seek coverage from mainstream health journalists.
7) **Nurses did that!** Nurses should tell their best stories, but make sure the role of nurses is clear. The media needs to learn more about the dramatic work of nurses. The Truth About Nursing has a story idea database on its website, and we encourage nurses to submit their most dramatic stories—good and bad. Too often we hear that important care just "happened" (as if the hospital walls did it) or that "we" did it—both of which obscure the fact that *nurses* did it.
8) **Consider formal training.** If you will be appearing before the media with any frequency, we recommend in-person media training. The Truth About Nursing's website has more information on how to obtain it.[27]
9) **Be nurse-identified.** Sometimes nurse experts appear in the media, but the piece simply identifies them as a PhD or as "Dr. Bivens"—without mentioning that the expert is a nurse. This leads the public to credit physicians or other nonnurses for this nurse's expertise or work. If forced to choose between RN and PhD identifiers, please choose the RN. In August 2012 nursing scholar Elizabeth Winslow, who has done important work on the overuse of preoperative fasting, published a piece in the *American Journal of Nursing* urging nurse scholars to ensure that both academic and mainstream publications identify them as RNs.[28] Some famous people downplay their status as nurses. *Three Cups of Tea* author Greg Mortenson, who works to improve the education and health of girls in Pakistan and Afghanistan, is a nurse. But as of mid-2014, we still did not find that fact in the detailed biography at his book's website.[29] As *Nursing Spectrum* editor Pam Meredith wrote in a 2002 editorial, "Pick up that RN flag and wave it."[30]
10) **Don't let HIPAA paralyze you.** The Health Insurance Portability and Accountability Act (HIPAA) is designed to keep patient information confidential.[31] *It does not forbid nurses to speak about their work.* Overreacting to HIPAA can mean that nursing will be cut out of the media picture. One Johns Hopkins media professional involved with the 2008 ABC

documentary *Hopkins* told us that the hospital used a standard release form to comply with HIPAA. He said that 95 percent of patients readily consented, in a process that sometimes took as little as twenty seconds.[32] The hospital also put the television crew that filmed *Hopkins* through the hospital's standard HIPAA training program, so they could get their own consents. Of course, even if nurses do not get patients to sign release forms, they can still talk to the media about their work and patient care, as long as they disclose no information that identifies any specific patient.

Catch the Media Being Good

Although we spend significant time trying to persuade the media to do a better job, we also try to provide as much positive reinforcement as we can. When we do see an accurate, enlightening depiction of nursing, we try to thank those responsible, sometimes in a detailed analysis on the Truth About Nursing's website, but if that is not possible, even in a short email. Every nurse should consider doing the same.

A more formal way of reinforcing good portrayals of nursing is through awards, such as the annual Truth About Nursing Awards, a list of the best and worst media portrayals of nursing we've seen in the previous year. When we led the Center for Nursing Advocacy, we called them the Golden Lamp Awards. Naturally, most people like to be recognized for good work. When Tim Green, editor of the poetry magazine *Rattle*, began to prepare a special nursing issue, he asked us how he could make the issue worthy of one of our "ten best media depictions of the year" awards. He listened carefully to our views, although we played no role in his editorial choices. The issue's nurse-penned poetry was powerful, insightful, and devoid of stereotypes—and it did win a Golden Lamp for one of the best portrayals of 2007.[33]

Different Ways to Persuade the Media to Reconsider Products

We have often asked media creators to reconsider their products, from Hollywood shows to print advertising. In some cases, we have persuaded media creators to address our concerns with relatively little effort. Other campaigns have required major efforts, including thousands of letters and global media coverage. Here are some ways to reach media creators in different situations.

Telephone Calls

Sometimes the only tool required to affect media content is the telephone. In most of our campaigns to improve poor portrayals of nursing, we first call media makers. Constellation Brands launched a multimedia naughty nurse advertising campaign for Hydra vodka water in 2006.[34] We called the company's vice president of corporate communications, who quickly decided to remove the nurse elements from the campaign.

When Bloomingdale's department store ran a radio advertisement in November 2007 featuring a "nurse" seducing a "physician" with a cashmere sweater, we called the company's senior vice president of public relations, who asked for something in writing. We sent an email about a half hour later. Two hours later, after the close of business on a Friday, Bloomingdale's told us that it had begun calling radio stations to prevent the advertisement from running over that busy holiday season shopping weekend.[35]

After *People* magazine ran a photograph of Poison singer and reality TV star Bret Michaels surrounded by naughty nurses in a December 2010 issue, as noted in Chapter 5, we had a telephone conversation with the magazine's editor. He apologized, promised to avoid such imagery in the future, and published the Truth About Nursing's letter about the damage such imagery caused.[36]

Of course, telephone calls alone are not always enough. In those situations, we move to letters or letter-writing campaigns.

Letters and Emails

Sometimes it just takes one email to make a difference. In September 2006 we asked ALR Technologies to change the informal name of its ALRT500 home health management device from Electronic Nurse to a name that did not suggest that the machine could replace a real nurse. In an email, we explained that the device does not make professional judgments and take skilled actions based on years of college-level science education, as nurses do. The company soon apologized and removed the nickname.[37]

Letter-Writing Campaigns

When the above efforts fail, it's usually time to turn up the heat. Letter-writing campaigns have been pivotal in many of our efforts to improve media on nursing. Sometimes a few letters are enough to get some result. When the quiz show *Jeopardy!* wrongly implied in 2004 that nurse practitioners treat only "minor ailments," a handful of letters were enough to persuade the producers to place a question on the show designed to improve understanding of nursing.[38] In July 2010, we learned of a casting call for *Cali Nurse*, a reality show planned by Lambert Productions that seemed likely to suggest that nurses and nursing students were good-hearted, fun-loving cuties looking for "dates with McDreamy."[39] It took just 78 emails for us to get a constructive call with the company's executive vice president, who promised to keep our concerns about stereotypes in mind as production moved forward. We sent copies of the first edition of this book to the production team; the show never appeared.

Some media creators require more than a few letters. When Skechers launched its global advertising campaign featuring Christina Aguilera as a dominatrix naughty nurse in 2005, the company was unresponsive to our calls. However, after our supporters sent 3,000 emails over two weeks, Skechers removed the advertisements.[40] In August 2008 the Registered Nurses Association of Ontario (RNAO) sent a letter asking Canada's Neilson Dairy to end use of naughty nurse models in advertisements and at a related extreme sports tour. RNAO's one letter did not move the company, but more than a thousand letters from RNAO supporters did. A week later the company apologized and promised to remove the naughty nurse imagery.[41]

In October 2013, MTV introduced the nurse reality show *Scrubbing In*. The show did not exactly fulfill the promise of *Cali Nurse* (no one dated McDreamy!). But as discussed in Chapters 2 and 5, *Scrubbing In* did offer plenty of degraded sexual imagery and reality show drama, with virtually no impressive clinical interactions. Milwaukee nursing student Milka Stojanovic started a Change.org petition to cancel the show and, with help from Ontario nurse Tyler Kuhk, ultimately got more than 30,000 signatures. At the same time, several prominent nursing groups called for the show's cancellation, including the Canadian Nurses Association, the Emergency Nurses Association, the RNAO, the American Nurses Association, and National Nurses United. The Truth About Nursing added a petition with an analysis of the show that gained 500 more signatures.[42] MTV executives contacted the Truth About Nursing and in the end agreed to air the remaining episodes at a less prominent time, re-edit later episodes, and take steps to convey accurate information about nursing, including working with us to create a web page about becoming a nurse and a "day in the life" web feature about a skilled New York City nurse.[43]

Press Releases

When we launched our campaign in 2006 to ask the Heart Attack Grill in Arizona to remove the nurse theme from its waitresses' sexy costumes, we started with telephone calls to the restaurant's owner. These interactions proved too much for him. We moved to emails and a letter-writing campaign, but those were not effective either.[44] Next we issued a press release to every print and broadcast media outlet in Arizona and to major media outside the state. A local television station picked it up, and the story quickly appeared in thousands of broadcast and major print media news outlets around the world.[45] Not everyone agreed with our position, and so far we have still not persuaded the Grill to end its use of the naughty nurse. But tens of millions of people heard our message about how nursing stereotypes affect nursing, helping to educate the public about the profession's value.

Consider the November 2010 weight loss segment of *The Dr. Oz Show* in which some "nurses" "got sexy" and danced with Oz, also discussed in Chapter 5. Our campaign about that generated hundreds of powerful letters, but it did not move the show to any real action. So we issued a press release.[46] The Associated Press did a story, which was soon picked up by 2,200 news entities across the world, including the *New York Times*, the *Los Angeles Times*, Online Nigeria, the *Times of India*, New Zealand Yahoo, and the Arabic language *Wael El-Ebrashy*. Oz issued a statement that closely resembled an apology and he promised to do better in the future.[47] A year later, his show broadcast the substantial, well-meaning "NURSES' SECRETS" segment discussed in Chapter 3.

Unorthodox Approaches

There are many ways to get the media's attention. For instance, in 2006 we sent a "worst portrayal of nursing" award to rock star Jack White, along with our analysis of his 2005 White Stripes song "The Nurse."[48] We explained how his lyrics associated a "nurse" with romantic love, mothering, and housekeeping. In response, White sent Sandy a satirical "Metaphorical Ignorance Award." White evidently did not grasp that we were actually objecting to his use of *metaphor* to reinforce nursing stereotypes: we did not imagine that his song was saying a real nurse rubbed salt in his physical wounds. But having gotten his attention, we issued a press release about our mock-award exchange and got coverage for our issues in the *Los Angeles Times, Salon*, and elsewhere.[49]

Options are greater for those with greater resources. In March 2014 the Nova Scotia Government and General Employees Union, which represented nurses at the Capital Health hospital group, ran television advertisements during a contract dispute to explain that patient safety is at risk when nurses are forced to care for too many patients.[50] The California Nurses Association (CNA) has used a wide variety of creative tactics, some controversial, to get its messages out. In the mid-2000s, after California governor Arnold Schwarzenegger opposed implementation of nurse staffing legislation that CNA had fought to pass, the union protested at his appearances across the United States and used various advertisements to tell the public about the dangers of high nurse-to-patient ratios.[51] After CNA won its campaign for minimum ratios,[52] it set its sights on universal health coverage.[53] In May 2008, CNA ran an advertisement in the *Washington Post* referring to Vice President Cheney's excellent federal government health insurance: "If Dick Cheney were anyone else, he'd probably be dead by now."[54] In June 2011, National Nurses United, the union CNA helped to found, held the first of many vigorous street protests calling on Congress to impose a 1 percent tax on Wall Street transactions to fund health care and other needs, predating the Occupy Wall Street protests held later in the year.[55] Not everyone applauded these positions and tactics, but they drew attention to CNA's issues.

Persuading Media Decision Makers in Direct Interactions

Let's say you want to affect what a specific media creator is telling the public about nursing right now. How would you do it? We have some suggestions.

Identify and Reach the Decision Maker

Many corporations have customer service telephone numbers, but those who staff them usually have little decision-making power, and they often seem to be trained to deflect concerns about their media rather than address them. We have found them receptive in only one instance, when the head of customer service at Coors in the US worked with us to convince the company's Canadian division to discontinue naughty nurse advertising in late 2006.[56]

When we reach the person who has the power to decide how a specific media product is made or shown to the public, that person will often listen and work with us. But identifying the decision maker is not always easy. That person's identity depends on the medium. For the news media, the person you want is usually the reporter or an editor. In commercial advertising, it's usually the vice president of marketing, consumer affairs, or corporate communications. In television, it is generally the executive producers. In film, it is usually the director and the writer.

In 2002, when we first tried to persuade the US government to reconsider the name of its Take a Loved One health campaign, Sandy called the main telephone line of the Department of Health and Human Services' Office of Minority Health. She was transferred to a low-level official. We got nowhere.

In 2004 we tried again, and this time we found the decision maker—the director of the Office of Minority Health—but his assistant would not set up a telephone call with him. So we launched a letter-writing campaign, and more than 300 supporters sent him emails.[57] The director's assistant then agreed to set up a call between the director and Sandy. In a constructive discussion, he vowed to explore a better name for the campaign, and it was later changed.

In 2006 CVS ran television advertisements suggesting that a pharmacist had transformed a patient's spouse into a "nurse" after a few hours of training in how to give medications.[58] We called CVS and were transferred to about fifteen different people and subdivisions of CVS over the course of four or five days. Finally we reached the company's vice president of customer service. He was very helpful in working with us to remove the nurse element of the advertisement.

In 2007 Seattle's Group Health launched advertisements for its "Ask the Doc" service that included the tag line "Nurse, hand me my laptop," suggesting that nurses are there to fetch things for physicians. Several nurses at Group Health, led by Carolyn Elliot, lobbied the company's marketing people to remove the spot, but they were told they had failed to appreciate the ad's "humor." The marketing director was "hopeful that [nurses] can let this go and we can all remember that we're all on the same team." So the nurses lobbied the CEO. He pulled the advertisement.[59]

In 2013, the urgent care chain American Family Care (AFC) aired television advertisements assuring the public that AFC patients got to see "a doctor, not a nurse," a baseless insult to advanced practice nurses, as noted in Chapter 9.[60] Sandy placed about seven calls, one per day, to the corporation's director of marketing. That person did not return the calls. Then Sandy called the CEO and left a detailed message. Finally, AFC's "chief medical officer," a physician, returned her call. After a long discussion in which the physician insisted that the physician care was better because physicians typically get more formal education, and Sandy explained that decades of actual evidence showed that advanced practice RN care was at least as effective,[61] the physician said AFC would pull the advertisement. Granted, he also said AFC would likely replace it with one that still told patients they would get to see a physician, which is not much better. It was not the most satisfying interaction, but at least we had found the decision-maker we needed.

Although assistants and receptionists do not have decision-making authority, it is vital that you treat them with respect. That is not just because it's the right thing to do, but also because assistants often control access. Although your goal is generally to get to their bosses, you should treat the assistants as if they *were* the decision makers. If you persuade them that your concern has merit—or at least that you are serious and will not waste their boss's time—you have a better chance of getting past them and maybe even influencing their presentation to their bosses to favor your view.

In general, if you're getting nowhere with the person you're dealing with, don't hesitate to politely go over his or her head. Just keep contacting people until you find the person who can make the decision. Be persistent!

Be Persistent!

If there is one tactic in getting the media to listen that supersedes all other tactics, it is *relentless persistence*. Make it clear that you will not go away until the person or organization you are dealing with fixes the media problem. It does not always work, but often it does.

In October 2013 nursing student Milka Stojanovic started a Change.org petition to persuade MTV to cancel *Scrubbing In*, as noted previously. But Milka did not just start the petition and wait; she undertook a multi-pronged social media offensive. That involved emailing the petition link to her academic contacts, Facebook-messaging major nursing schools, and posting the link on discussion forums everywhere from the MTV website to a leading social-networking site for nurses—which soon banned her for supposedly spam-posting the link. Then she really boosted the campaign by targeting prominent nursing blogs on the Tumblr platform and contacting those whose Tumblr tags indicated they had issues with the show. Milka also noticed that the show was starting to generate a lot of Twitter activity, including prodigious tweeting by nurse Tyler Kuhk, who even managed to engage with some of the show's cast members. Tyler also discussed the show with well-placed contacts at the Ontario Nurses Association, which started a campaign, as did other prominent Canadian and US nursing organizations. These collective efforts led to online and television reports in Canada—and more than 31,000 signatures on Milka's petition. MTV noticed.

In November 2009 the Lung Cancer Alliance (LCA) launched a major public awareness campaign built on a satirical rap video featuring a "Dr. Lung Love" character surrounded by naughty nurses, as explained in Chapter 5.[62] Early that month, the Truth About Nursing posted an analysis and started a campaign, which generated more than 100 letters to LCA. At the same time, we began calling LCA daily, trying to reach the group's executive director. When that route was fruitless, we began calling the group's board, which included some prominent figures from the fields of health care and government, leaving detailed voicemail messages. After a couple of weeks, we finally got a letter from LCA's executive director. She detailed LCA's good works and past support for nursing, and she said she understood nurses' concerns about the "perceived misrepresentation." But LCA did virtually nothing to address them. So we urged supporters to call her directly. At the same time, we had issued a press release, and *Modern Healthcare*, the influential magazine for healthcare executives, soon ran a substantial story about our concerns. Before the end of the month, LCA had quietly removed the video from its website.[63]

In 2007 Cadbury Schweppes Canada ran television commercials featuring female nurses hopping into bed with male patients who chewed Dentyne Ice gum.[64] We called to discuss the advertisement. The company's director of corporate communications in Canada was notably unreceptive to our concerns. ("We test marketed it and no one complained that it was offensive!"). For over a week we had daily conversations that yielded no positive result. So we launched a letter-writing campaign. The RNAO joined us and launched its own letter-writing campaign. But even after a combined 1,500 letters from our two groups, the communications director would not budge. In the meantime Sandy found the work telephone numbers of the top seven Cadbury Schweppes executives in the world and began calling them daily, connecting exclusively with their voicemail. She left them lengthy, detailed messages about the complex role media undervaluation plays in the global nursing shortage. After a week, the CEO of Cadbury Schweppes called Sandy from London to apologize, discuss her concerns, and to tell her he was pulling the advertisement.[65]

Study the Media Product and Anticipate Arguments

Before contacting media creators, look closely at the media product. Are parts of it ironic? Is it actually criticizing a stereotype rather than endorsing it? Media creators are more likely to listen if you show that you understand their work but still have an issue with it. Likewise, if a counter-argument is almost certain to be made, it may make sense to address it up front. This tactic may lessen resistance, or at least show that you have thought carefully about the issue. For example, when dealing with naughty nurse imagery, you can count on being told that it's "just a joke," though "jokes" are one of the most common ways to spread harmful stereotypes, as discussed in Chapter 5. We try to convey that we get the joke, or would appreciate a joke that was not so tired and offensive. When we contacted Fox News Channel's *Redeye* about an April 2008 show celebrating the naughty nurse stereotype, we presented our analysis in a satirical letter pretending to praise the show for embracing the stereotype.[66] Our press releases about such imagery, like the one we did about the naughty-axe film *Nurse 3D* in February 2014, typically include humorous elements to show that we understand the joking element in the imagery.[67]

Play Good Cop/Bad Cop

Advocates may confront choices about whether to focus more on the "inside track" (such as by offering gentle private suggestions that might move powerful media creators slightly in the right direction) or the "outside track" (such as by offering rigorous public analysis of the meaning and effects of specific media products, which makes collaboration with creators less likely). We have adopted different approaches in different contexts, although we are better known for the outside approach. Of course, not everyone has to approach things the same way. We've noticed that nursing has no shortage of "inside track" adherents.

In some cases, a combination of these approaches may be effective. We started asking *ER* to improve its portrayal of nursing in 2001. For some time in the early 2000s, it was rare for the minor nurse characters to appear on the show. In contrast to the many physician characters, the one major nurse character had little clinical role, and she spent most of her time engaged in romances with physicians or enduring family tragedies. We had a lengthy, cordial conference call with an *ER* producer and the show's "medical" adviser in late 2001, but it was pretty clear the show did not want our advice on an ongoing basis. So we began sending the show our critical analyses of its episodes and urging our supporters to pressure it to improve, and we did so until the show ended in 2009.[68] We understand that the show did not like these efforts, but a stronger major nurse character named Sam Taggart was introduced in late 2003, and she was ultimately featured in many of the show's best nursing plotlines.[69]

In March 2005 we urged advertisers to withhold their advertisements until *ER* improved. The next month, the senior vice president of global medical affairs for pharmaceutical giant Schering-Plough, physician Hans Vemer, responded to our campaign by asking the show to help address the nursing shortage by developing "stories that highlight accurate roles, responsibilities, skills and contributions of today's modern nursing profession."[70]

We understand that Sojourn Communications, a Hollywood-based communications company, played a key role in helping *ER* develop the Eve Peyton plotlines of late 2005, which addressed some of our concerns about nursing skill and autonomy; indeed, some scenes might easily have been crafted by us. Peyton's exit drew heavily on the battle-axe image, but on the whole the episodes were helpful.

After 2005, *ER* at times made a point of displaying nursing autonomy and skill. In the show's final season, Taggart even started a nurse anesthetist program, breaking the show's tradition of having major nurse characters aspire to medical school when they pursue graduate studies. There was little more about nursing leaders or managers, and the physician-centric show still fell well short of a good portrayal of nursing, but on the whole, it made a clear improvement.[71]

Move Fast

It is often easier to get the attention of media figures if you're able to connect with them soon after a troubling portrayal appears. That's especially true of talk radio. In June 2007, when radio host Stephanie Miller and sidekick Jim Ward had some fun with naughty nurse stereotyping, we sent them an analysis, and they promptly read and mocked parts of it on the air. Within minutes, a supporter called Sandy and she quickly called the show, which allowed her on the air briefly to explain her concerns.[72]

In January 2006, on Sean Hannity's radio show, one caller asked a US soldier who had been an inpatient at Walter Reed Army hospital whether there were any "hot nurses" there. The soldier reportedly replied that there were "a few pretty ones" but that most were "motherly." A supporter immediately notified us, and Sandy called Hannity's office. Twenty minutes later, Sean Hannity called us back, and we talked about nursing stereotypes for some time. Hannity made supportive comments about nurses on the air in the following days.[73]

Use the Media's Own Process

Some media creators have procedures for challenging their conduct. For example, in 2007 Heineken began running Dos Equis advertisements in which "the most interesting man in the world" bench-pressed two young women in short white dresses and nurses' caps.[74] Following the advice of a Heineken corporate relations officer, we appealed to an independent board that handles such matters for Heineken, using codes of marketing that Heineken follows. Among other things, we argued that the spot violated the Heineken International Commercial Communication Code, which required that advertisements "be prepared with due regard for our social responsibility" and that they not "impugn human dignity and integrity." The review board, which included former US vice presidential candidate Geraldine Ferraro, agreed that the advertisement should be changed. Heineken then digitally altered the women's clothing to remove the nurse elements and proceeded to air that version.

Collaborate

In various campaigns, we have collaborated with the American Nurses Association, Canadian Nurses Association, National Nurses United, the American College of Nurse Midwives, and the RNAO, as well as many other groups and individuals. Collaboration has enabled us to mount much larger and more effective campaigns. It was clearly a critical factor in the MTV campaign, as well as in our work successfully challenging the US government's Take a Loved One to the Doctor campaign and the Dentyne Ice advertisement. In January 2014, after the American Academy of Nurse Practitioners had joined us and more than 1,500 Truth About Nursing supporters in protesting the mockery of nurse practitioners on *Lab Rats*, Disney agreed to alter the troubling episode to eliminate the insult to nurse practitioners in future airings and to take steps to avoid similar issues in the future.[75] Sometimes we have been able to get help from companies outside the nursing community, as we did when Schering-Plough wrote to *ER*. When Mattel released its Nurse Quacktitioner doll, we convinced Walmart to sell the dolls back to Mattel, as a way of adding pressure on Mattel. Unfortunately, Mattel did not agree to the buy-back.[76]

Suggest Alternatives

Media creators may be receptive if they are presented with an alternative way they can achieve their goals without reinforcing nursing stereotypes. In the 2013 *Scrubbing In* campaign, we proposed several things that MTV might do besides simply canceling the show, which was a long shot given the network's investment and the advanced stage the show had reached, with all filming complete. We urged MTV to try to maximize the use of clinical segments, and the network agreed to do what it could with the few episodes on which editing was not complete, although we can't claim to have seen great improvement. Among our ideas was that MTV provide information to its young audience about nursing careers and practice. The network obliged by working with us on the online efforts described previously. We also asked MTV to consult with us should it decide to produce a second season of *Scrubbing In* or any other program featuring nurses, so we could try to help them create a better portrayal of nursing. MTV agreed to do so.[77]

In 2005 Walmart placed an advertisement in nursing journals featuring a "nurse" and the tag line "It doesn't take a brain surgeon to recognize a good deal on scrubs." We contacted Walmart to object to the suggestion that nurses aren't all that smart. The company not only agreed to change the advertising copy, but also took us up on our offer to help.[78]

Sometimes it can be helpful to propose a specific alternative course to the media, even if there is little chance the media creator will adopt it. After reading our analysis of a damaging January 2007 episode of *Grey's Anatomy*, nurse Mandy Mayling of Los Angeles wrote and sent the show an alternative script. The inventive script showed how the episode might have featured at least as much drama while accurately representing nursing.[79]

Expect Resistance

Change can be scary. So changing the way people think is not easy or quick. Since the beginning, we have faced vigorous opposition from some media creators and supporters. Naughty nurse fans can be especially committed, but Hollywood shows and pop musicians also enjoy a good deal of blind loyalty. Some wonder how we keep going in the face of this. But we believe that US nurses and supporters have a special obligation to reduce negative stereotyping of nursing because US media often has so much global influence. We recall Mahatma Gandhi, who described the path to social change this way:[80]

First they ignore you;
Then they laugh at you;
Then they attack you;
Then you win.

Nursing has been largely absent from serious discussions of health care in the media for decades. It's not exactly encouraging to be laughed at or attacked, but we believe those are huge steps up from being ignored. In some cases these reactions have been a prelude to achieving our immediate goal of improving a given media product—and, we believe, our larger goal of changing the way people think about nursing. In December 2013, *Forbes* posted a piece by contributor Leah Binder that recognized writing on health care that produced "disruptive innovation," creating change by "gor[ing] somebody's ox."[81] Binder, CEO of the respected hospital-safety organization The Leapfrog Group, titled her piece "The Best Disruptive Writings of 2013—Health Care Edition." She recognized the Truth About Nursing's work under the heading "Gored Oxen Four: Conventional Wisdom About Delivering Care."

Organize Chapters of the Truth About Nursing

As of early 2014, the Truth About Nursing has local chapters throughout the United States and in 14 other nations, but we are always looking to start more. Chapters meet periodically and consider ways to encourage local media to improve its treatment of nursing. One active Truth About Nursing chapter has been our Las Vegas affiliate, under the leadership of copresidents Dee Riley and Michele Nichols. In May 2010 the chapter held an event at the Jet Nightclub in the Mirage Hotel to protest a naughty nurse costume contest. Our members cheerfully spoke with club patrons about the value of nursing and the problems with the naughty nurse image. In November 2011 the chapter held a peaceful protest outside the Heart Attack Grill, which by that time had made its way to Las Vegas with its naughty nurse servers. Members handed out hundreds of flyers to Grill customers and passersby.[82] If nurses in every media market worked together to implement the ideas in this book, media all over the world would change the way it treats nursing. There is more information about starting a chapter on the Truth About Nursing's website.[83]

Message in a Bottle: Create Your Own Media

Nurses know best what nursing is and what nurses do, so they should explain their work to the world directly. Some nurses have actually become media professionals, and some media professionals have become nurses, both of which we encourage. But you don't need to be a media professional to create compelling media: you can use a personal blog to improve understanding. Depending on their interests, nurses might use written work; visual, performance, and tactile media; and video, broadcast, and film.

Writing about Nursing

Writing has many benefits as a way to help others understand nursing. It allows for precise, detailed explanation that can be very helpful for a profession that needs to convey complex skills and thought processes.

Letters to the Editor

Letters to the editor are a great place for anyone to start. Letters can be as short as one paragraph, and they are easier to get published than some other types of traditional print media. Letters are often used to persuade the media to do better, but they can influence the public in their own right. For example, in March 2011 the widely read *People* magazine published Sandy's short letter explaining why the publication's recent printing of a photograph of reality television star Bret Michaels surrounded by naughty nurses was a problem.[84]

A February 2006 issue of *Good Housekeeping* included an effective letter from nurse Berni Martin protesting a feature from a past issue that had included a health tip from an anonymous emergency department physician that readers should lie to triage nurses in order to be seen faster.[85]

Not all letters need to respond to specific past media items; some discuss issues of the day. In May 2005 the *Wawatay News* in Ontario published a Nurses Week letter to the editor by Canadian federal health nurse Lyn Button of the Sioux Lookout Zone. The letter provided special insight into what nurses do for patients in remote rural communities. [86]

Don't be discouraged if your first letter doesn't get published. Many of ours don't get published either. But some do, and none would ever get published if we were discouraged by every rejection. Be persistent!

Op-eds

We urge nurses to write op-eds (opinion-editorial pieces), which can show that nurses have valuable perspectives on a wide variety of health issues. In October 2010 the *Washington Post* ran an excellent op-ed by nurse practitioner Veneta Masson explaining why she no longer got annual mammograms.[87] Reviewing the research, Masson found no evidence that the test saved lives, but she noted the severe harm many had suffered from unnecessary treatment following false-positive results. In August 2009 nurse Linda Record Srungaram wrote a strong op-ed for the *Houston Chronicle* arguing that Texas nurses needed better whistle-blower protection, noting that two nurses had actually been indicted after filing a complaint about a physician with the state medical board.[88] (After a long ordeal, the nurses were not convicted.)[89] Nurse Kathleen Bartholemew's powerful March 2009 piece in the *Seattle Post-Intelligencer* urged the public to reconsider the allocation of healthcare resources, citing recent layoffs at a local hospital.[90] In December 2005 the *Milwaukee Journal Sentinel* published Gina Dennik-Champion's persuasive op-ed supporting pending legislation to authorize medical marijuana use.[91] That same month the Toronto *Globe and Mail* ran a moving op-ed by Calgary maternity nurse Raewyn Janota, who described the care she provided to a couple whose baby was stillborn.[92]

Getting op-eds published can be challenging, especially if you are trying for a major periodical or have a message that editors do not expect. When we got our op-ed arguing for a Nobel Prize in nursing published in the *Baltimore Sun* in December 2006, it was the culmination of *three years* of work. We revised the draft many times, sought out a noted coauthor (ultimately persuading the prominent nursing professor Kristine Gebbie to join us), and submitted the op-ed to many publications before we succeeded. So be tenacious, revise, seek advice, and keep pitching your message.

Feature Articles

Nurses don't need to depend on reporters to cover them, because they can write about their own work! One common way to do that is through features, which describe interesting events or ideas that are not breaking news. In March 2010 nurse Laura Stokowski published a powerful "Letter to Hollywood" on Medscape, the prominent website for health professionals, outlining the common myths about nursing that Hollywood promotes and explaining what nurses really do for patients.[93] Another example is John Blanton's excellent April 2007 *Wall Street Journal* article about his post-9/11 journey from *WSJ* editor to intensive care unit nurse and back again.[94]

Advertisements

Placing advertisements in the mainstream print media can be expensive. We have managed to get significant media coverage without paying for it (and needless to say we have also tried and failed to do so many times). For most nurses that is probably the best avenue for media attention. However, those with resources have placed paid advertisements that give the public helpful information about nursing. In 1997 the British Columbia Nurses' Union put out an advertisement featuring a photograph of a nurse taking her patient's pulse. The text read: "He thinks he's having a conversation about the hospital jello. She's actually midway through about 100 assessments."[95] Of course, there was no room to articulate everything nurses assess, plan, and decide, and at the right time we might hope the nurse would also consider some "nursing out loud." But the advertisement told the public that nursing is complex and important, with a sly reference to the continuing invisibility of nursing expertise.

Nonfiction Books

Many nurses have written nonfiction books to explain their nursing experience or help people with their expertise. Writing and publishing a book can be a serious project, but books can have a lasting impact. Consider keeping a journal of dramatic events that have happened to you over the previous shift. Do this for a year—or for a week, depending on where you work—and you may have enough fodder for a book!

Memoirs can be an effective way for nurses to tell people about nursing. Echo Heron is well known for dramatic nonfiction books about her work, starting with the best-selling *Intensive Care: The Story of a Nurse* (1988).[96] Claire Bertschinger published *Moving Mountains* (2005) about caring for children in the 1980s Ethiopian famine—work that reportedly inspired the 1985 Live Aid benefit.[97] More recent memoirs about the work of strong, autonomous nurses include Jennifer Culkin's *A Final Arc of Sky* (2009), an account of critical care and emergency flight nursing that was both powerfully written and very specific in its descriptions of nursing expertise,[98] and *The Nightingale of Mosul* (2010) by Susan Luz (with Marcus Brotherton), in which a high-ranking military reserve nurse related her adventures in Iraq and challenging nursing positions around the world.[99]

Some nurses have written books to educate the public about health issues. Nurse Pat Carroll's *What Nurses Know and Doctors Don't Have Time to Tell You* (2004) effectively explained important health principles to the lay public, although it was marred by a title that managed to both celebrate and denigrate nurses.[100] Nurses Gloria Mayer and Ann Kuklierus have written four influential "plain talk" books for the public, including 1999's *What to Do When Your Child Gets Sick*, which is sent to the parents of every newborn child in California and South Dakota courtesy of the state.[101] Nurse Serita Stevens, a prolific author and screenwriter, wrote *Forensic Nurse* (2004) to explain that growing field to the public.[102] Nurse Cheryl Dellasega, an expert in relational aggression, writes books to help women, girls, and nurses improve their relationships, including *Forced to Be Family* (2007).[103]

Nurses can also contribute to books edited by others. For example, *Nurse—Past, Present, and Future: The Making of Modern Nursing* (2010), edited by Kate Trant and Susan Usher, is a short but striking book of text and photographs. With short essays and stories by nurses from around the world, the book combines basic concepts and cutting-edge issues to highlight the history, diversity, and importance of modern nursing.[104]

Novels

Novels can be a very powerful way to convey the nursing experience. One of the highest-profile novelist nurses is Echo Heron, who has written several hospital thrillers, including *Fatal Diagnosis* (2000).[105] Nurse Elizabeth Ann Scarborough wrote *The Healer's War* (1989), a mystical novel about a US military nurse in the Vietnam War that won the Nebula Award for best US science fiction or fantasy novel of the year.[106] Nurse Richard Ferri's *Confessions of a Male Nurse* (2005) was a funny account of a gay man in nursing, although we were uneasy with the way it presented the main character's love affair with a physician, which seemed to suggest that medicine had far greater value than nursing.[107] Other nurses have written novels, but few prominent ones seem to focus on nursing. The world is waiting for yours!

Other Literature and Storytelling

Nurses participate in compelling dramas every day: write about them! There are many avenues for nurses who want to write about nursing. Veneta Masson has published books of poetry that reflect her years as a nurse in Washington, DC; the most recent was *Clinician's Guide to the Soul* (2008).[108] The poetry magazine *Rattle*'s 2007 special issue on nursing also included many impressive nurse poets who explored the healthcare experience from a nurse's perspective. In December 2008 forensic nurse and poet Carmen Henesy got publicity for a poem begging San Francisco Mayor Gavin Newsom not to slash funding for nurses who treat child-sex abuse victims.[109] Nurses can also tell the public something of what they do through short fiction, which is published in a variety of magazines.

Even satirical pieces can convey something of the nursing experience. In 2005 we issued a satirical April Fool's Day press release about a groundbreaking study published in the *Journal of the American Medical Association* concluding that nurses are skilled, autonomous professionals who do vital work to improve public health. We included fake reaction from a variety of prominent media sources who professed shock. The "study"—which we invented—was entitled "Who Knew?"[110]

Kids' Literature

A compelling series of children's books about modern nursing could be very effective, especially since many children's books, like Holly Hobbie's *Fanny* (2008),[111] suggest that medicine is the really desirable healthcare career—particularly for ambitious girls. We need books to highlight the value of nursing for toddlers, preschoolers, elementary kids, tweens, and teenagers.

One series of novels that inspired many children to become nurses was the *Cherry Ames* series, originally published from 1943 to 1968.[112] Springer Publishing reissued the series in 2005–2007, but the gender and nurse-physician relations are antiquated and unlikely to impress today's young readers. Nurse Serita Stevens wrote *Charlie London, RN* in 2004 to try to update the Cherry Ames series.[113] The main nurse character was bright and positive, but we found that her reverence for physicians undermined the message about nursing. We need works that show nursing is as valuable and challenging as medicine.

Of course, J. K. Rowling's Harry Potter books do include the very minor nurse character Madam Poppy Pomfrey, who is skilled at healing in a supernatural setting. But we need nurses to put nursing center stage.[114] Maybe Harry Potter could become a flight nurse; that broom would be pretty quick to accident scenes!

The Internet: Websites, Blogs, and Discussion Boards

In 2012 the Internet was estimated to have more than 2.4 billion users worldwide, including most of the public in the developed world, and there were estimated to be 634 million websites.[115] Virtually all the written media forms discussed previously are now available online. The Internet is the main way the Truth About Nursing interacts with the media and the public. The Internet offers countless communication avenues that might help nurses tell the public what they do.

Many nursing discussion boards and blogs are available to all Internet users. They are important ways to spread information about nurses to the public. Some do a good job of exploring current nursing issues. However, some popular nursing discussion boards do not always convey to members of the public who stumble upon them that nurses are well-educated professionals. Of course, these are places nurses go to vent and discuss their very real work difficulties. But we urge nurses to consider if their posts would inspire decision makers to give nursing the resources it needs.

Websites have become an essential communication tool. Some nurse-created sites try to give the public information about what nursing is, including the Truth About Nursing's www.truthaboutnursing.org. Johnson & Johnson's Campaign for Nursing's Future has significant information about nursing on its website, www.discovernursing.com.

Nurses should consider creating or enhancing websites to explain nursing, including the sites of their employers and professional groups. Websites are now the public face of an organization. Nursing schools often profile their faculty, letting the public know about professors' credentials and interests. But it is still rare to find much about nurses on hospital websites, as we explained in Chapter 10 in discussing the Truth About Nursing's 2012 analysis of the sites of leading US hospitals.[116] As we noted, few websites highlight nursing care or the people who deliver it in any detail, much less the detail devoted to physicians. Site sections that do describe nursing seem to be aimed mostly at nurses themselves. For example, we have seen no websites that advertise a hospital's Magnet status as a draw to patients—we have only seen it used as a nursing recruitment tool.

Massachusetts General Hospital's site (www.massgeneral.org) does list the credentials of a small number of nursing leaders in some detail and it describes the work of many nursing teams, units, and programs. However, the descriptions appear with those of other nonphysician professions under "Patient Care Services." They appear to be directed at nurses rather than patients. They are brief and bland, paling in comparison to the extensive, high-production-value promotion of the hospital's medical departments, which boast about the qualifications and care of physicians. The site also has a page with links to information about the hospital's Magnet Recognition, but little effort to make it comprehensible to anyone outside nursing; it's hard to imagine a lay person spending time there.[117]

Make sure that your institution's website conveys *to the public* the key role nurses play in patient care. To develop a website, ask media relations professionals for help. You might profile each nursing service and individual nurses. The public should be able to learn who is doing the nursing, including the nurses' educational background and credentials, as well as contact information so families and the public can get answers to their questions. Include headshots and contact information for each nurse, not just the top executives. What innovations have your nurses played a role in? Have their achievements been in the news or recognized by nursing groups? Explain how your institution is working to improve nursing care. Consider including photographs, audio, and video. Be sure it is easy to get to the nursing material from the site's main page. It may be more effective to integrate information about nursing in the site areas that promote the institution's health field–specific institutes, centers, and departments—you know, where the sites tend to boast about their great physicians and suggest the physicians are doing or directing everything that matters. Some sites have a "Find a Physician" link from the main page. Consider adding a "Find a Nurse" link right next to it, so visitors can contact any nurse in the hospital.

Many people look for general health information on the Internet. Nurses can create websites to educate their patients or communities about health, and in doing so, illustrate nursing expertise. In today's managed care environment, many patients get home after a hospital visit with little idea how to manage their conditions. They may not understand how to use their crutches, monitor their wounds, test their blood sugar levels, exercise, or avoid foods that put them at risk. Even when hospital nurses manage to give patients this information, patients may forget or simply be overwhelmed. The Internet can be a great way to fill this need and perhaps prevent future hospitalizations. If you do set up an informational website, consider becoming certified by

Health on the Net Foundation, an international nongovernmental organization that guides consumers to reliable health websites.[118]

Visual, Performance, and Tactile Media

Nurses can also use many exciting types of media to *show* the world what they do and why it matters. Memorials, exhibits, and other media can help shape the public's view of nursing and its history. We have already proposed an international museum of modern nursing, which nurses should play the key role in establishing.

Some nurses have taken the lead in developing effective visual displays. When nurse Diane Carlson Evans realized that the two US Vietnam war memorials in Washington, DC, failed to include nurses' contributions, she spent nine years lobbying legislators and the public. The result was the US Vietnam Women's Memorial, dedicated in 1993, a statue of three nurses and a patient involved in a hopeful rescue operation.[119]

In 2003 nurses at the University of Pennsylvania played a key role in organizing the Philadelphia Fabric Workshop and Museum's exhibit "RN: The Past, Present and Future of the Nurses' Uniform." This exhibit was the source of the RN patches discussed previously, which enable nurses to identify themselves to patients and colleagues.[120]

Some have tried to capture the nursing experience in photographs. It can be hard for still images to convey what most people really need to learn about nurses: that they are life-saving professionals with advanced skills. Without the full context, it's also easy for some photographs of nurses providing emotional support to their patients to reinforce the angel stereotype. Still, photographs are worth trying, especially when accompanying words can provide that context.

In 2005 and 2007, the *American Journal of Nursing* sponsored Faces of Caring: Nurses at Work, a contest designed to capture the best photographs of nurses.[121] Some winning photographs were among the best still images of nurses we have seen. Only some of the photographs were taken by nurses themselves; we encourage more nurses to take photographs of their colleagues at work.

And in 2012, photographer Carolyn Jones published *The American Nurse*, a coffee table book of portraits that received a lot attention from nurses and even a *PARADE* magazine feature in May 2013.[122] On the whole, the portraits and brief accompanying interview text gave a sense of the wide-ranging work of nursing, and a few even suggested how nurses use their skills to help patients. Jones also made a fine feature-length documentary film called *The American Nurse: Healing America* (2014) about five of the profiled nurses.[123] The nurses came off as strong, committed people who think holistically and make their own clinical decisions. Nurses who have made their mark in pop music include Naomi Judd, as well as John Darnielle of the Mountain Goats. But we are not aware that many nurses have created music that addresses nursing directly, as Sonic Youth's *Sonic Nurse* (2004) did.[124] Nurses should consider it. They Might Be Giants's *Here Comes Science* (2009) shows that clever pop music can teach listeners about science.

Plays and other spoken performances are compelling media that more nurses should consider. *Nurse!* was a one-woman off-Broadway play sponsored by the New York State Nurses Association.[125] Based on actual nurses' strikes, the 2003 play's characters faced the dilemma of working mandatory overtime or losing their jobs. Some nurses also do comedy performances that convey some of the nursing experience. Hawaii's Hob Osterlund, a clinical nurse specialist in pain management, has a comic alter ego called Ivy Push who hosts the "Chuckle Channel," which aims to improve patient health through laughter.[126] Neonatal intensive care unit nurse Greg Williams does nurse-themed stand-up comedy in Atlanta, Georgia, and around the nation.[127]

Stamps and other collectible items can help nursing. A number of nations have paid tribute to the profession in stamps, and not surprisingly, Florence Nightingale has appeared on many of these stamps. The US Postal Service has also issued stamps honoring nurses Clara Barton, Mary Breckinridge, Dorothea Dix, Phoebe Pember, and Clara Maass, as well as nurse-author Louisa May Alcott, nurse-pilot Amelia Earhart, nurse-abolitionist Harriet Tubman, and the nursing profession as a whole.[128] In October 2008 the American College of Nurse-Midwives worked with the Postal Service to create a stamp series about nurse midwife care.[129] Since the Postal Service began allowing others to design their own stamps, several vendors now sell them. Zazzle's collection of nurse stamps is certainly not free of generic and angel-oriented options, but it also includes stamps with messages like "Nursing is the hardest job you'll ever love" (featuring a stack of textbooks with impressive titles) and "I can fix it! I'm a nurse!" We're also happy to say someone (not us) offers "save a life: be a nurse."[130] We encourage nurses to create or lobby for more stamps to help educate the public about nursing. Of course, what the stamps alone can convey is limited—the 1976 US stamp honoring yellow fever research nurse Clara Maass said only "She gave her life"—but a message like that can entice people to learn more.[131]

Even toys and games can teach about nursing. When our son was four years old, he told us that boys couldn't be nurses. We were mortified. So we gave him the Archie McPhee "Male Nurse Action Figure," and he changed his mind. Sadly, Archie McPhee no longer makes these action figures, so we encourage you to make one![132]

Nurses should also consider designing board games and video games to educate kids about nursing. Nurses might design a counterpart to Milton Bradley's legendary Operation game. How about Post-Operation, in which "nurse" players prevent dehiscence and evisceration, cardiovascular collapse, infections, and other complications by observing shifting patient conditions and responding with quick actions? Or a new version of the video game *Grand Theft Auto* in which nurse players take on the challenge of teaching a gravely wounded crime boss how to do his complex self-care, embrace a healthy lifestyle, and motivate his low-life cronies to set up a community health program? Welcome to Vice-Free City!

Video, Broadcast, and Film

The broadcast media (television and radio) and film are traditionally harder for novice creators to make use of than are some other media. But with the explosion of information technology in recent decades, nurses can now create and post on the Internet helpful video and audio with far less effort.

Video

Videos can now be created and made available to the world with minimal equipment and technical expertise. Web videos posted on YouTube are extremely popular, especially among young people we need to recruit to nursing. Nurse-created video could range from short recruiting videos to longer discussions of nursing or general health topics. One example is the University of North Dakota's 2008 CD *Follow your dreams – Make a Difference – Become a Nurse*, which included several short videos and other features to attract potential nurses from the American Indian and Alaskan Native communities. Unfortunately, recent children's videos—most notably the ones aimed at girls—have been especially likely to present medicine as the only career worth pursuing in health care. So countering that myth would be especially helpful.

Nurses have already created some compelling Web video. One of the best short works we've seen is the irreverent 2004 rap video created by emergency department nurse Craig Barton at the University of Alabama, as we mentioned in Chapter 7.[133] In 2004 Liz Dubelman posted a gripping, innovative "VidLit" (literature-based flash animation) based on nurse Veneta Masson's poem "The Arithmetic of Nurses," about a home care nurse's work with a "sick old man."[134] Masson's matter-of-fact text charted the human spirit straining to break through physical decay and social neglect. In 2006 students at Binghamton University posted a recruiting video called "We're Bringing Nursing Back," based on Justin Timberlake's electrofunk hit "SexyBack," with new lyrics that extolled nursing.[135] The video had its problems—it failed to get across that nurses use advanced skills to save lives—but the students deserve credit for an audacious effort to attract career seekers. And consider the 2012 video "Mama Said Be a Nurse," a gleefully immature ode to nursing school graduation that student C-Ham and her cohorts at Azusa Pacific University set to LL Cool J's rap classic "Mama Said Knock You Out."[136] We can't endorse everything in there, but among the questionable bits the video included bursts of wit and technical nursing information that would surprise anyone who thought nurses were unskilled handmaidens.

In October 2011 the Truth About Nursing created and posted on YouTube a short video called "Nursing: Isn't That Sweet?!"[137] Made using Xtranormal software, the five-minute video explores nursing stereotypes through a look at what happens when a nurse named Wendy encounters her old high school classmate Jim, many years later. The two characters have a spirited exchange of views!

Radio

Radio remains a very effective way to communicate, especially now that even a small station's programming can be delivered globally on the Web. Almost every community has radio stations, and every station needs a health show hosted by nurses. The gold standard of nurse-hosted radio shows is *HealthStyles*, hosted by Diana Mason and Barbara Glickstein, on WBAI in New York.[138] It features nurses as experts on nearly every show, and when physicians are on, the hosts treat them as colleagues, not gods. In addition, nurse Maureen McGrath hosts the *Sunday Night Sex Show*, a wide-ranging look at sexual health and related issues on Vancouver's CKNW that features nurses and other experts.[139] McGrath told us that she has invited many nurses to appear, "but they are shy to come on. Physicians, on the other hand, welcome the invite." Even so, one of McGrath's 2014 shows that did have a nurse expert was "Please Knock Before You Enter: Sexuality and Intimacy in Care Homes." Further south, the irreverent California nurses Casey Hobbs and Shayne Mason host *Nurse Talk*, which offers health advice, including the idea that "laughter is the best medicine."[140]

Television and Film

As we have seen, television and film remain powerful forces throughout the modern world. In recent years there have been some films and television shows with helpful portrayals of nursing. Examples include *Nurse Jackie, Call the Midwife, 24 Hours in A&E, Angels in America*, and the *Nursing Diaries* installment by Richard Kahn.[141] Nurses were instrumental in the creation of some of these media. However, as we have explained, most influential television and film products—such as popular Hollywood television dramas—remain very troubling. Nurses with the resources and skills should consider taking a more active role in producing, writing, and advising on broadcast media.

Some nurses have already made feature films. Florida nurse David Burton's 2009 documentary *InGREEDients* examined the perils of trans fats. Nurse Kathy Douglas directed *Nurses: If Florence Could See Us Now* (2012). As discussed in Chapter 7, that film included some good information about nursing, although it was dominated by vague caring language and generic uplift, and it had fairly little about nurses' specific skills or tangible contributions to patient outcomes.[142]

Other nurses have made television programming. In November 2013 Oregon nurse Sonya Justice launched a new television show called *The Reel Nurses Talk Show* (or *RNTV*) on Portland Community Media and YouTube.[143] The interview-oriented show conveys valuable information on such topics as pain management and hospital-acquired infections, using nurse experts exclusively. Justice has said that she also wants to counter global stereotypes of nurses as flunkies. Nurse practitioner Ruth Tanyi produced and hosted a television series about diabetes called *Bad Sugar*, broadcast on California's KHIZ-TV in 2006 and 2007.[144] Tanyi explained how to avoid or at least control the disease by focusing on lifestyle, including diet, rest, and exercise. Nurses are well placed to convey the health expertise these projects require—and in the process, to show the public that they *are* health experts.

Nurses should also consider developing ideas and writing scripts for the full range of entertainment programming. Almost anything can affect how nursing is perceived, from reality shows to adult and teenage dramas to children's programs, such as *Sesame Street* and *Dora the Explorer*.

Consider the popular Disney preschool show *Doc McStuffins*, which started in 2012. The show features an African-American girl (Doc) who wants to be a physician like her mother and gets ready by fixing her ailing toys and dolls, which come to life when Doc is there. Each episode sends a basic health message, usually in a narrow, physician-centric "diagnosis and treatment" framework.[145] But wait! One of the *dolls*, Hallie the Hippo, is "Doc's nurse." At different points the Hallie character reflects most of the major nursing stereotypes, from low-skilled handmaiden to motherly angel to crusty battle-axe. Her main job often seems to be fetching the *Big Book of Boo-Boos* for Doc. The show's creator has noted that she originally saw the Hallie character as a "fumbling, bumbling mess," though the voice actress has supposedly brought more confidence to the role.[146] The show has been lauded for its positive role-modeling, telling girls of color that they can be physicians.[147] Presumably it would not occur to most in the media that such a contemptous portrayal of nursing aimed at the next generation in its formative years is harmful. We can do better, and we must.

It's Up to Us

When the public does not understand the value of what nurses do—when nurses seem to have written in invisible ink—nursing cannot get the respect and resources it needs, and people suffer and die. We can all help resolve this global public health crisis, especially by improving the media portrayals that play such a critical role. *We can change things*. We live in a world in which women and racial minorities can hold the highest public offices, a reality that would have shocked many people a hundred years ago. These changes are the result of sacrifice, relentless persistence, and hard work. As we said at the start of this book, achieving that kind of change may seem to require a "superhuman" effort, but that simply means it takes a long time to complete.

Together we can create a world in which parents encourage bright children of both genders to become nurses, a world that gives nursing the resources needed to save the lives of millions. We can create a world that understands what one nurse's aunt learned, in a story the nurse later told us:

> I remember my aunt, who was an author, telling me I "could do better than that," and be a physician or a writer, as I so love to write. She would often say, "Why be just a nurse? You are wasting yourself in such a lowly profession." But you know, when she was dying of breast cancer, I stayed at her house with her (she lived alone) for her last two weeks. I felt honored to be able to be there as her favorite niece . . . and as her nurse. The night before she died she said this: "What would I do without you? Thank God you are a nurse." This was the last thing she said to me.

Notes

1. Charles William Heathcote, "Franklin's Contributions to the American Revolution as a Diplomat in France," US History.org (February 22, 1956), http://tinyurl.com/d79ysqj.
2. James Carney and John F. Dickerson, "The Rocky Rollout of Cheney's Energy Plan," *Time* (May 19, 2001), http://tinyurl.com/lve3y6g.
3. TAN, "Would You Like a Free Bumper Sticker?," accessed June 27, 2014, http://tinyurl.com/kgzfl7y.
4. TAN, "Nursing: The Best Career on Earth. How You Can Become a Nurse," accessed June 27, 2014, http://tinyurl.com/nherw5c.
5. Jim Bell, executive producer, "What Your Hospital Doesn't Want You to Know," *Today Show*, NBC (September 21, 2006).
6. Patricia Raymond, "Nursing Image = Nursing Power," *Real Life Healthcare*, a publication of the *Sacramento Bee* (June 2004), http://tinyurl.com/kt2k786.
7. Virginia Linn, "Concerns Over Patient Confusion Spawn a Small Movement Back to One-Color Nursing Uniforms: Back to White?" *Pittsburgh Post-Gazette* (October 12, 2004), http://tinyurl.com/lu7vzgy; CFNA, "Professional Recognition and Wet Snowballs," TAN (October 12, 2004), http://tinyurl.com/mlam8qf.
8. Lisa Gutierrez, "Uniform Prescription," *Kansas City Star* (October 6, 2004), http://tinyurl.com/oj7wwll; CFNA, "Is the Patch Right for You?," TAN (October 6, 2004), http://tinyurl.com/n8fwxjr.
9. Children's Hospital Los Angeles, "Caregiver Roles," accessed March 8, 2014, http://tinyurl.com/ovmyc3v.
10. J. Morgan Puett and Mark Dion, "RN: The Past, Present and Future of the Nurses' Uniform," Exhibit at the Fabric Workshop and Museum (October 3, 2003–February 14, 2004), http://tinyurl.com/n34a2lt; CFNA, "RN: The Past, Present and Future of the Nurses' Uniform," TAN (November 14, 2003), http://tinyurl.com/plnt63h; TAN, "Wear the RN Patch!," accessed March 30, 2014, http://tinyurl.com/l2ycoez.
11. Ani Burr, "Yes, I'm the Student Nurse.... All in White," *Scrubs Magazine* (June 18, 2012), http://tinyurl.com/ouypmvn.
12. Margaret Helminiak, personal email communication (June 15, 2008).
13. Rhea Sanford, "Practicing Out Loud: Connecting Patient Education and Bedside Care," Presentation to Connecticut League for Nursing, "CLN to Host Nursing Leadership Conference" (October 23, 2001), http://tinyurl.com/kxazukq or http://tinyurl.com/lqvw5pg.
14. Susan Frampton, Sara Guastello, Carrie Brady, Maria Hale, Sheryl Horowitz, Susan Bennett Smith, and Susan Stone, "Patient-Centered Care Improvement Guide," Planetree and Picker Institute (October 2008), http://tinyurl.com/lw8jk2m.

15. J. Buss, "Associations between Obesity and Stress and Shift Work Among Nurses," *Workplace Health & Safety* 60, no. 10 (October 2012): 453–458, http://tinyurl.com/n9xsbde.
16. Robert Wood Johnson Foundation, "Tobacco Cessation Success: Smoking Rates Drop for Registered Nurses" (February 18, 2014), http://tinyurl.com/jw5oqt5.
17. Marianna Klebanov, "NAPNAP Calls for an End to Corporal Punishment of Children," *The Examiner* (August 25, 2011), http://tinyurl.com/m9fdljp; TAN, "Cycles of Abuse" (September 18, 2011), http://tinyurl.com/lufv97b.
18. Channel 39, "New Zealand Nurses Organisation Celebrate World Smokefree Day" (Dunedin, May 28, 2010), http://tinyurl.com/ozg43bg; TAN, "A Smokefree World" (May 28, 2010), http://tinyurl.com/mskaumo.
19. Margaret Helminiak, personal email communication (June 15, 2008).
20. TAN, "I Am Your Registered Nurse," accessed May 9, 2014, http://tinyurl.com/k8qppcw.
21. Bernice Buresh and Suzanne Gordon, *From Silence to Voice*, 3rd ed. (Ithaca: Cornell University Press, 2013).
22. *Southern Reporter*, "Borders General Takes Starring Role on Danish TV" (December 31, 2013), http://tinyurl.com/lqvldrh.
23. Sarah Deeth, "New Campaign Aims to Raise Awareness and Reduce Alcohol-Facilitated Sexual Assaults," *Peterborough Examiner* (August 29, 2012), http://tinyurl.com/mktlfgn; Sexual Assault Voices of Edmonton, "We Dream of a World without Sexual Assault," accessed March 9, 2014, http://www.savedmonton.com; TAN, "Just Because She's Drunk . . . Doesn't Mean She Wants To . . . " (August 29, 2012), http://tinyurl.com/o6p9lfo.
24. John Leland, "In 'Sweetie' and 'Dear,' a Hurt for the Elderly," *New York Times* (October 6, 2008), http://tinyurl.com/l2gyqj7.
25. "Music Found to Decrease Blood Pressure of Catheter Test Patients," *Mainichi Daily News* (March 8, 2006), http://tinyurl.com/m7m7wt5; CFNA, "Music Has Charms To Soothe Those Having a Catheter Test," TAN (March 8, 2006), http://tinyurl.com/k55qwu6.
26. Marc Siegel, "The Unreal World: How Appropriate Was Girl's Treatment On 'Mercy'?," *Los Angeles Times* (March 22, 2010), http://tinyurl.com/mqpfdvo; Marc Siegel, "The Unreal World: A Good Nurse Has 'Mercy,'" *Los Angeles Times* (October 19, 2009), http://tinyurl.com/ycxb2n5; Marc Siegel, "The Unreal World: 'HawthoRNe': Treatment Depends on When the Stroke Started," *Los Angeles Times* (August 24, 2009), http://tinyurl.com/y8mqfgk; Marc Siegel, "The Unreal World: Few Nurses Are 100% 'Jackie,'" *Los Angeles Times* (June 29, 2009), http://tinyurl.com/mlhys5u.
27. TAN, "Get Media Savvy and Media Training," accessed June 27, 2014, http://tinyurl.com/kuohz8d.
28. Elizabeth Winslow, "We Silence Our Profession When We Fail to Identify Ourselves as Nurses," *American Journal of Nursing* 112, no. 8 (August 2012): 11, http://tinyurl.com/ngfvxn6.

29. Greg Mortenson, "Greg Mortenson Bio," Three Cups of Tea, accessed June 27, 2014, http://tinyurl.com/pc8sta2.
30. Pam Meredith, "Pick up That RN Flag and Wave It," *Nursing Spectrum* (December 2, 2002), http://tinyurl.com/psajzae.
31. US Department of Health and Human Services, Office for Civil Rights, "HIPAA Medical Privacy—National Standards to Protect the Privacy of Personal Health Information," www.hhs.gov/ocr/hipaa/; US Department of Health and Human Services, Office of the Secretary, "Health Insurance Portability and Accountability Act of 1996, Public Law 104–191" (August 21, 1996), http://tinyurl.com/kezocbp.
32. Gary Stephenson, Johns Hopkins University Hospital, telephone conversation (2008).
33. Tim Green, ed., "Tribute to Nurses," *Rattle* (Winter 2007), http://tinyurl.com/n6o3sy7; CFNA, "Tribute to Nurses: Unusual Access to Us," TAN (May 16, 2008), http://tinyurl.com/m284jar.
34. CFNA, "Water Made Less Naughty," TAN (September 2006), http://tinyurl.com/neoljk3.
35. CFNA, "Cashmere Mafia Nurses in Bondage," TAN (November 16, 2007), http://tinyurl.com/pjyahh3.
36. TAN, "Open Up and Say . . . Naah!" (March 7, 2011), http://tinyurl.com/l98sh9x.
37. CFNA, "Debugging the 'Electronic Nurse,'" TAN (September 20, 2006), http://tinyurl.com/qxh22wd.
38. *Jeopardy*, syndicated television show (September 7, 2004); CFNA, "What Are Nurse Practitioners?," TAN (September 7, 2004), http://tinyurl.com/otoxgzt.
39. TAN, "Going Back to Cali Nurse" (July 2010), http://tinyurl.com/k8v2rhj.
40. CFNA, "Skechers Pulls Christina Aguilera 'Nurse' Ad after Receiving More Than 3,000 Letters from Nursing Supporters," TAN (August 17, 2004), http://tinyurl.com/lfz2ebb.
41. CFNA, "Your Ultimate Recovery Team," TAN (August 2008), http://tinyurl.com/nxgj7p2.
42. TAN, "Scrubbing Out" (October 24, 2013), http://tinyurl.com/nwb8zn9.
43. TAN, "Scrubbing Less" (November 12, 2013), http://tinyurl.com/k6otvht.
44. CFNA, "Worth Dying For," TAN (October 2006), http://tinyurl.com/c5ouw9m.
45. CFNA, "Real Nurses Want 'Naughty Nurse' Off the Menu," TAN (October 26, 2006), http://tinyurl.com/6v4r4l9; CFNA, "Press Coverage: Heart Attack Grill Coverage," TAN (May 2, 2007), http://tinyurl.com/n25o59o.
46. TAN, "Dr. Oz's Sexy 'Nurse' Backup Dancers" (December 6, 2010), http://tinyurl.com/q5qoagh.
47. TAN, "Thinking Right, Thinking Bright" (December 6, 2010), http://tinyurl.com/2cucb5r.
48. Jack White, composer, The White Stripes, performer, "The Nurse" from the album *Get Behind Me Satan*, V2 Records (2005); CFNA, "Boy You Have No Faith in Nursing," TAN (April 21, 2006) http://tinyurl.com/kmgw6sx.

49. CFNA, "Jack White Slams Nursing Group for 'Metaphorical Ignorance': Rock Star and Nurses Trade Mock 'Awards,'" TAN (April 21, 2006), http://tinyurl.com/n3c2974; CFNA, "Press Coverage of the Jack White Exchange of Mock Awards," TAN (May 31, 2007), http://tinyurl.com/nxlr687.
50. CTV Atlantic, "Halifax Nurses Warn of Patient Safety Risks in New TV Ads" (March 14, 2014), http://tinyurl.com/px57t7j.
51. Margot Roosevelt, "Nursing a Grudge," *Time* (February 27, 2005), http://tinyurl.com/kec6fcd.
52. National Nurses United, "National Campaign for Safe RN-to-Patient Ratios," accessed March 30, 2014, http://tinyurl.com/7hk2sdf.
53. National Nurses United, "Medicare for All," accessed March 24, 2014, http://tinyurl.com/pvf5vzn.
54. Rose Ann DeMoro, "If Dick Cheney Were Anyone Else, He'd Probably Be Dead by Now," *Huffington Post* (December 11, 2007), http://tinyurl.com/mmkgfp4.
55. TAN, "Nursing the Debt Machine" (October 10, 2011); *Daily Kos*, "Nurses Take on Wall Street" (June 22, 2011), http://tinyurl.com/kbp37vr.
56. CFNA, "Coor Slight," TAN (December 2006), http://tinyurl.com/l8wmgwp.
57. CFNA, "Center Urges HHS to Modify Name of 'Take a Loved One to the Doctor' Campaign," TAN (December 7, 2004), http://tinyurl.com/mn46m5a.
58. CFNA, "CVS Pharmacist Returns From Matrix; Can Now Download Entire Nursing Curriculum into Your Brain in Four Hours!," TAN (January 24, 2006), http://tinyurl.com/mwvx9bj.
59. CFNA, "Nurse, Fetch Me the Ball," TAN (November 15, 2007), http://tinyurl.com/p56k8n5.
60. CFNA, "American Family Care Clinics—You Get To See a Physician, Not a Nurse!," TAN (May 31, 2013), http://tinyurl.com/pkfg5pz.
61. TAN, "Do Physicians Deliver Better Care Than Advanced Practice Registered Nurses?," accessed March 11, 2014, http://tinyurl.com/yd7r3yv.
62. TAN, "To Serve Dr. Lung Love" (November 2, 2009), http://tinyurl.com/lrej4bs.
63. *Modern Healthcare*, "Outliers: Sure We've Heard of Bad Raps . . . But This Is Ridiculous" (November 23, 2009), http://tinyurl.com/nkghksw; TAN, "Lung Cancer Alliance Quietly Removes Dr. Lung Love Video after Truth's Campaign Covered in *Modern Healthcare*" (November 30, 2009), http://tinyurl.com/m5z2fwu.
64. CFNA, "Don't You Think I'm So Sexy—I'm Just So Fresh, So Clean," TAN (September 27, 2007), http://tinyurl.com/mue2geq.
65. CFNA, "Getting Fresher," TAN (October 6, 2007), http://tinyurl.com/lm2rwwk.
66. Tom O'Connor, writer, "Episode Dated March 31, 2008," *Red Eye*, Fox (March 31, 2008); CFNA, "Wear the Miniskirts and Just Save Some Lives!," TAN (April 1, 2008), http://tinyurl.com/l7moqow.
67. TAN, "Real Nurses Not So Thrilled by *Nurse 3D*'s Extra Dimension" (February 8, 2014), http://tinyurl.com/n822x8h.
68. TAN, "Letters to ER," accessed March 11, 2014, http://tinyurl.com/k3cvsty.

69. TAN, "*ER* Episode Analyses" (2009), http://tinyurl.com/odsbmqw.
70. CFNA, "Schering-Plough Asks 'ER' to Portray Nursing Accurately," TAN (April 26, 2005), http://tinyurl.com/p2symb3.
71. TAN, "The Extubating Babysitter" (March 29, 2009), http://tinyurl.com/mavyu3b.
72. CFNA, "We Must Stop the Naughty Scandinavian Porn Nurses from Infiltrating America!," TAN (June 13, 2007), http://tinyurl.com/jw9mhk5.
73. CFNA, "Are There Any Hot Nurses at Walter Reed? Sean Hannity Is on the Case!," TAN (January 18, 2006), http://tinyurl.com/kanxna6.
74. CFNA, "The Most Interesting Nurse Ad in the World," TAN (October 25, 2007), http://tinyurl.com/lf2ch7z.
75. Bryan Moore and Chris Peterson, writers, Victor Gonzalez, director, "Bionic Showdown," *Lab Rats*, Disney XD (August 5, 2013); TAN, "Nurse Practitioner Evil!" (August 5, 2013), http://tinyurl.com/mzuzud9; TAN, "Lab Rats Experiment a Success!" (February 2014), http://tinyurl.com/njtnk46.
76. CFNA, "Duck Soup," TAN (December 2005), http://tinyurl.com/l2fj2ej.
77. TAN, "Scrubbing Less" (November 12, 2013), http://tinyurl.com/k6otvht.
78. CFNA, "Wal-Mart Changes Brain Surgeon Ad," TAN (April 2, 2005), http://tinyurl.com/m553h35.
79. Mandy Mayling, "The Soft Bigotry of Low Expectations: New Script Idea," TAN, http://tinyurl.com/nqyrte4.
80. Mohandas Gandhi, quoted in "Gandhi Quotes," WorldofQuotes.com, accessed March 24, 2014, http://tinyurl.com/lpaw7l8.
81. Leah Binder, "The Best Disruptive Writings of 2013—Health Care Edition," *Forbes* (December 30, 2013), http://tinyurl.com/qjgqwfm.
82. TAN, "Las Vegas, Nevada Chapter of the Truth About Nursing," accessed June 27, 2014, http://tinyurl.com/n74os9t.
83. TAN, "Chapters of the Truth About Nursing," accessed June 27, 2014, http://tinyurl.com/n8bshpz.
84. TAN, "Open Up and Say . . . Naah!" (March 7, 2011), http://tinyurl.com/l98sh9x.
85. Janet Bailey, Janice Graham, and Leslie Pepper, "What Doctors Wish You Knew . . . 75 Surprising Tips—From Heading Off a Headache to Avoiding a Heart Attack," *Good Housekeeping* (November 2005); CFNA, "Paging Dr. X to the Triage Booth," TAN (February 2006), http://tinyurl.com/nzlgt4d.
86. CFNA, "Letter from Sioux Lookout: 'Nurses Help Communities Thrive,'" TAN (May 19, 2005), http://tinyurl.com/ko77v7s.
87. Veneta Masson, "Nurse Practitioner Explains Why She Refuses to Endorse Routine Mammography," *Washington Post* (October 11, 2010), http://tinyurl.com/24dvr2q; TAN, "Pride and Prejudice" (October 11, 2010), http://tinyurl.com/ko7klkc.
88. Linda Record Srungaram, "When Nurses Are Prosecuted for Patient Advocacy, We All Lose," *Houston Chronicle* (August 23, 2009), http://tinyurl.com/k6qczwa; TAN, "Messing with Texas" (September 11, 2009), http://tinyurl.com/pzklorl.

89. Kevin Sack, "Whistle-Blowing Nurse Is Acquitted in Texas," *New York Times* (February 11, 2010), http://tinyurl.com/mdvy889; TAN, "Remain in Light" (February 11, 2010), http://tinyurl.com/o9khkr7.
90. Kathleen Bartholomew, "We All Hurt When Hospitals Shrink Themselves into Budgetary Compliance," *Seattle Post-Intelligencer* (February 15, 2009), http://tinyurl.com/k3lckxg; TAN, "The Disease Care Industry" (March 17, 2009), http://tinyurl.com/l5ot2kn.
91. Gina Dennik-Champion, "Nurses Back Medical Marijuana," *Milwaukee Journal Sentinel* (December 10, 2005), http://tinyurl.com/m6kdaps; CFNA, "Powerful Op-Ed Explains Why Wisconsin Nurses Back Medical Marijuana," TAN (December 10, 2005), http://tinyurl.com/kar3rhk.
92. Raewyn Janota, "The Unique Gifts That Nurses Receive," *Globe and Mail* (Toronto: December 21, 2005); CFNA, "'The Unique Gifts That Nurses Receive,'" TAN (December 21, 2005), http://tinyurl.com/lc23hqb.
93. Laura Stokowski, "Letter to Hollywood: Nurses Are Not Handmaidens," Medscape (March 12, 2010), http://www.medscape.com/viewarticle/718032.
94. John Blanton, "Care and Chaos on the Night Nursing Shift," *Wall Street Journal* (April 24, 2007), http://tinyurl.com/25kgyw; CFNA, "There and Back Again," TAN (April 24, 2007), http://tinyurl.com/ndu5dx8.
95. British Columbia Nurses' Union, "Jello Ad" (1997), http://tinyurl.com/nz2wnus.
96. Echo Heron, *Intensive Care: The Story of a Nurse* (Raleigh: Ivy Books, 1988).
97. Claire Bertschinger, *Moving Mountains* (New York: Bantam, 2005).
98. Jennifer Culkin, *A Final Arc of Sky* (Boston: Beacon Press, 2009).
99. Susan Luz with Marcus Brotherton, *The Nightingale of Mosul* (New York: Kaplan Publishing, 2010).
100. Pat Carroll, *What Nurses Know and Doctors Don't Have Time to Tell You* (New York: Perigee Trade, 2004).
101. Gloria Mayer and Ann Kuklierus, *What to Do When Your Child Gets Sick* from the *What to Do for Health Series* (LaHabra, California: Institute for Healthcare Advancement, 1999), http://tinyurl.com/luzv8oe.
102. Serita Stevens, *Forensic Nurse: The New Role of the Nurse in Law Enforcement* (New York: St. Martin's Press, 2004).
103. Cheryl Dellasega, "Books: Nonfiction," accessed March 28, 2014, http://tinyurl.com/p2gpypu.
104. Kate Trant and Sue Usher, eds., *Nurse—Past, Present, and Future: The Making of Modern Nursing* (London: Black Dog Publishing, 2010).
105. Echo Heron, *Fatal Diagnosis* (New York: Ballantine Books, 2000).
106. Elizabeth Ann Scarborough, *The Healer's War* (E-Reads, 2010).
107. Richard Ferri, *Confessions of a Male Nurse* (New York: Harrington Park Press, 2005).

108. Veneta Masson, *Clinician's Guide to the Soul* (Washington, DC: Sage Femme Press, 2008).
109. Heather Knight, "The Rhyming Nurse at S.F. General," *San Francisco Chronicle* (December 8, 2008), http://tinyurl.com/lv2szxo; TAN, "Children of the City" (December 8, 2008), http://tinyurl.com/lyfrlv8.
110. CFNA, "Landmark JAMA Study Finds Nurses to Be Autonomous, Skilled; Nation Reels," TAN (April 1, 2005), http://tinyurl.com/k7mspvn.
111. Holly Hobbie, *Fanny* (New York: Little, Brown Books for Young Readers, 2008); TAN "Fanny" (June 4, 2010), http://tinyurl.com/klpmcpv.
112. Helen Wells, *Cherry Ames Nurse Stories* (New York: Grosset & Dunlap, 1943–1968).
113. Serita Stevens, *Charlie London, RN* (Norwalk, Connecticut: Palm Publishing, 2004).
114. Margaret Comerford Freda, "Nurses in the Strangest Places," *American Journal of Maternal Child Nursing* 31, no 4 (2006): 214, http://tinyurl.com/l7gzu6q.
115. Internet World Stats, "Internet Usage Statistics" (2012), http://tinyurl.com/7mswb; Pingdom, "Internet by the Numbers" (December 2012), http://tinyurl.com/a3t2pjr.
116. TAN, "Nursing Representation on the Websites and Boards of Directors at the Top 17 Hospitals Ranked by *U.S. News and World Report* in 2012" (March 2012), http://tinyurl.com/n8hp4kr.
117. Massachusetts General Hospital Patient Care Services, "Magnet Recognition," accessed March 24, 2014, http://tinyurl.com/mglwxu3.
118. Health On the Net Foundation, "About Health On the Net Foundation," accessed March 14, 2014, http://tinyurl.com/ms4dmjg.
119. Diane Carlson Evans, "Moving a Vision: The Vietnam Women's Memorial," Vietnam Women's Memorial, accessed March 14, 2014, http://tinyurl.com/4llllkg.
120. J. Morgan Puett and Mark Dion, "RN: The Past, Present and Future of the Nurses' Uniform," Exhibit at the Fabric Workshop and Museum (October 3, 2003–February 14, 2004), http://tinyurl.com/n34a2lt; CFNA, "RN: The Past, Present and Future of the Nurses' Uniform," TAN (November 14, 2003), http://tinyurl.com/plnt63h.
121. *American Journal of Nursing*, "*AJN*'s Photo Exhibit: Faces of Caring: Nurses at Work," accessed March 30, 2014, http://tinyurl.com/l6utxkz; CFNA, "The Faces of Caring: Nurses at Work," TAN (May 2007) http://tinyurl.com/mkhn55x; CFNA, "The Faces of Caring, Nurses at Work," TAN (May 6–31, 2005), http://tinyurl.com/kngsqbw.
122. Carolyn Jones, *The American Nurse* (book) (New York: Welcome Enterprises, 2012), http://tinyurl.com/ml7mhpa.

123. Carolyn Jones, director, *The American Nurse: Healing America* (film) (2014), http://tinyurl.com/na5yunw; TAN, "The American Nurse" (May 2, 2014), http://tinyurl.com/otdyl8z.
124. Sonic Youth, *Sonic Nurse*, Geffen/Interscope (2004), http://tinyurl.com/8tua6bb; CFNA, "Sonic Youth, Sonic Nurse," TAN (July 12, 2004), http://tinyurl.com/kzgl476.
125. Lisa Hayes, playwright and actor, *Nurse!* (2003). See Diana J. Mason and Diane Roux-Lirange, "Review of 'Nurse!,'" TAN (June 21, 2003), http://tinyurl.com/mtso3c6.
126. Hob Osterlund, "Ivy Push," accessed March 14, 2014, http://tinyurl.com/pe29z4k.
127. Greg "G" Williams, "2TallRN," accessed March 14, 2014, http://2tallrn.com.
128. U.S. Postal Service, "Women on Stamps" (2003), http://tinyurl.com/o4bthta.
129. Birth Activist, "Hug Your Midwife—National Midwifery Week Oct. 5–11" (October 7, 2008), http://tinyurl.com/k3kxmsv.
130. Zazzle, "Nurse Postage Stamps," accessed March 14, 2014, http://tinyurl.com/ppzjwhk.
131. American Association for the History of Nursing, "Clara Louise Maass," accessed March 14, 2014, http://tinyurl.com/6lt82s.
132. CFNA, "Archie McPhee Male Nurse Action Figure," TAN (October 5, 2004), http://tinyurl.com/o4y7x4k.
133. Caperton Gillett, "Faces of UAB: Heart Beats: Craig Barton—Nurse | Rapper," *UAB Magazine* (Fall 2011), http://tinyurl.com/kpucn77; Craig Barton, "We're ER Nurses, Medications We Disburses" (2004), http://tinyurl.com/lwksdax; CFNA, "Rap Recruiting Video," TAN (2004), http://tinyurl.com/l7oo4tf.
134. Veneta Masson, author, Liz Dubelman, director, "The Arithmetic of Nurses," VidLit (2004), http://tinyurl.com/lxqeq32; CFNA, "The Arithmetic of Nurses," TAN (July 1, 2005), http://tinyurl.com/phgtv6x.
135. Binghamton University Students, "Nursing Back," YouTube (November 14, 2014), http://tinyurl.com/mhw8xuf; CFNA, "We're Bringing Nursing Back," TAN (2007), http://tinyurl.com/orqg8g7.
136. Christie Hamilton and Thomas Lee, lyrics, LL Cool J, music, Christie Hamilton, performer, "Mama Said Be a Nurse," YouTube (April 1, 2012), http://tinyurl.com/pkfbb37.
137. TAN, "Nursing: Isn't That Sweet?," YouTube (October 25, 2011), http://tinyurl.com/pomtxz6.
138. Diana Mason and Barbara Glickstein, producers and hosts, *HealthStyles*, WBAI (1986–), http://tinyurl.com/orznqmg.
139. Maureen McGrath, *Sunday Night Sex Show*, CKNW (2012–), http://tinyurl.com/pc8nwox.
140. Casey Hobbs and Shayne Mason, *Nurse Talk* (2011–), http://nursetalksite.com.

141. Richard Kahn and Linda Martin, directors, *Lifeline: The Nursing Diaries*: Part 1: *The Rookies*, Discovery Health Channel (2004); CFNA, "Part 1: The Rookies," TAN (December 16, 2004), http://tinyurl.com/ob9df8c.
142. David Burton, writer and director, *InGREEDients* (2009), http://www.ingredientsmovie.com/
143. Sonya Justice, creator and host, *The Reel Nurses Talk Show*, Portland Community Media (2013–), http://tinyurl.com/ny8lt82.
144. CFNA, "Good Sugar," TAN (November 6, 2006), http://tinyurl.com/oop5qxk.
145. Chris Nee, creator, *Doc McStuffins*, Disney Junior (2012–), http://tinyurl.com/le9dk9e.
146. Ari Karpel, "How the Creator of 'Doc McStuffins' Bucked the Norm and Created 'Cheers' for Preschoolers," Fast Company (March 20, 2012), http://tinyurl.com/mdbz7z3.
147. Lynn Elber, "'Doc McStuffins' TV Show Gives Black Girls, Aspiring Doctors Hope," Associated Press (June 12, 2012), http://tinyurl.com/cfhya9e.

ABOUT THE TRUTH ABOUT NURSING

Registered nurses are the critical front-line caregivers in health care today. For millions of people worldwide, nurses are the difference between life and death, self-sufficiency and dependency, hope and despair. Yet a lack of true appreciation for nursing has led to a shortage that is one of our most urgent public health crises. The nursing shortage has claimed countless lives and is overwhelming the world's health systems. It is no exaggeration to say that the future depends on a better understanding of nursing.

The Truth About Nursing is an international nonprofit organization working to meet that challenge. It pursues an advocacy program started by five graduate students at Johns Hopkins University School of Nursing in 2001. The Truth About Nursing tells the media and the public what nurses really do. It analyzes the media's treatment of nurses, helping nurses stand together to end harmful depictions and encourage accurate ones. Better public understanding of nursing will lead to more social, political, and financial support for the profession, which will in turn relieve the nursing shortage and improve the health of all people.

To contact the authors or the Truth About Nursing, visit www.truthaboutnursing.org.

All royalties from this book go to support the Truth About Nursing.

ABOUT THE AUTHORS

Sandy Jacobs Summers has served as executive director of the Truth About Nursing since its founding, pursuing work she started in 2001 with other graduate nursing students at Johns Hopkins University. She frequently speaks to the media and at conferences. In 2002, Summers earned master's degrees in community health nursing and public health from Johns Hopkins. She holds a BSN degree from Southern Connecticut State University. Prior to her graduate work, Summers practiced nursing for fifteen years in the emergency departments and intensive care units of major US trauma centers, including public hospitals in San Francisco, New Orleans, and Washington, DC. In the mid-1990s, she worked in Phnom Penh, Cambodia, where she taught nursing teachers at the Central Nursing School. She also practiced intensive care nursing for a year at a hospital on St. Thomas in the US Virgin Islands.

Harry Jacobs Summers has been senior adviser to the Truth About Nursing since its founding, also serving as the group's main writer. He has an undergraduate degree from Columbia University and a law degree from Georgetown University. Summers studied for a year on a Fulbright scholarship in New Zealand. He also taught commercial law to government officials for three years in Phnom Penh, Cambodia. Since 1998 he has been a litigation attorney at the Federal Election Commission in Washington, DC.

Sandy and Harry have coauthored articles on nursing and the media for major nursing journals, textbooks, and mainstream publications. They live in Baltimore with their two children.

INDEX